THE PSYCHOLOGY OF INTIMACY

THE GUILFORD SERIES ON PERSONAL RELATIONSHIPS

Steve Duck, Series Editor
Department of Communication Studies,
The University of Iowa

To my husband,
George Gregory Eaves,
with love

Acknowledgments

I would like to thank some of the people whose efforts and ideas have enriched this book. Duane Buhrmester read a significant portion of an earlier draft, and provided invaluable insights and support. I am also grateful to Duane for hours of "co-constructive dialogue," the results of which are woven into this book.

I thank Steve Duck for commissioning me to write this book. He has shared with me his wide-ranging expertise in the field of personal relationships, as well as his reactions, criticisms, and unfailing support and encouragement. Peter Wissoker, at Guilford Press, was always helpful and never intrusive. Nancy Tuana generously read an earlier draft of the book and shared her comments with me. Twelve years of intimate friendship and collegiality with Nancy have kept my views on gender and intimacy continuously evolving. Paula England was also kind enough to read and make helpful comments on an earlier draft of the book. Margaret Owen provided wisdom and expertise on development and close relationships in infancy. I am also grateful for my productive and rewarding association with Monica Basco. Through our collaborative work and our friendship, my understanding of intimate relationships has been truly enriched. I have learned much about developmental approaches to understanding relationships from our group discussions with Duane Buhrmester, Teresa Nezworski, Margaret Owen, Elizabeth Tingley, and Ann Minnett. I would also like to thank Paula England, Robin Jarret, Nancy Jellinek, Holly Silk, Deborah Stott, Marilyn Waligore, and Gwen Raaberg. Our reading group broadened and deepened my awareness of gender as a determinant of human experience. I also appreciate Rebecca Johnson's hours in the "stacks" of the library, which ensured that Table 2.2 was complete and attractively presented.

I owe a special debt of gratitude to Greg Eaves, whose love and support consistently nourished the often grueling effort a book like this requires. He listened and commented patiently on the hazy beginnings of ideas through many long walks in the park. Last, but hardly least, I would like to thank my parents, Morton and Lois Prager. They taught me unerringly, through word and example, that a thing can most definitely be done if one puts one's mind and the sweat of one's brow to the task.

Contents

EPILOGUE

Introduction

Care in the heart . . . bows it down;
But a good word makes it glad.
—Prov. 12:25

If any reason needs to be given for devoting an entire book to intimacy, it
is that intimacy is good for people. Intimate involvement seems to promote human well-being. Consider the following:

*Intimate relationships seem to buffer people from the pathogenic effects of
stress.* In the face of stressful life events people who have intimate relationships have fewer stress-related symptoms, faster recoveries from illness, and a lower probability of relapse or recurrence than those who do
not have intimate relationships. Evidence for the buffering effect of intimate relationships has been found when stress is due to pregnancy (Dimitrovsky, Perez-Hirshberg, & Itskowitz, 1987); the birth of a child
(Collins, Dunkel-Schetter, Lobel, & Scrimshaw, 1993; Robinson, Olmsted, & Garner, 1989); the illness of one's child (Hobfoll & Lerman,
1988); one's own illness, particularly, heart disease (Coyne & Smith,
1991; Hobfoll, Nadler, & Leiberman, 1986; Waltz, 1986; Waltz, Badura,
Pfaff, & Schott, 1988); retirement (Salokangas, Matilla, & Joukamaa,
1988); and death of a spouse (Lewittes, 1989; Lopata, 1979).

*Intimate interactions may account for many of the health benefits that in-
timate relationships provide.* Intimate relationships are often differentiated
from other personal relationships by the presence of confiding interactions between the partners. It is therefore possible to conclude that these
intimate, confiding interactions account for the beneficial effects of intimate relationships. Research suggesting that confiding carries its own
health benefits (e.g., Brown & Harris, 1978; Lewittes, 1989; Reis, Wheeler, Kernis, Spiegel, & Nezlek, 1985), even without an intimate relation-

1

ship, supports this conclusion. For example, survivors of the Nazi Holocaust showed improved health after disclosing traumatic material when compared to a group of survivors who did not disclose (Pennebaker, Barger, & Tiebout, 1989), Similar health benefits have been found following disclosures by American college students (Greenberg & Stone, 1992; Pennebaker & Beall, 1986; Pennebaker, Colder, & Sharp, 1990). Some studies have shown that confiding stressful (as opposed to trivial) material brings measurable *physiological* benefits (Esterling, Antoni, Fletcher, Margulies, & Schneiderman, 1994; Lutgendorf, Antoni, Kumar, & Schneiderman, 1994).

People are more likely to seek intimate interactions when they can benefit from them. People seek all kinds of social support when they are stressed or ill or can otherwise benefit from assistance from others (Duck, 1993b). A tendency to seek intimate communication when distressed has been noted especially among the depressed (Duckro, Duckro, & Beal, 1976; Rotenberg & Hamel, 1988; Stiles, Shuster, & Harrigan, 1992). Confiding and other forms of conversational intimacy may be critical predictors of perceptions of social support (Reis, 1984a).

The foregoing research suggests that intimate contact with others enhances well-being, often when people need it most, that is, when they are under stress. Conversely, the absence of intimacy seems to have deleterious effects on health and well-being. Consider the following:

People who lack intimate relationships are at risk for a variety of ills. They have higher mortality rates, more accidents, and higher risks for developing illnesses than those who have intimate relationships (Berman & Margolin, 1992; House, Landis, & Umberson, 1988). They show depressed immunological functioning (Kiecolt-Glaser et al., 1988). They are more vulnerable to feelings of loneliness (Wheeler, Reis, & Nezlek, 1983) and are more likely to develop symptoms of psychological disturbance (Chamberlaine, Barnes, Waring, & Wood, 1989; Peterson et al., 1993; Reisman, 1985; Steil & Turetsky, 1987).[1]

Self-concealment has been associated with illness and symptoms of distress. Self-concealment refers to the withholding of personal material about the self from others. It has been associated with the presence of such psychological symptoms as anxiety and depression (Larson & Chastain, 1990) and such physical symptoms as hypertension (Handkins & Munz, 1978).

Relationships that do not allow confiding fail to provide the beneficial effects of those that do (Coffman, Levitt, Deets, & Quigley, 1991; Hobfoll & Lerman, 1988). Even people with sizable social networks are likely to develop symptoms of psychological disturbance in the face of stressful events if they lack confiding relationships (e.g., Brown, Bhrolchain, &

Harris, 1975; Cohen & Hoberman, 1983; Lowenthal & Haven, 1968; Miller & Lefcourt, 1983). Support from nonintimate relationship partners has even been predictive of negative outcomes (Hobfoll & Lerman, 1988; Hobfoll & Lieberman, 1989; Lewittes, 1989).[2]

Finally, an *increased* risk of distress, illness, and poor adjustment seems to accompany poorly functioning personal relationships (i.e., those that are unsatisfying, unstable or heavily conflicted):

Poorly functioning relationships with parents, spouses, and friends have been associated with negative outcomes. People who have conflicted or unsatisfying close relationships are more likely to demonstrate poor self-efficacy (Coyne & Smith, 1994; Fisk, Coyne, & Smith, 1991); psychological symptomatology (Rhodes, Ebert, & Meyers, 1994), especially depression (Keitner & Miller, 1990; Peterson et al., 1993; Vinokur & van Ryn, 1993); and physical complaints (Waring & Russell, 1980). Interpersonal conflicts may account for as much as 80% of people's daily negative affect (Bolger, DeLongis, Kessler, & Schilling, 1989). Conversely, relationship-focused psychotherapy can, under certain conditions, ameliorate depressive symptoms (Jacobson, Dobson, Fruzzetti, Schmaling, & Salusky, 1991).

In sum, beneficial effects of intimacy on health and well-being are widely evident. Satisfied intimate relationship partners are less vulnerable to the negative outcomes of stress than are those who are less satisfied or lack intimate relationships. Confiding, and the relationships in which confiding occurs, seems to bestow special advantages to the people involved.

As evidence of the beneficial effects of intimate relationships accumulates, scholars are seeking a deeper understanding of how these effects are realized. The purpose of this book is to encourage this deeper understanding by promoting three specific objectives. The first objective is to develop a concept of intimacy that stimulates theory and research on the interrelationships among its components. The current concept recognizes two components: (1) *intimate interactions*, which are dyadic communicative exchanges, and (2) *intimate relationships*, in which people have a history and anticipate a future of intimate contact over time. Intimate interactions themselves have two components: (1) *intimate behavior*, in which people share that which is private and personal; and (2) *intimate experiences*, which are individual experiences of intimacy, closeness, bonding, and so forth.

The second objective is to use the current conception to organize the diverse theoretical, empirical, and clinical literatures on intimacy. The purpose of this organizational effort is to raise new questions, or to frame familiar questions in new ways, by pulling together works that initially had divergent purposes. This book's final product should be a set of new (and not so new) directions for intimacy research.

The third objective is to develop a framework for understanding the effects of context on intimate interactions and relationships. This book outlines ways that different relational contexts either directly affect intimate interactions and relationships or modify the effects of the various intimacy components on one another.

ORGANIZATION OF THE BOOK

My major emphasis in this book is on the interplay between intimate interactions and relationships on the one hand and individual needs and well-being on the other. I argue that when we share that which is most personal (and authentic) about ourselves, we open ourselves up to the influence of those with whom we have shared. This influence may be nurturant, benign, or obstructive. A nurturant influence can result in experiences of being liked, understood, and appreciated; important psychological needs are momentarily fulfilled, and our well-being is enhanced. Further, a nurturant influence enhances our relationship, contributing to its stability and minimizing the impact of conflict. At worst, however, the intimacy process fails, leaving us vulnerable to betrayal and psychological injury.

This book has three parts, the first of which creates a definition of intimacy and uses it to organize existing definitions. The first chapter in Part I formulates the two-part definition of intimacy described earlier. The theory of natural concepts originated by Rosch, Mervis, Gray, Johnson, and Boyes-Braem (1976) guides this formulation. It suggests that intimacy itself is too broad a concept to unify a systematic body of scientific work. It therefore recommends that the more specific components defined above serve to guide research. Chapter 2 then organizes existing conceptions of intimacy according to those intimacy concepts from Chapter 1 that receive the most emphasis. It also reviews methods of measuring intimacy and classifies them according to the definitions that seem to best capture their content. The chapter concludes by considering the advantages (and disadvantages) of the current conception, its roots in existing definitions, and measurement issues involved with each of its components.

In Part II, I approach intimacy from a life span perspective and address three related propositions:

1. Intimate interactions and intimate relationships exert their effects on individual well-being in part by responding to the needs, con-

cerns, and stresses that arise with each stage of development. The chapters in Part II discuss various life-stage-related needs, concerns, and stresses that, through theory and/or research, affect or have been affected by intimate interactions and relationships. They consider the processes and mechanisms by which intimate interactions and relationships might exert their effects on individual adaptations to life-stage-related concerns.

2. Life-stage-related needs, concerns, and stresses affect behavior in intimate interactions and thereby affect the quality of intimate relationships. In line with Erikson (1963), this proposition assumes that each stage of development has its own set of needs and stresses. It further assumes that intimate behavior inevitably reflects the efforts made to cope with these needs and stresses. People then bring these adaptive, coping efforts into interactions with others, thus shaping those interactions and relationships.

3. Interactions and relationships experienced earlier in life can modify expectations of and behavioral adaptations to intimate interactions and relationships later on. Consider this example: In her first marriage Gabriella adapted to a volatile, explosive husband by avoiding conflict and concealing her true feelings. Now in her second marriage, Gabriella expects explosiveness and uses the same adaptations, although her husband's behavior does not warrant them. Through expectations developed from her previous experience Gabriella has generalized learning from one relationship to another. Developmental theorists have long recognized the potential impact of early childhood relationships on later adaptations (e.g., Klein, 1935). This book takes its cue from this example, however, and assumes that experiences throughout life can modify later adaptations.

Chapters 3–7 each review the literature on life-stage-related changes in intimate relating. Following a detailed discussion of these propositions in Chapter 3, Chapter 4 discusses ways that intimate interactions and relationships influence and are influenced by life-stage-related needs, concerns, and stresses in infancy and the preschool years. Chapter 5 does the same for early and middle childhood and preadolescence. Chapter 6 addresses adolescence and young adulthood, and Chapter 7 focuses on middle and late adulthood. Each chapter suggests research directions likely to shed light on the three propositions presented above.

Part III considers the processes by which intimate experiences and intimate relationships arise from and affect intimate behavior. Each of the three chapters in Part III considers a specific aspect of the conceptual model of intimacy described in Chapter 1. Chapter 8 explores interrelationships among the components of intimate interactions. It proposes that intimate experiences are intrinsically rewarding to the individual and that these experiences may explain links between intimate interactions and well-being. Its objective is to identify processes by which intimate behavior generates intimate experiences. Chapter 9 investigates interrelationships between intimate interactions and intimate relationships. It proposes that frequent intimate interactions between relationship partners (or relational intimacy) should exert beneficial effects on the functioning of that relationship. Its objective is to identify interrelationships between relational intimacy, intimate relationship functioning, and important components of intimate relationships (i.e., affection, trust, and cohesiveness).

Chapters 8 and 9 also address a third proposition, namely, that the effects of intimate interactions and relationships can only be understood in context. These chapters suggest that no behavior or adaptation is effective in all contexts. Context affects behavior directly and modifies its impact on interactions and relationships. Chapter 8 identifies four levels of contextual influences: immediate, personal/relational, group, and sociocultural. The purpose of identifying levels of context is to encourage thorough and explicit study of contextual effects. Both Chapters 8 and 9 use this typology of contexts to systematically identify relevant contextual variables.

Although most contextual variables can be classified by level, some seem to exist at all four levels. Gender is one of these and receives special attention. At the immediate level, gender means sex, which refers *only* to the categories of female and male and the accompanying reproductive functions that define organisms as such. Gender is more than sex, however. It refers here to the personal, interpersonal, group, and sociocultural correlates of the categories of female and male. These correlates include personality characteristics, subgroup memberships, lifestyle, economic opportunities, and potential power and influence. The effects of gender, therefore, cannot be attributed solely to individual characteristics, as they often have been.

Chapter 10 considers how intimate relationships fulfill (or fail to fulfill) our needs for intimate contact. It proposes that partners' compatibility (regarding need strengths) and negotiating skills (regarding how they should fulfill one another's intimacy needs) together determine the likelihood that their needs will be met. It proposes further that intimacy needs do not exist alone but exist in conjunction with other needs. The fulfillment of some of these may seem, on the surface, to be in opposition to the fulfillment of intimacy needs. Negotiations about intimate contact may only be effective when negotiations about fulfilling other needs are effective as well.

In the Epilogue, which summarizes the book's major themes, I make the following proposals for future study: First, because individual well-being and intimate relationship functioning are closely intertwined, the study of intimacy should address the impact of intimate interactions on both. This dual focus is most likely to yield a complete picture of how intimacy affects individual well-being. Second, the study of intimacy must consider how contextual factors modify the impact of intimate interactions on individual well-being and intimate relationships. Potent contextual factors such as relationship type, life stage, and gender deserve explicit examination by researchers. Third, researchers should draw on social-cognitive concepts like schemas to discover links between behavior and experience in intimate interactions and relationships. The carry-over of expectations and adaptive behaviors from earlier experiences may explain continuity while the impact of new experiences on these expectations and adaptations can help explain change. Fourth, an understanding of individual development should enhance and be enhanced by research on intimacy. It is likely that intimate interactions and relationships exert their beneficial effects on individual well-being by fulfilling important psychological needs and addressing individual concerns. The better we understand the interplay between intimacy and individual concerns and needs, the more complete our understanding of intimacy's beneficial effects will be.

CONCEPTIONS
OF INTIMACY

What Is Intimacy?

> The life of human beings . . . does not exist in
> virtue of activities alone which have some *thing*
> for their object. . . . This and the like together
> establish the realm of *I–It*. . . . But the realm of
> *I–Thou* has a different basis. . . . When *Thou* is
> spoken, there is no thing. *Thou* has no bounds.
> —MARTIN BUBER, *I and Thou*

Consider whether the following scene between Mira and Val, who are
friends, seems intimate:

> [Val] sighed, and turned to Mira. "So how are you and Ben?" . . . [Mira
> answered,] "I don't know why I'm feeling so low. . . . [Ben] wants a
> baby." [Mira] watched Val's face. It did not change. "How do you feel
> about that?" [Val asked]. "Well, it may seem strange coming from me
> but I'm not sure I even like the idea of marriage." [Mira] developed it;
> Val watched her intently. . . . "What would I do? . . . I know I should-
> n't have a baby, I know that for myself. But I love Ben so much, I
> might give in. Just the thought of being without him gives me the sen-
> sation of being on an elevator that suddenly drops ten floors. . . ." Mira
> saw in Val's face what it was that made her so extraordinary. . . . Val's
> expression at this moment had everything in it; understanding, com-
> passion, the knowledge of pain, an awareness of the impossibility of
> what, when we are young, we consider happiness, and at the same
> time, an amused, ironic gaiety, the joy of the survivor who knows the
> value of small pleasures. . . . They laughed together heartily. "Fuck the
> future!" Val crowed, and Mira grabbed her hand and they sat looking
> at each other's not-young faces . . . grinning at a joke that in this
> young place was not widely shared. (French, 1977, pp. 558–560)

At times it is easy to decide when an experience or exchange between people is intimate. A friend discloses her most personal fears, joys,
and struggles to another (as Mira does here). The other listens intently,
responding with "understanding, compassion, the knowledge of pain" (as
Val does). One friend appreciates that the other is "extraordinary." Two
friends laugh together about a private meaning that may or may not be
understood by others who are present. These are intimacy's modal characteristics, the first to occur to scholars and laypersons alike when they
are asked to define intimacy (e.g., Helgeson, Shaver, & Dyer, 1987; Monsour, 1992). The conversation between Mira and Val therefore is easily
classified as an intimate interaction.

It is also easy to imagine scenarios that are more on the boundary of
commonly held conceptions of intimacy. Consider the following:

> Two people who have just met come together for a sexual encounter,
> learning much about one another's bodies but still knowing little about
> each other's values, beliefs, preferences, and secrets.

> Two strangers, each enjoying a solitary hike through the mountains,
> stop to enjoy an especially beautiful vista in silence. Their eyes meet
> momentarily in mutual acknowledgment of the overwhelming majesty
> of the scene before them, but they do not speak.

Unlike the example with Mira and Val, these examples of intimacy seem
to occur (1) outside of a relationship context and (2) without words. Lay
conceptions of intimacy, however, emphasize verbal self-disclosure and
an ongoing relationship between people (Monsour, 1992; Waring &
Chelune, 1983; Waring, Tillman, Frelick, Russell, & Weisz, 1980). Consider another example:

> A mother listens carefully and compassionately to her 5-year-old son's
> tearful description of an encounter with the neighborhood bully. To
> show him that she understands his dilemma, she shares with him her
> own experiences with bullies when she was a child.

Although this interaction is intimate, there may be limitations to the intimacy that this mother and son can share. Intimacy might be limited
when two partners do not have the same psychological relationships with
one another (Duck, 1994a). According to Duck, different psychological
relationships occur when partner A has more knowledge about partner B
than B has about A. If partners must have the same psychological relationship with one another to be considered intimate, then the relation-

ship between a parent and a child or between a psychotherapist and a client would be excluded. Yet, as the example suggests, much about these relationships is intimate.

These examples of boundary cases illustrate why no single definition of intimacy can be found in the theoretical, research, or clinical literature. This chapter, as a consequence, is devoted to articulating a definition that can meaningfully encompass existing definitions.

FUNCTIONS OF A DEFINITION OF INTIMACY

I propose four functions that a working definition of intimacy should serve. First, a definition of intimacy should integrate the various perspectives that currently exist about what intimacy is (Montgomery, 1984b). Different definitions of intimacy come from different theories of personality and interpersonal relations, each of which has made contributions to our understanding of intimacy. A good definition of intimacy should illuminate the linkages between existing theoretical perspectives.

Second, a good definition of intimacy should define the relationship between one locus of intimacy and another. Acitelli and Duck (1987) noted that definitions of intimacy often fail to specify whether intimacy is an individual capacity, a property of interactions, or a characteristic of a relationship. A good definition of intimacy, then, should facilitate understanding of the conceptual links between intimacy in dyadic interactions and intimate relationships. It should also incorporate the common usage of the word, which refers to individual experience. Lay conceptions of intimacy often consider experiences of transcendence and/or intense emotion (Register & Henley, 1992), experiences that involve another person in an important way, to be integral to intimacy.

Third, scholarly definitions of intimacy must distinguish between the concept of intimacy and related concepts (Perlman & Fehr, 1987). Intimacy clearly overlaps with concepts such as love, closeness, self-disclosure, support, bonding, attachment, and sexuality. While a good definition will never eliminate the overlapping nature of concepts, it should allow scholars to distinguish between studies that address intimacy and those that, for example, address love.

Fourth, a good working definition of intimacy recognizes that the ultimate definition is unobtainable. A definition of intimacy must allow for the kind of concept intimacy is. Intimacy is a "natural" or "fuzzy" concept, which means that it is characterized by a shifting template of features rather than by a clearly bounded set (Fehr, 1993; Helgeson et al.,

1987; Rosch et al., 1976). Clear distinctions between the features of intimate relationships and the features of other kinds of relationships will not
always be possible, particularly regarding peripheral features and border-
line examples.

To these four requirements, I add a fifth. Ideally, a definition scholars use should be reconcilable with (if not identical to) lay definitions. A
scholarly definition clearly needs more precision than do lay definitions,
but it may not be useful if it excludes many of the experiences the average
layperson would call intimate. The risk of deviating too much from lay
definitions is that research will be undertaken that has little relevance to
people's everyday experiences with intimacy.

INTIMACY AS A NATURAL CONCEPT

Intimacy is a natural concept (Helgeson et al., 1987). A natural concept
is one in which the boundaries that separate category members from non-
members are fuzzy (Rosch et al., 1976). As a result of these fuzzy boundaries, natural concepts are organized so that some examples of the concept are more central (e.g., a central example of intimacy is a mutually
supportive heart-to-heart talk between two adolescent girls) while others
are more peripheral (e.g., two preschool girls having fun playing together
in the sandbox). Peripheral members are distinguished by the disagreement that comes up regarding their membership in the category. Because
this uncertainty regarding membership is inherent, intimacy and other
natural categories have been called fuzzy concepts.

If scholars lack consensus about what the definition of intimacy is, it
is in part because it is difficult to specify the features of a natural concept.
Such concepts are organized differently than are classical or logical concepts (Cantor & Mischel, 1979; Medin, 1989). Logical concepts have
summary lists of features or properties that are necessary for membership
in the category defined by the concept and sufficient to determine membership. While some concepts qualify as logical concepts by these criteria
(concepts like triangle, for example) most concepts do not. Scientific research, however, has traditionally relied on the precision of logical concepts. It is in the interest of precision that scholars have directed their efforts toward identifying a set of defining features for intimacy (e.g.,
Orlofsky, 1988; Prager, 1983a; Reis & Shaver, 1988; Schaefer & Olson,
1981). Natural concepts like intimacy, however, are not characterized by
finite lists of necessary and sufficient features.

The probabilistic nature of category membership, then, complicates
efforts to study intimacy scientifically (Fehr & Russell, 1991; Medin,

1989; Rosch et al., 1976) and becomes a problem when examples are at the periphery of the concept. Peripheral examples may be equally qualified for membership in two related categories. As Buss (1988) put it, "[because] category members are not sharply demarcated . . . each category blends into adjacent ones. Thus, the category of love may blend into the categories of liking, lust, friendship, affection, or passion" (p. 109). In the case of fuzzy concepts, category membership is more continuous or probabilistic than discrete.

If a natural concept like intimacy has no single set of defining features and if the boundaries between intimacy and related concepts are blurry, it might seem that an organized body of research on intimacy could never accumulate. The picture is not so grim, however, because, natural categories have their own predictable structure despite their probabilistic character (Medin, 1989). One way to use this structure to increase generalizability across paradigms and across studies is discussed in this chapter.

Research on intimacy can take advantage of the fact that natural categories are structured hierarchically (Rosch et al., 1976). Specifically, there is a nested hierarchy of abstraction within concepts. At the *basic level*, a category is one that has achieved a balance between two principles of categorization: (1) it effectively discriminates phenomena in the category from phenomena in similar but not identical categories, and (2) it reduces trivial differences among members within the category so that the most important attributes of category members overlap, leaving only less important attributes to distinguish them. At the next higher level of abstraction are *superordinate* categories whose members share only a few attributes. At a lower level of abstraction than the basic level (i.e., a more specific level) are *subordinate* categories, or categories whose members share most attributes and are differentiated only on more trivial or less central attributes. Guitar, piano, and drum are all basic level categories. Musical instrument is the superordinate category, while folk guitar, grand piano, and kettle drum are subordinate categories (Rosch et al., 1976, p. 388).

The basic level of a conceptual hierarchy maximizes its *cue validity*, which refers to its differentiation from other categories. The higher the cue validity of a category, the more differentiated it is from similar categories. Superordinate categories have low cue validity because category members share too few attributes, while subordinate categories lack cue validity because category members share too many attributes (Rosch et al., 1976).

Attributes of concepts are also organized on a scale of *prototypicality* (Fehr, 1988). Any attribute shared by members of a category can be

ranked according to how many members of the category possess that attribute. The greater the proportion of members possessing the attribute,
the more prototypical the attribute is (Rosch & Mervis, 1975).

This hierarchy of attributes is important in understanding natural
concepts because members of these categories often do not possess all of
the defining features of the category. Rather, they overlap with one another in a pattern that Wittgenstein (1953) called a "family resemblance
structure." A family resemblance structure can be depicted as a set of concentric circles. The largest proportion of cases share the features in the
center circle. For example, the center circle would contain those features
that serve as the most salient cues for signalling intimacy. The outer circles contain less salient feautures; they are often present, but are less pervasive. They are therefore not particularly salient in signaling intimacy.
Moreover, features in the outer circles overlap more frequently with features of related concepts (e.g., love, trust) and are therefore less serviceable in distinguishing examples of intimacy from related phenomena. A
hypothetical family resemblance structure of the features of intimacy is
depicted in Figure 1.1.

When features characterizing a concept are organized in concentric

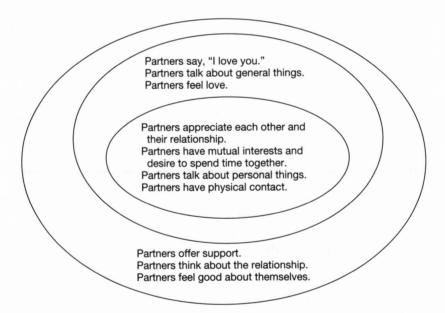

FIGURE 1.1. Hypothetical family resemblance structure for features of intimacy.
(Features taken from Helgeson, Shaver, & Dyer, 1987.)

circles, examples that possess many or most of the features in the center circle can be identified as *prototypes*. When concepts are organized around prototypes, an example's resemblance to the prototype decides category membership (Fehr, 1988; Fehr & Russell, 1991; Rosch & Mervis, 1975; Rosch et al., 1976). Prototypic members of a category are those that "most reflect the redundancy structure of the category as a whole" (Rosch, et al., 1976, p. 433). By this logic, both examples mentioned above—the supportive, self-disclosing adolescent girls and the preschoolers enjoying sandbox play—could be examples of intimacy. Evidence from research on laypeople's definitions of intimacy suggests that the first example, "that of the adolescent girls talking, incorporates more features that are higher in the hierarchy (i.e., are in the center circle) than does the second example. This is because, for laypeople, self-disclosure serves as a more salient intimacy cue than sharing activities (Helgeson et al., 1987; Monsour, 1992). The adolescent girls' conversation appears more prototypical because it incorporates features of intimacy shared by many other examples of the concept. Moreover, the children's sandbox play would be judged as an example of intimacy to the extent that the features of sandbox play are similar to the adolescent girls' conversation (Medin, 1989). As Buss (1988) put it, "[examples will] differ in their status from highly central or prototypical to progressively more peripheral until the fuzzy borders are reached and the adjoining categories are entered" (p. 110).

A MULTITIERED CONCEPT OF INTIMACY

Scholars are still left with the important task of defining intimacy. How can information about natural concepts help us define intimacy in a way that is helpful to researchers hoping to explore a distinct aspect of human experience? First, scholars should decide whether to retain intimacy as a superordinate, basic, or subordinate concept. I will argue momentarily that while intimacy may serve the lay public well as a basic concept (Helgeson et al., 1987), it will serve scholars better as a superordinate concept. Second, by recognizing the fuzzy boundaries inherent in natural concepts, scholars may be better off defining one or more of the essential features of intimacy instead of trying to establish the boundaries around it. Scholars could determine how the prototypical attributes of related concepts such as intimacy, love, trust, affection, and closeness differ while recognizing that peripheral features and cases are likely to overlap. Third, scholars may wish to define prototypes that can guide decisions about what kinds of cases will be included in the study of intimacy.

Intimacy as a Superordinate Concept

Intimacy may serve scholars best as a superordinate concept under which certain basic concepts are subsumed. The reason intimacy works better as a superordinate concept than as a basic one is that there are too few attributes that all instances of intimacy share to lend the concept much cue validity. For example, each of the following seems to be an instance of intimacy:

- When Jorge looks at Mariano, he feels a rush of warmth and love (intimacy seems to be an emotion).
- Jerry holds his infant close and strokes his skin (intimacy seems to describe tender physical contact).
- Yan Chang tells Alice a secret, and Alice promises not to reveal it to anyone (intimacy seems to involve sharing private information).
- Kareem is married to Aretha (intimacy seems to describe a kind of relationship).
- Marta knows that when Dwight purses his lips and looks away, he's feeling nervous (intimacy describes how well two people know each other).
- Wilma and Betty reminisce about their many shared experiences (intimacy seems to describe a kind of interaction).
- Felicia caresses Alex (intimacy seems to describe sexual contact).
- Mark feels close to Greg while they are fishing in silence (intimacy requires no communication).
- Marion stands close enough to Edward for him to feel her breath on his face (intimacy describes how two people occupy space together).

While each of these could be an example of intimacy in its common usage, there are few features these examples have in common. Intimacy researchers have faced the undesirable choice of talking simultaneously about all of the phenomena represented in the above examples or implicitly ignoring some aspects of intimacy. Intimacy is too broad a concept, with too little cue validity, to be of much value to scholars.

Basic Intimacy Concepts

For scholarly purposes, I suggest that the superordinate concept of intimacy be parceled into two basic concepts: intimate interactions and intimate relationships. Hinde's (1981) distinction between these two concepts can be useful here. Hinde has argued that interactions are dialogues between people and do not require the presence of a relationship to occur. Relationships, in contrast, imply "a series of interactions between two individuals known to each other." In the context of a relationship, an "interaction is affected by past interactions [and] is likely to influence future ones" (p. 2). Intimate interactions, then, are dialogues between people that have certain specific characteristics (to be discussed momentarily), and intimate relationships involve multiple dialogues over time.

Intimate interactions and intimate relationships, then, may serve researchers well as basic intimacy concepts because they each refer to a different and clearly distinguishable notion of *space and time*. Interactions refer to dyadic behavior that exists within a clearly designated space-and-time framework. Once that particular set of dyadic behavior has ceased, the interaction is over. Relationships, however, exist in a much broader, more abstract space-and-time framework. Their beginnings and endings are more difficult to mark. They continue in the absence of any observable behavior between the partners.

A clear distinction between intimate interactions and intimate relationships is important for several reasons. First, those factors that affect intimate interactions may not necessarily be the same ones that most affect intimate relationships (Duck & Sants, 1983). For example, characteristics of the immediate context (time of day, nature of occasion, physical surroundings) may strongly affect a particular interaction but have minimal effect on a relationship (see Chapters 8 and 9). Second, only a fraction of the interactions in an intimate relationship is intimate (Clark & Reis, 1988). Intimate partners argue, have fun together, and advise, consult, inform, and ignore one another. None of these interactions need be intimate, yet the partners may nevertheless have an intimate relationship. Finally, intimate interactions clearly do not always occur in relationships. Wynne and Wynne (1986) note that intimate disclosures may occur in interactions between strangers precisely "*because* of the unlikelihood of a further relationship and the attendant opportunities for betrayal" (p. 385; emphasis in original). For these reasons, intimate interactions and intimate relationships are best understood as separate, although related, phenomena.

Intimate interactions serve as the starting point for a definition of intimacy in this book. In part, this is because intimate relationships, both conceptually and in fact, are built on multiple intimate interactions. It is difficult to imagine referring to the friendship between Mira and Val as intimate, for example, without assuming that these friends have engaged, at some point and probably frequently, in intimate interactions. In contrast, although intimate interactions can exist without intimate relationships, the presence of an intimate relationship surely influences the probability and frequency of such interactions.

Intimate interactions serve as an excellent starting point for a second reason as well: The concept of intimate interaction can serve as a conceptual bridge between discrete behaviors and experiences on the one hand and intimate relationships on the other. This is because intimate interactions themselves can be broken down for heuristic purposes into two components: intimate behavior and intimate experience. Intimate behaviors refer to the actual observable behaviors people engage in when interacting intimately, whether these are verbal or nonverbal (e.g., self-disclosure, attentive listening). Intimate experiences are the feelings and perceptions people have during and because of their intimate interactions (e.g., warmth, pleasure, affection). Intimate interactions, then, are composed of behaviors and experiences, while intimate relationships are composed of multiple intimate interactions and their experiential by-products. This multitiered concept of intimacy is depicted in Figure 1.2.

Intimate Interactions

When is an interaction intimate? All conceptions of intimate interactions (see Chapter 2) seem to center on the notion that intimate behav-

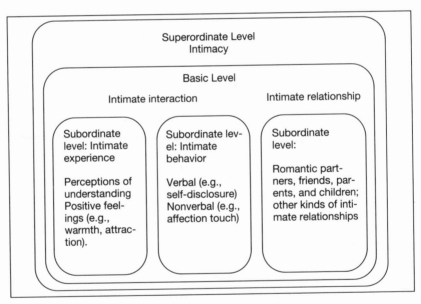

FIGURE 1.2. Multitiered concept of intimacy.

ior consists of sharing that which is personal.[1] Each conception suggests that whether partners share a touch or a verbal expression of emotion, reveal information about themselves, or acknowledge mutual understanding, they would not do so under impersonal circumstances.

This attribute of intimate interactions is so important to the concept of intimacy that the word *intimate* has been used to describe the information itself (e.g., an intimate revelation). As several scholars have suggested, however, equating intimacy with conversational topics omits too much about intimacy that matters to people (e.g., Montgomery, 1984a, 1984b; Reis & Shaver, 1988; Wynne & Wynne, 1986). The sharing of intimate interactions, then, need not be confined to the verbal disclosure of personal facts (Morton, 1978).

Conceptions of intimate sharing have referred to both verbal and nonverbal behaviors (Reis & Shaver, 1988). Verbal sharing can involve self-disclosure of personal facts, opinions, and beliefs; it can also include emotional expressiveness. Nonverbal sharing can include a shared meaningful glance; an affectionate touch; shared emotional expression, such as tears or laughter; and shared sexuality. Some scholarly conceptions of intimate interaction have suggested that sharing must contain a "revelation" in order to be intimate (Beach & Tesser, 1988; Reis & Shaver, 1988). This view may unnecessarily eliminate such intimate moments as squeezing hands under the dinner table or gazing into the eyes of a beloved infant. These moments involve sharing something deeply personal with another, even though the message may be one that the other is already aware of ("I love you") and even though the message is not verbalized.

Conceptions of intimate interactions have at times been limited to those that are reciprocal in some way (e.g., M. S. Davis, 1973). I suggest that this is also an unnecessary constraint that eliminates many people's experiences of intimacy. A more comprehensive notion of sharing includes both reciprocal and complementary sharing. When sharing is reciprocal, each partner in an interaction shares something similar with the other, verbally or nonverbally. For example, when self-disclosure is reciprocal, each partner divulges personal information to the other. When reciprocal sharing is nonverbal, for example, each lover may stroke the other while each gazes into the other's eyes. Other examples might include friends walking with linked arms or a parent and child watching television with their arms wrapped around one another.

Sharing can also be complementary. In this type of intimate interaction, partners engage in different kinds of participation. For example, in many interactions, one partner will self-disclose while the other sensitively responds to what is disclosed (as in Reis and Shaver's model and in

Miller's, [1990] model). Interactions between a psychotherapist and client, often experienced as intimate (Fisher & Stricker, 1982), are complementary in that the partners do not have equal amounts of knowledge about one another. Socially supportive intimate interactions can be complementary when one partner asks for advice, support, or reassurance about a personal matter and the other provides it sensitively (e.g., Duck, 1990).

Intimate interactions, however, are best defined not only by the kinds of behavior that characterize them but by the intimate experiences of the partners during or as a result of the interaction. Intimate experiences themselves can be usefully defined as having affective and cognitive/perceptual components. The affective component consists of positive involvement in, interest in, or feelings about oneself, the interaction, and the partner. The cognitive/perceptual component consists of each partner's perception that there is an understanding between the partners.

In this book I have restricted the affective component of intimate experience to *positive experiences* because conversations that generate negative affect between the partners are not usually experienced as intimate (Derlega & Chaikin, 1975). As Clark and Reis (1988) aptly noted, "It does not seem appropriate to describe the consequences of fighting or emotional withholding in a marriage, for example, as a negative effect of intimacy, because it is precisely the failure to adequately provide components of the intimacy process per se that is problematic" (p. 637). People can, of course, experience intimacy while sharing unpleasant emotions with another person; for example, combat veterans talk of intimacy on the battlefield (L. Rubin, 1985). Here, negative emotion is not directed at the partner or the interaction but to an external target. Positive affect and perceiving oneself as understood by another together might constitute *validation* (see Sullivan, 1953, and Reis & Shaver, 1988).

The multitiered concept of intimacy in this book therefore begins with a definition of intimate interactions. Intimate interactions are conceptualized as having two components: intimate behavior and intimate experience. An intimate interaction, then, is one in which partners share personal, private material; feel positively about each other and themselves; and perceive a mutual understanding between them. In order to avoid excluding intimate moments, sexual encounters, shared silence, and other interactions commonly experienced as intimate, this definition goes beyond the traditional social psychological one (i.e., beyond verbal self-disclosure and sympathetic responsiveness). It still includes, however, the lengthy verbal exchanges that theorists such as Sullivan (1953), Rogers (1980), and Jourard (1968) envisioned.

By defining intimacy primarily in terms of interactions, I have conceptualized intimacy as dyadic. A difficulty with dyadic notions of intimate interactions, raised by Acitelli and Duck (1987), arises when researchers and clinicians wish to consider the separate points of view of each person participating in the interaction. While one partner may have experienced an interaction as intimate, the other partner may not have had that experience. This raises the question of whether an interaction is intimate if only one partner experiences it as such. For example, if either party is deceiving or exploiting the other, is feeling abused or used, or is dissembling in any way, then it would be difficult to define the interaction as intimate, even if one party is fooled into thinking it is so. Duck (1994a) has argued that in such cases, the partners are in two completely different psychological relationships. When intimacy researchers have only one partner's perspective, we may therefore need to acknowledge that our information about a particular interaction is incomplete (Acitelli & Duck, 1987).

Intimate Relationships

When intimate interactions serve as the starting point for a definition of intimacy, intimate relationships can then be defined in relation to intimate interactions. The nature of the association between intimate interactions and intimate relationships is far from clear, however. At the simplest level, an intimate relationship is one in which intimate interactions occur on a regular and predictable basis. There is a history of repeated intimate interactions, and each partner in the relationship can count on and expect intimate interactions with the other at acceptable intervals. *Relational intimacy*, in this book, refers to the presence of frequent intimate interactions between the relationship partners.[2]

As noted by Reis and Shaver (1988), however, we rarely imply so narrow a definition of an intimate relationship. Indeed, most would argue that the existence of these frequently occurring interactions themselves create other dimensions of intimate relationships that become part of our definition of an intimate relationship in their own right (Acitelli & Duck, 1987; Reis & Shaver, 1988).

If intimate relationships are defined by the presence of relational intimacy, and if relational intimacy alone does not suffice to define an intimate relationship, what else should we include in a definition? There are two approaches to addressing this question that are worth considering. One is to include the by-products of intimate interactions in a definition of intimate relationships. These by-products arise from the intimate experiences that both generate and are generated by intimate behavior. Intimate experiences, however, are momentary (by definition). They exist in a space-and-time framework immediate to the interaction itself. It is likely, however, that these experiences can evolve into more long-term states or characteristic patterns of feeling and thinking in relation to a particular interaction partner. For example, I have argued that intimate interactions by definition involve partners having warm feelings toward one another. It seems reasonable to presume that over time these warm feelings would develop into a more enduring affection, regard, or love for the partner that would persist even when the partners are in conflict. Enduring affection may, therefore, reasonably be included among the defining characteristics of intimate relationships.

A second approach would define the characteristics of intimate relationships as those that are necessary for sustaining relational intimacy. Because the presence of relational intimacy is necessarily a defining feature of an intimate relationship, then those characteristics of relationships that are necessary for sustaining relational intimacy reasonably become defining features of intimate relationships as well.

Using a combination of these two approaches, I argue here for the inclusion of three relationship features in a definition of intimate relationships: (1) sustained affection (or love) between the partners, (2) mutual trust, and (3) partner cohesiveness. Each of these relationship characteristics is a by-product of intimate interaction and contributes to the maintenance of relational intimacy.

Intimacy and Affection. The literature on love has addressed, in both theory and empirical research, how intimacy and affection are associated in personal relationships. Research has revealed an intimacy component in love relationships (Hendrick & Hendrick, 1986; Sternberg & Grajek, 1984). Similarly, people who regularly engage in intimate interactions are more likely to love one another than those who do not. Measures of love often encompass intimacy.

In this book, affectionate relationships are a broader class of relationships within which intimate relationships fall. There are relationships in which the partners feel affection for one another but do not engage in intimate interactions (e.g., relationships in conflict, relationship partners separated by distance). In contrast, it is difficult to imagine an intimate relationship in which partners do not feel affection for one another. If intimate interactions, by definition, involve partners having positive feelings for one another, then intimate relationships should principally include those in which there is some affection between the partners.

Intimacy and Trust. Intimate relationships create the framework of trust that makes intimate interactions more likely (Reis & Shaver, 1988). Trust is an attitude or expectation that one partner has toward another that allows that partner to take the risks involved in intimate interaction.

Deutsch (1973) defined trust as "confidence that one will find what is desired from another, rather than what is feared." A trusting partner believes that she or he faces little risk of harm, exploitation, betrayal, or deceit from another as a result of any intimate encounter the two partners may have (Gurtman, 1992). Since intimacy involves revealing the vulnerable parts of the self, partners must trust one another to continue to interact intimately, almost by definition. Conversely, it is also likely that intimate interactions establish trust (Altman & Taylor, 1973). Intimate interactions provide partners with the opportunity to demonstrate their trustworthiness. Early in relationships, intimate behavior is necessarily based on the hope that this partner will turn out to be trustworthy rather than on any evidence from experience (J. Holmes, 1991).

Intimacy and Cohesiveness. I suggest that intimacy and cohesiveness may best be thought of as two classes of overlapping, but not identical, experiences people can have in their relationships. Cohesiveness is the togetherness, sharing of time, and sharing of activities in a relationship (Beach, Sandeen, & O'Leary, 1990; Spanier, 1976). I would argue further that intimacy in relationships requires cohesiveness. To engage in intimate interaction, people have to be together in positive ways (including telephoning or writing, when these are the only ways available to be together).[3] Experiences of cohesiveness, in contrast, may or may not include intimate experiences. Two people can enjoy completing a task together (agentic cohesiveness) or watching a ball game together (communal cohesiveness) without also engaging in intimate interaction (Robins, 1990). However, cohesive activity, such as sharing a meal, may often serve as a backdrop for intimate interaction.

An intimate relationship, then, is one in which the partners share regular intimate interactions, feel affection for one another, trust one another, and have cohesiveness. Affection, trust, and cohesiveness seem to be necessary conditions for sustaining intimacy in a relationship. They are also by-products of intimate interactions. Most intimate relationships, of course, have many other characteristics that are important to sustaining intimacy and that undoubtedly result from intimate interactions. Relationships that lack affection, cohesion, or trust seem unlikely, however, to sustain intimate interactions.

Intimate versus Nonintimate Relationships

To make meaningful predictions about intimate relationships, we must distinguish them from nonintimate relationships. Nonintimate relationships include relationships that are impersonal or role-bound (e.g., physicians and patients, students and teachers), more casual or distant personal relationships (e.g., casual friendships, friendly neighbors, schoolmates, "tennis buddies"), and relationships that once were but are no longer intimate (e.g., ex-spouses, former friends). In contrast to nonintimate relationships, then, intimate relationships are less role-bound and more involved and are characterized by frequently occurring intimate interactions *in the present*.

Intimate relationships should also be distinguishable from *close relationships* that lack intimacy. Kelley et al. (1983) described close relationships as those characterized by "strong, frequent, and diverse interdependence" (p. 38). They noted that "relationships need not involve the exchange of intimate information or produce regular intense positive feelings in order to be tightly interconnected in the ways we would regard as defining closeness" (p. 39). Marital, parent–child, and sibling relationships exemplify relationships that are nearly always close but not always intimate. Close relationships that are low in intimacy would include Cuber and Haroff's (1965) devitalized marriages, Fitzpatrick's (1988) "separates," and the pseudointimates described by Orlofsky, Marcia, and Lesser (1973). They would also include those relationships that are chronically discordant (e.g., Cuber and Haroff's conflict-habituated couples) if that discord precludes intimate interactions. Intimate partners differ from partners who are close but not intimate, then, because they frequently engage in personal, affectively positive interactions that convey and promote mutual understanding.

SUMMARY AND CONCLUSIONS

In this chapter, I have created a multitiered concept of intimacy. I have identified intimacy as a superordinate concept, and suggested that intimacy, as a concept, cannot be defined precisely enough for research purposes. Rather, basic intimacy concepts, within a clearly delineated superordinate structure, can be defined with more precision and are therefore more likely to be serviceable for the study of intimacy.

The two basic intimacy concepts that are addressed in this book are *intimate interaction* and *intimate relationship*. This book's working definition of intimate interaction includes both *intimate behavior* and *intimate experience*. The former is any behavior in which partners share that which is personal and/or private with each other. Intimate experience is the positive affect and perceived understanding that partners experience along with or as a result of their intimate behavior.

My definition of intimate relationships begins with *relational intimacy*, which refers to the presence of ongoing, frequently occurring intimate interactions between the partners. A complete definition of intimate relationships should go further, however, to include partners' enduring feelings or attitudes that result from their intimate interactions. By the same token, a definition of intimate relationship should also include characteristics of the relationship that are necessary for sustaining continued relational intimacy. I have proposed three characteristics that appear to meet these criteria: affection, trust, and cohesiveness. Each of these seems to both emerge from and sustain relational intimacy.

Existing Conceptions of Intimacy: An Overview

Chapter 1 identified two basic intimacy concepts: intimate interactions and intimate relationships. *Intimate interactions* are dyadic verbal or non-verbal exchanges in which one or both partners share something private or personal with the other.[1] Intimate interactions leave partners feeling positively about one another and about themselves. Intimate partners perceive that they know and/or understand each other. Intimate relationships exist over time and are characterized by a history of intimate interacting. Intimate partners expect to continue having intimate interactions in the future. Intimate relationships are also characterized by affection, trust, and cohesiveness between the partners. (See Chapter 1 for a more detailed discussion of these concepts.)

The current chapter uses these two basic intimacy concepts as lenses through which to view and organize existing conceptions of intimacy. These intimacy concepts are useful for this purpose in several ways. First, they allow existing conceptions to be systematically differentiated from one another, based on which basic intimacy concept receives the most emphasis. Second, they reveal areas of overlap among conceptions. While different conceptions may emphasize different basic intimacy concepts, few are pure types. Rather, most conceptions attempt to address more than one intimacy concept. Because the multiple intimacy concepts being addressed are not clearly articulated, however, most conceptions are fuzzier than they need to be. A third way in which the two basic intimacy concepts are useful, then, is in clarifying existing conceptions.

These intimacy concepts may also be useful because of what they leave out. They do not include intimacy capacity as a type of intimacy. They therefore distinguish between conceptions of intimacy and conceptions of individual differences in intimacy capacity.

Conceptions of intimacy capacity are concerned with defining individual differences in needs, desires, or capacities for intimacy. They describe individual characteristics that increase the likelihood that an individual will participate in intimate interactions and/or relationships. They also make predictions about who will find satisfaction in intimate relationships and who will be able to sustain those relationships. This review includes conceptions emphasizing individual differences because of their important influence on theory and research on intimacy. However, conceptions emphasizing individual differences are not treated as conceptions of intimacy per se.

Each section in this chapter addresses a group of definitions from the existing literature. These definitions are grouped on the basis of which basic intimacy concept seems to receive the most emphasis. Each section also reviews the theoretical underpinnings of the definitions in that group. Some of these definitions, organized by intimacy concept, are presented in Table 2.1. Finally, each section describes measures of intimacy that seem to reflect the conception of intimacy being discussed. Sample measures of intimacy, organized in this fashion, are presented in Table 2.2.

TABLE 2.1. Conceptions of Intimacy

Conceptions emphasizing intimate interactions: Intimate behavior	
Sullivan (1953, p. 246)	"clearly formulated adjustments of one's behavior to the expressed needs of the other person"
M. Patterson (1976, p. 235)	"a product of eye contact, distance, smiling and other behaviors"
Fruzzetti & Jackson (1990, pp. 126–127)	"an interaction that . . . is self-revealing and/or relationship-focused in its content . . . one partner does or says something [that] . . . is readily discriminated . . . by the partner, who responds in a positive, understanding and/or self-revealing way her- or himself"
Reis & Shaver (1988, p. 375)	"an interpersonal process that involves communication of personal feelings and information to another person who responds warmly and sympathetically. This response validates the first person's experience"

(continued)

TABLE 2.1 (*continued*)

Conceptions emphasizing intimate interactions: Intimate experience	
Chelune, Robinson, & Krommor (1984, p.13)	"a subjective appraisal, based upon interactive behaviors, that leads to certain relational expectations"
Sexton & Sexton (1982, p .2)	"closeness, love, caring, and affection"
L'Abate & L'Abate (1979, p. 178)	"the sharing of hurt and of fears of being hurt"
Conceptions emphasizing intimate relationships	
Sternberg (1986, pp. 120–121)	"(a) a desire to promote the welfare of the loved one, (b) experienced happiness with loved one, (c) high regard for the loved one, (d) being able to count on the loved one in times of need, (e) mutual understanding with the loved one, (f) sharing of one's self and one's possessions with the loved one, (g) receipt of emotional support from the loved one, (h) giving of emotional support to the loved one, (i) intimate communication with the loved one, and (j) valuing the loved one in one's life"
Tolstedt & Stokes (1983, p. 574)	"reflects feelings of closenesss and emotional bonding including intensity of liking, moral support and ability to tolerate flaws in the significant other"
S. Gilbert (1976, p. 221)	"a deep form of acceptance of the other as well as a commitment to the relationship"
Waring (1981, p. 34)	"a composite of . . . affection . . . expressiveness . . . compatibility . . . cohesion . . . sexuality . . . conflict resolution . . . autonomy . . . and identity"
Perlman & Fehr (1987, p. 16)	"the closeness and interdependence of partners, the extent of self-disclosure, and the warmth or affection experienced [within the relationship]"
Clinebell & Clinebell (1970, p. 1)	"the degree of mutual need-satisfaction within the relationship"

TABLE 2.2. Selected Measures of Intimacy and Related Constructs

Authors	Measure name	Construct assessed	Subscales and reliability	Appropriate population	Validity
		Measures of intimate interaction: Intimate behavior			
Furman & Buhrmester (1985); Buhrmester & Furman (1987)	Network of Relationships Inventory (NRI)	Companionship and Intimacy	(α = .54–.95) No subscales; ratings on global intimacy and dyadic intimacy	Developed with elementary and middle school children	
Jourard & Lasakow (1958)	Jourard Self-Disclosure Inventory (SDI)	Depth and breadth of self-disclosure	Five disclosure targets; mother, father, male friend, female friend, spouse	Developed with college students	
Mannarino (1976)	Chumship Checklist	Intimacy with a best friend or "chum"	No subscales; assesses three criteria of friendship: friendship stability, honest communication and sensitivity to friend's needs, preference to spend time with friend	Developed with 60 6th grade boys	
Snell, Miller, & Belk (1988)	Emotional Self-Disclosure Scale (ESDS)	Self-disclosure	(α = .83–.95; test–retest r = .35–.72) Depression, Happiness, Jealousy, Anxiety, Anger, Calm, Apathy, Fear	Developed with college students	

(continued)

TABLE 2.2. (continued)

Authors	Measure name	Construct assessed	Subscales and reliability	Appropriate population	Validity
Snell, Belk, & Hawkins (1986)	Masculine and Feminine Self-Disclosure Scale	Self-disclosure of sex-typed personality characteristics	Four subscales: Masculine Traits, Masculine Behaviors, Feminine Traits, Feminine Behaviors ($\alpha = .80–.94$)	Developed with college students	Measure showed positive correlations with Jourard Self-Disclosure Questionnaire.
Taylor & Altman (1966); Strassberg & Anchor (1975)	Intimacy Rating Scale	Depth/intimacy of self-disclosure	($\alpha = .82–.96$) Thirteen topical categories: Religion, Love and Sex, Own Family, Parental Family, Hobbies and Interests, Physical Appearance, Money and Property, Current Events, Emotions and Feelings, Relationships with Others, Attitudes and Values, School and Work, Biography	Developed with college students	Eight of 16 student judges agreed on depth rating of over 2/3 of disclosing statements. Measure differentiated among targets students were willing to disclose to.
Vondracek (1969)	Amount and Intimacy of Self-Disclosure	Intimacy of self-disclosure	Amount and intimacy of self-disclosure (interrater reliability = .71–.76)	Developed with college students	
		Measures of intimate interaction: Intimate experience			
Burgoon, Buller, Hale, & de Turck (1984); Burgoon & Hale (1988)	Relational Communication Scale	Eight themes underlying relational communication	($\alpha = .70–.86$) Immediacy/Affection Subscales (Intimacy I; $\alpha = .81$), Similarity/Depth (Intimacy II; $\alpha = .77$), Receptivity/Trust	Developed with college students	Repeated factor analytic studies determined subscales. Measure predicted variations in interactive behavior.

Source	Measure	Construct	Psychometrics	Sample	Validity/Notes
			(Intimacy III; α = .76); other subscales: Composure, Formality, Dominance, Equality, Task Orientation	Developed with college students	
Duck, Rutt, Hurst, & Strejc (1990); Leatham & Duck (1990)	Iowa Communication Record (ICR)	Components of communication	Subscales (or communication components): Quality (α = .88), Value (α = .77); Change (α = .81); Control (Kendall's W = .102)	Developed with college students	
Wheeler & Nezlek (1977)	Rochester Interaction Record (RIR)	Social interaction, intimacy, and satisfaction	(α = .67–.84) No subscales	Developed with college students	Roommate pairs agree on when they interacted. κ = .76–.81.

Measures of intimate relationships: Relational measures

Source	Measure	Construct	Psychometrics	Sample	Validity/Notes
Aron, Aron, & Smollan (1992)	Inclusion of Others in Self Scale (IOS)	Interpersonal closeness	One pictorial item	Developed with college students	Measure correlated in predicted direction with Subjective Closeness Index and Sternberg Intimacy Scale and predicted relationship maintenance 3 months later.
Hetherington & Soeken (1990)	Intimate Relationship Scale (IRS)	Intimacy	Whole scale: (α = .85–.95) Three dimensions: Personal or Emotional; Physical; Cognitive	Married couples in early to middle adulthood	A panel of nurse-midwives judged content. Measure showed positive correlations with Dyadic Adjustment Scale and Relationship Change Scale.

(continued)

TABLE 2.2. (*continued*)

Authors	Measure name	Construct assessed	Subscales and reliability	Appropriate population	Validity
Maxwell (1985)	Close Relationship Questionnaire (CRQ)	Closeness in relationships	Separation Distress, Naturalness, Touching, Following, Imitation, Reciprocity and Synchrony of Behavior, Help, Similarity, Disclosure	Developed with adults ages 19–74	Close relationship partners tend to agree on closeness. Measure predicted amount of time spent together and marital satisfaction.
Moss & Schwebel (1993)	Relationship Intimacy Styles Questionnaire (RISQ)	Components of romantic intimacy	Four subscales: Cognitive, Affective, Physical, and Commitment Intimacy	Developed with "partners in enduring romantic relationships"	Content was judged by Ph.D. scientist/practitioners in health and science fields.
Schaefer & Olsen (1981)	Personal Assessment of intimacy in Relationships (PAIR)	Perceived and expected intimacy ($\alpha > .70$ for all scales)	Emotional, Social, Intellectual, Sexual, and Recreational Intimacy; Conventionality Scale	Developed with adults ages 18–61	Positive correlations were obtained with Locke–Wallace Marital Adjustment Test.
Sharabany (1974); Sharabany & Wiseman (1993)	Intimate Friendship Scale	Dimensions of intimate friendship	Eight dimensions: Frankness and Spontaneity, Sensitivity and knowing, Attachment, Exclusiveness and Uniqueness, Helping and Sharing, Degree of Being Able to Take from and Impose upon the Friend, Common Activities, Trust and Loyalty ($\alpha = .72–.89$)	School-age children to adolescents	Psychologists classified items into scales; ratings tend to be reciprocated between friends. Measure discriminates between best and "other" friend.

Study	Measure	Description	Content	Sample	Findings
Snyder, Wills, & Keiser (1981)	Marital Satisfaction Inventory (MSI)	Dimensions of marital interaction (α = .88; test–retest r = .89)	Intimacy-related: Affective Communication, Sexual Dissatisfaction, Global Affection; also Problem-Solving Communication, Quality and Quantity of Leisure Time Together, Disagreement about Finances, Sex Role Orientation, History of Family and Marital Disruption, Dissatisfaction with Children, Conflict over Childrearing; Validity Scale	Developed with married couples from community and clinic	Individual subscales differ significantly from one another in their level of behavioral specificity.
Tolstedt & Stokes (1983, 1984)	Intimacy Questionnaire	Affective and physical intimacy	Affective Intimacy (α = .78), Physical Intimacy (α = .89)	Adults, couples	Items clustered together and around an item asking about intimacy. Positive correlations were obtained with the Jourard Self-Disclosure Questionnaire.
Waring, McElrath, Mitchell, & Derry (1981)	Victoria Hospital Intimacy Interview (VHII)	Intimacy (α = .51–.66; interrater reliability = .68–.83)	Affection, Commitment, Compatibility, Expressiveness, Identity, Sexuality, Conflict Resolution, Autonomy	Couples	

(continued)

TABLE 2.2. (continued)

Authors	Measure name	Construct assessed	Subscales and reliability	Appropriate population	Validity
Waring & Reddon (1983); Reddon, Patton, & Waring (1985); Wood, Barnes, & Waring (1988)	Waring Intimacy Questionnaire (WIQ)	Marital intimacy (test–retest r for subscales = .73–.90; Kuder–Richardson 20 = .52–.87; total = .86–.89)	Conflict Resolution, Affection, Sexuality, Identity, Compatibility, Expressiveness, Autonomy, Cohesion	Developed with married couples	Confirmatory factor analysis substantiated subscale structure. Correlations were in predicted directions with Schaefer & Olson's Personal Assessment of Intimacy in Relationships.

Measure of intimate relationships: Affective-cognitive measures

Authors	Measure name	Construct assessed	Subscales and reliability	Appropriate population	Validity
Christensen & Sullaway (1984); Christensen (1987)	Relationship Issues Questionnaire	Differences in spouses' desires for intimacy and independence (α = .86 [wife], .79 [husband])	Intimacy, Independence	Married couples	Positive correlations were obtained with the Love Scale and the Dyadic Adjustment Scale.
Davis & Todd (1985); Davis & Latty-Mann (1987)	Relationship Rating Scale	Types of love (α = .96)	Viability; Intimacy; Passion; Caring; Satisfaction; Conflict	Those in a love relationship, friendships, romantic relationship	
Miller & Lefcourt (1982)	Miller Social Intimacy Scale (MSIS)	Social intimacy (α= .86–91; test-retest r = .84-96)	No subscales; 17 items	Developed with college students and married couples in therapy	Correlations were in predicted directions with Schlein, Guerney, & Stover's Interpersonal Relationship Scale, UCLA Loneliness Scale, Tennessee Self-Concept

(continued)

Source	Scale	Construct	Dimensions	Sample	Validity
					Scale, and Jackson's Personality Research Form.
Olson & Portner (1983)	Family Adaptability and Cohesion Scale (FACES II)	Cohesion and adaptability (mean α = .90; test–retest r = .84)	Emotional Bonding	Developed with 2,082 parents and 416 adolescents	Confirmatory factor analysis established construct validity.
Sternberg (1986); Chojnacki & Walsh (1990)	Triangular Love Scale	Three components of love (α = .79–90; test–retest r = .75–.81)	Three subscales: Intimacy, Commitment, Passion	Developed with college students	Positive correlations were obtained with Jourard Self-Disclosure Questionnaire.
Walker & Thompson (1983)	Intimacy	Intergenerational intimacy (α = .91–.97)	Five dimensions: General Intimacy/Affection; Attachment; Disclosure; Tension; Worry	Developed with three generations of women, ages 20s through 80s	
Measures of intimate relationships: Behavioral measures					
Stover, Guerney, Ginsberg, & Schlein (1977a, 1977b)	Self-Feeling Awareness Scale, Acceptance of Other Scale	Speaker's expression of feelings/thoughts in clear, specific, subjective terms (SFAS); responder effectiveness conveying understanding and acceptance (AOS)	Interrater reliability: Self-Seeking and Awareness κ = .84; Acceptance of Other κ = .88	Established couples	

TABLE 2.2. (continued)

Authors	Measure name	Construct assessed	Subscales and reliability	Appropriate population	Validity
Holt (1977)	Inventory of Intimacy Development	Intimacy, maturity	Three subtasks: Intellectual, Physical, Emotional	Young adults (ages 21–31)	Content was judged by "6 judges with expertise in human development theory and practice."
King & Christensen (1983)	Relationship Events Scale (RES)	Courtship progress, including increasing intimacy. Partner agreement assessed by Cohen's $\kappa = .55$	No subscales	Developed with college students and married couples	Significant associations found with respondent's classification of the relationship's status (e.g., going steady), relationship length, expectations of permanence, Rubin's Love Scale, relationship outcome, and extent of sexual activity.
Kobak & Hazan (1991)	Ratings of confiding communication	Depth of disclosure and acceptance of distress	Disclosing ($\alpha = .91$) and Acceptance of Distress ($\alpha = .92$)	Adult couples	Self-ratings, spouse ratings, and observer ratings converge.
Measures of individual differences					
Constantinople (1969)	Inventory of Psychosocial Development	Erikson's first six stages of psychosocial development ($\alpha = .88$)	Basic Trust vs. Basic Mistrust, Autonomy vs. Shame and Doubt, Initiative vs. Guilt, Industry vs. Inferiority, Identity vs. Identity	Developed with college students	A review by Waterman & Whitbourne (1981) reported correlations in predicted directions with the Marlowe–Crowne

		Diffusion, Identity vs. Isolation ($\alpha = .77$)			Social Desirability Scale, positive mood states, - adaptive personality traits, successful social functioning, and positive academic attitudes and behaviors.
Descutner & Thelen (1991); Doi & Thelen (1992)	Fear of Intimacy Scale	Anxiety experienced in or at the prospect of close relationships ($\alpha = .93$)	No subscales; 35 items	Validated with college students and again with middle-aged adults	Correlations were in predicted directions with the Jourard Self-Disclosure Questionnaire, the Miller Social Intimacy Scale, the UCLA Loneliness Scale, Cacioppo, Petty, & Kao's Need for Cognition Scale, the Bem Sex-Role Inventory, and dating partners' reports that subjects were difficult to get close to.
McAdmas (1980, 1984)	TAT–Intimacy Motive Scoring System	Intimacy Motive (interscorer reliability = .88)	No subscales; Five pictures; high interscorer reliability and peering ratings	Developed with college students	Correlations were in expected direction with subjects' open-ended reports of intimacy themes in satisfying experiences, and with the open-ended recollections of significant events containing intimacy themes.

(continued)

TABLE 2.2. (*continued*)

Authors	Measure name	Construct assessed	Subscales and reliability	Appropriate population	Validity
Miller, Berg, & Archer (1983)	Opener Scale	Tendency to open up and encourage others to be open (test–retest $r = .69$; $\alpha = .79–.93$)	Preceived Reaction of Others, Interest in Listening to Others, Interpersonal Skill	Developed with college students	Correlations were in predicted directions with the Jourard Self-Disclosure Questionnaire, Perspective-taking and Shyness.
Orlofsky, Marcia, & Lesser (1973); Tesch & Whitbourne (1982)	Intimacy Status Interview	Intimacy capacity (interrater agreement ranged from 70% to 94%)	Interview (20–30 minutes) covering quality of intimacy with romantic partner and close friend	College students and young adults	Correlations were in predicted directions with Yufit Intimacy/Isolation Checklist, Edwards Personal Perference Schedule, Ford's Social Desirability Scale.
Rosenthal, Gurney, & Moore (1981)	Erikson Psychosocial Stage Inventory (EPSI)	Resolution of first six stages of Erikson's theory (including intimacy)	Trust, Autonomy, Initiative, Industry, Identity, Intimacy ($\alpha = .62–.75$)	Developed with secondary school students	Correlations were in predicted directions with Psychosocial Maturity Inventory.
Shadish (1984, 1986)	Interpersonal Relations Scale (IRS)	Intrapersonal and interpersonal intimacy ($\alpha = .92–.96$; test–retest $r = .77$)	No subscales; 66 items	Developed with college students	Convergent validity was established via method of contrasted groups. Negative correlations were found with MMPI F-scale, Eysenck Inventory Lie Scale, Spielberger's State–Trait Anxiety Inventory.

Author(s) (Year)	Measure	Construct (reliability)	Description	Sample	Validity
Tesch (1985)	Psychosocial Intimacy Questionnaire (PIQ)	Psychosocial intimacy (internal consistency: α = .97–.98; test–retest r = .69–.84)	No subscales; 60 items	Developed with college students; intended for both adults and adolescents	Correlations were in predicted directions with Dyadic Trust Scale, Love Scale, Constantinople's Inventory of Psychosocial Development Intimacy versus Isolation Scale, Marlowe–Crowne Social Desirability Scale.
White, Speisman, Jackson, Bartis, & Costos (1986)	Intimacy Maturity Scale	Intimacy maturity	Five components: Orientation to the Relationship; Caring/Concern; Sexuality; Commitment, Communication (correlations between subscale scores and total score: r = .82–.86)	Married couples in their mid- to late 20s	Correlations were in the predicted directions with the Spanier Dyadic Adjustment Scale, Locke–Wallace Mental Adjustment Test, and the Bem Sex-Role Inventory.
Selected measures of related constructs					
Berscheid, Snyder, & Omoto (1989)	Relationship Closeness Inventory (RCI)	Closeness, interdependence (α = .56–.90)	Frequency of Interaction, Diversity of Activities, Strength of Partner's Influence	Developed with college students	Measure discriminates between close and not close relationships and is modestly correlated with subjective closeness index.
Hatfield & Sprecher (1986)	Passionate Love Scale	Passion, love (α = .56–.90)	No subscales	Adults	Construct validity has been shown to be high.

(continued)

TABLE 2.2. (*continued*)

Authors	Measure name	Construct assessed	Subscales and reliability	Appropriate population	Validity
Hendrick & Hendrick (1986)	Love Attitudes Scale	Types of love (α = .70+ for 5 of 6 subscales)	Eros, Ludus, Storge, Pragma, Mania, Agape (test–retest r= .60–.78)	Developed with college students	Positive correlations were obtained between each subscale and measures reflecting the theoretical conception of each love style.
Johnson-George & Swap (1982)	Specific Interpersonal Trust Scales (SITS)	Trust (α = .78– .83)	Overall Trust; Emotional Trust; Reliableness	Developed with college students	Discriminant validity was established via factor analysis of subjects' responses to the Rubin Liking and Loving Scales.
Rempel, Holmes, & Zanna (1985)	Trust Scale	Trust in close relationships (α = .81 overall)	Faith (α = .80), Dependability (α = .72), Predictability (α = .70)	Married couples, young to middle adult	Subscales were consistent with theoretical constructs. Discriminative validity was shown by differential correlations among the subscales.
Z. Rubin (1970)	Rubin's Loving and Liking Scale	Love and liking (α = .84 for females, .86 for males)	Attachment, Caring, Intimacy, Self-disclosure	Developed with adults	Negative correlations were obtained with Marlowe–Crowne Social Desirability Scale.

CONCEPTIONS EMPHASIZING INTIMATE INTERACTIONS

I suggested in Chapter 1 that intimate behavior and intimate experience are the components of intimate interactions. Definitions that emphasize one or the other or both of these components, then, are conceptions of intimate interactions.

Intimate Behavior

Conceptions of intimate interactions have historically emphasized intimate *behavior*. Initially, this focus was largely on confiding and self-disclosure. Jourard (1968) gave birth to this focus when he suggested that taking another into one's confidence through self-disclosure, and the concomitant trust involved, were prerequisites to forming a loving relationship. He asked, "How can I love a person whom I do not know?" (p. 25). Similarly, S. Gilbert (1976) saw self-disclosure as central to intimacy because self-disclosing exchanges imply "a deep form of acceptance of the other as well as a commitment to the relationship" (p. 221). A focus on self-disclosure made good sense considering how central self-disclosure is to lay conceptions of intimacy (Monsour, 1992). Scholars and laypeople alike, then, have viewed self-disclosure as the *sine qua non* of intimate behavior.

It is important not to equate intimate behavior with self-disclosure, however. Not all self-disclosures are intimate. Even those authors who emphasize the important role played by self-disclosure have agreed that negative disclosures, particularly those containing negative feelings about the partner, do not promote intimate experience (Derlega & Chaikin, 1975; Gilbert, 1976). Some nonintimate self-disclosures may serve an impression management function. These are carefully selected and worded disclosures, and are minimally self-revealing (Derlega & Grzelak, 1979; Gitter & Black, 1976; Prager, Fuller, & Gonzalez, 1989).

Interest in self-disclosure began with questions about its impact on individual well-being; it then expanded to include its role in intimate relationships. This interest had its roots in humanistic conceptions of personality and social behavior, particularly from Carl Rogers's theory. Rogers (1980) proposed that all human beings are intrinsically endowed with a self-actualizing tendency, a tendency to strive toward being the best self they can be. He argued further that full awareness of oneself was critical to the self-actualization process because it allowed one to symbolically represent experience (through verbalization) and to learn from it (Rogers, 1959). Finally, Rogers (1951) insisted that full awareness and acceptance of oneself was dependent upon the "conditions for growth"—specifically, genuineness, unconditional acceptance, and empathy—provided by important relationships. Following Rogers, Jourard (1971) argued that the optimum use of these growth conditions in a relationship required self-disclosure. He said, "When a person has been able to disclose himself utterly to another person, he learns how to increase his contact with his real self, and he may then be better able to direct his destiny on the basis of this knowledge" (p. 6).

Humanistic conceptions of intimacy, then, with their emphasis on self-disclosure, addressed the potentially positive impact of intimate behavior on individual growth and self-actualization. Later, as it became apparent that the most positive experiences with self-disclosure were frequently within the context of personal and/or psychotherapeutic relationships, self-disclosure research expanded its focus to self-disclosure within relationships (e.g., Derlega et al., 1993).

Not all interactional conceptions of intimacy have centered on self-disclosure. In one research tradition, intimate interaction was conceived solely in terms of nonverbal behavior (M. L. Patterson, 1976). Intimate nonverbal behavior is synonymous with what Mehrabian (1969) called "immediacy" behaviors, which include maintaining close physical proximity, and eye contact, forward lean, and smiling. These behaviors have been linked to subjects' reports of a positive attitude toward their interaction partner. Nonverbal intimacy is one among many clusters of nonverbal behaviors that have been found to affect interaction process and to reflect how the people interacting feel and think about one another. Interest in the nonverbal aspects of interaction was therefore not initially driven by theory so much as by efforts to identify determinants of systematic patterns of nonverbal behavior within interactions (M. L. Patterson, 1976).

Sample Measures

The assessment of behavior in intimate interactions has largely been based on self-reports of patterns of self-disclosure (see Table 2.2). The most widely used of these self-report self-disclosure measures is the Jourard Self-Disclosure Inventory (SDI; Jourard & Lasakow, 1958). This measure asks subjects to reveal how much they disclosed (from "not at all" to "have discussed fully") to several partners about various topics (in a list of 20) of a personal nature. This scale and others like it (Chelune, 1976; Cozby, 1973; Taylor & Altman, 1966; Worthy, Gary, & Kahn, 1969), ask participants to make inferences about their behavior—how they usually behave, how they believe they would behave, or how they remember behaving in a variety of situations.

One self-report measure that assesses intimate behaviors other than self-disclosure is King and Christensen's (1983) Guttman scale of progress in courtship.[2] The Relationship Events Scale (RES) contains 19 items reflecting behaviors of increasing intimacy that commonly serve as indicators of relationship progress. Research participants are asked whether each behavior or event has occurred in their relationship at least once. Behaviors assessed include "My partner has called me an affectionate name," "I have said 'I love you' to my partner," and "We have spent a vacation together that lasted longer than three days."

Self-report measures of behavior have also been used to assess children's intimate interactions. From Sullivan's (1953) interpersonal theory of psychiatry Mannarino (1976) derived a primarily behavioral measure of intimacy called the Chumship Checklist. This 17-item self-report inventory asks children about behaviors that are potentially validating, such as how honestly they can communicate with their friends and how sensitive they are to their friends' needs and interests. Another measure of children's intimate behavior is Buhrmester and Furman's (1987) Network of Relationships Inventory, which includes a 3-item self-report intimacy scale for children that asks "How much do you share your secrets and private feelings with other people" and "How much do you have people to tell everything to?" At this time few measures are available to assess children's intimate interactions.

Self-report measures of self-disclosure coexist with rating scales designed to code actual self-disclosure in interactions (e.g., Klos & Loomis, 1978; Vondracek, 1969). Chelune's (1976) coding scheme organizes verbal behavior in interviews, and rates self-disclosure on the dimensions of amount, number, and percentage of self-references; intimacy ("personalness"); congruence of affective manner of presentation; and rate per minute. Morton's (1978) scheme codes self-disclosure along two dimensions: description, the privacy or personalness of facts disclosed, and evaluation, or the depth of emotion, judgment, or opinion expressed. Combining the two dimensions resulted in four categories of behavioral self-disclosure: high on both dimensions, high on description only, high on evaluation only, and low on both dimensions. Schemes for coding valence, or the positiveness or negativeness of self-disclosure, have also been developed (Tolstedt & Stokes, 1984).

Behavioral measures of self-disclosure have had only modest correlations with self-report inventories (Cozby, 1973; Prager, 1989; Vondracek, 1969). Perhaps this is because the latter are more like trait inventories and thereby require inferences about patterns of behavior across time and situations. There is evidence, however, that if behavioral measures thoroughly sample the behavior from which people draw their inferences, correlations between behavioral and self- report measures increase.

Intimate Experiences

Most conceptions of intimate interactions consider intimate experiences as well as behavior. These conceptions define intimacy as a combination of dyadic behavior and individual experience. Sullivan (1953) was the first to stress the importance of both intimate experience and behavior. He was also the first to suggest that intimate interpersonal interactions play an important role in shaping individual psychological development. He believed that children have needs for acceptance and validation and that these needs can be met in intimate interactions with close friends during preadolescence. Sullivan believed that *sensitivity* and *responsiveness* in intimate interactions, more than self-disclosure, were behavioral prerequisites to validation experiences and that in preadolescence youngsters "develop a real sensitivity to what matters to another person . . . [and learn what they can do] to contribute to the happiness or to support the prestige and feeling of worthwhileness of [their] chum" (1953, pp. 245–246). According to Sullivan, when children learn to adjust their own behavior in response to the needs of another person, they are on their way to developing intimate relationships.

Conceptions of intimate experience include both affective and cognitive components, although the emphasis they place on each varies. Cognitively oriented definitions focus on the meanings individuals impart to their experiences in interactions with others (see Duck, 1994). Cognitive social learning theory provides a precedent fo this focus. Cognitive social learning theorists advocated a focus on cognition in social interaction over 20 years ago (Bandura, 1978; Mischel, 1973; Rotter, 1982). These theorists argued that people form *expectancies*, based on prior experiences of their vicarious or direct reinforcement, about which behaviors will be reinforced and how (Mischel, 1973).

Although they might not have claimed cognitive social learning theory as the root of their approach, Chelune, Robison, and Krommor (1984) constructed a definition of intimacy that emphasized expectations and the cognitive aspects of intimate experience. Chelune et al. proposed that intimacy is the result of individuals using data collected from their experiences interacting with another person to construct expectations about the future of the relationship. According to Chelune et al., intimacy is the result of "a relational process in which we come to *know* the innermost, subjective aspects of another, and are known in a like manner" (Chelune et al., 1984, p. 14; emphasis added). Chelune et al., then, emphasized two cognitive (or perceptual) aspects of intimate experience: (1) the expectation that intimate contact with a particular partner can be counted on and (2) the experience of knowing and being known, understanding and being understood.

Definitions that emphasize the *meaningfulness* of interaction and *mutual understanding* are also concerned with the cognitive aspects of intimate experience (Nezlek, Wheeler, & Reis, 1983; Sexton & Sexton, 1982). Duck (1994a) argued recently that that the communication and sharing of meaning "either symbolically or directly in the social interactions of everyday talk" (p. 147) is central to interaction processes. Intimacy, in Duck's view, would be inseparable from the shared meanings that relationship partners create in their ongoing interactions.

Some conceptions of intimacy place more emphasis on the affective aspects of intimate experience. According to Beach and Tesser (1988), intimate experience requires emotional intensity, or interaction participants will not perceive themselves as having experienced intimacy. L'Abate and L'Abate (1979) argued that verbalizing emotions, such as the hurt feelings and fear that underlie anger, is the essence of intimate experience. Intimate experience, in their view, involves peeling away layers of defenses to reveal the true feelings and vulnerabilities of relationship partners.

Capturing the essence of intimate experience, according to most conceptions (e.g., Jourard, 1971; Hatfield, 1988; Reis & Shaver, 1988; Sullivan, 1953), seems to require an acknowledgement of both cognitive and affective aspects of that experience. Theorists have done this by combining these two aspects of experience into one concept, like validation (Sullivan, 1953). Validation seems to combine within it the experiences of understanding, acceptance, and warmth. Understanding refers to the perception interaction partners have that one partner has received the second partner's meaning correctly. Understanding is a relatively cognitive aspect of intimate experience. Acceptance refers to an attitude toward the understood material on the part of the listener. An accepting partner makes no effort to change the other partner's views, personality, or behavior, but rather remains in relationship with that partner the way she (or he) is. Acceptance, then, is also a relatively cognitive aspect of intimate experience. Both understanding and acceptance would be relatively hollow, however, without each partner experiencing positive affect toward the other. It is this combination of experiences—being understood and accepted by someone who feels positively about one—that seems to capture what is important and rewarding about intimate experience.

Two conceptions of intimate interactions pointedly distinguish the emotions of intimate experience from intimate behavior. The first is Hatfield's (1988) model. Hatfield developed separate definitions of cognitive, emotional, and behavioral intimacy. She defined cognitive intimacy as partners' willingness to reveal themselves and "share profound information about one another . . ." (p. 205). Emotional intimacy is their deep caring for one another and the intense emotions that the intimate relationship generates in them. Behavioral intimacy refers to partners' seeking out and enjoying close physical proximity and touch. Hatfield's notion of emotional intimacy corresponds to my notion of affective intimate experience, while her cognitive and behavioral intimacy both fit into my notion of intimate behavior. Reis and Shaver's (1988) conception of intimate interactions also clearly distinguishes the behavioral and experiential aspects of intimate interactions. In their conception intimacy is a process that begins when one partner reveals personally meaningful feelings or information to another person and the other person responds empathically and supportively. Their definition refers to two critical components of intimate interaction behavior: self-disclosure and verbal responsiveness. In addition, according to Reis and Shaver, the discloser's feelings of being "understood, validated, and cared for by the listener" (Reis, 1990, p. 16) are an important part of the process (this component of their definition seems to refer more to intimate experience).

My own definition of intimate interaction in Chapter 1 is aligned with these conceptions, which emphasize and distinguish behavior and experience. This review of existing conceptions of intimate interactions indicates that this approach to defining intimacy has precedents in the literature.

Sample Measures

Measures assessing intimate experience focus on the cognitions and emotions that individuals have as a result of their interactions with others. Knowledge about the other person is one likely outcome of intimate behavior. Mutual knowledge has been the focus of cognitively-oriented assessments of intimate experience (Diaz & Berndt, 1982; Orlofsky, 1976; Orlofsky & Ginsburg, 1981). For measures of mutual knowledge, participants are asked to anticipate a close friend's responses to an attitude or personality inventory. Assessments of intimate experience have arisen from the premise that mutual knowledge and understanding are important outcomes of intimate interaction.

Other researchers have asked subjects to rate the *feelings* they have about their daily interactions with others. With the interaction record methodology (Duck, Rutt, Hurst, & Strejc, 1991; Wheeler & Nezlek, 1977) participants are asked to make a few quick ratings of any interaction they had that was over 10 minutes in length. Because subjects are rating specific interactions on the same day that they participated in them, they are theoretically better able to remember and capture their feelings about those interactions. Further, they are recording their subjective reactions to interactions, data to which they have ready access (Nez-lek, Wheeler, & Reis, 1983). This methodology is particularly useful for documenting the affective component of intimate interactions as they occur.

CONCEPTIONS EMPHASIZING INTIMATE RELATIONSHIPS

Most conceptions of intimacy address intimate relationships. These seem to fall into three categories. First are those that attempt a comprehensive description of intimate relationships in all their aspects. I call these *relational conceptions*. The second type includes those that emphasize the affect, or feelings, people have about each other and their relationship. These definitions often address intimate experiences in the context of relationships. I have called these *affective conceptions*. The third type emphasizes patterns of behavior within an intimate relationship. These definitions, which I have called *behavioral conceptions*, are concerned with interactions in the context of intimate relationships.

Relational Conceptions

The relational conceptions of intimate relationships have in common their attempt to capture the many ways relationship partners can be intimate and the many aspects of intimate relationships. Unlike conceptions emphasizing interactions, relational conceptions attempt to define a *relationship* that exists over time and space. Relational definitions differ from interactional definitions in that the latter are more concerned with intimacy as a here-and-now phenomenon that does not necessarily require an ongoing relationship.

Relational definitions seem to have one or both of the following objectives. One, they attempt a comprehensive, multidimensional definition of an intimate relationship; they are concerned with everything about a relationship that contributes to its inclusion in the category of intimate relationships. Because they are concerned with patterns of behavior over time, these definitions sometimes resemble lists of trait-like characteristics of relationships. Clinebell and Clinebell's (1970) conception for example, defined intimacy as "the degree of mutual need-satisfaction within the relationship" (p. 1). These authors presented a conception of intimate relationships that encompasses as many ways of being intimate as there are needs to satisfy—sexual, emotional, aesthetic, creative, recreational, work, crisis, conflict, commitment, spiritual, and communicative. Schaefer and Olson (1981) took a similar approach. They distinguished intimate relationships from nonrelational intimate experiences on the basis of participant's expectations in the former, that they share many different kinds of intimacy. In Schaefer and Olson's view, intimate relationships are defined by seven types of intimate contact: emotional, social, intellectual, sexual, recreational, spiritual, and aesthetic. They argued further that relationship satisfaction depends on partners sharing intimate experiences in a variety of domains inasmuch as individual partners want differing degrees of each kind of intimacy. Waring and his colleagues (Reddon et al., 1985; Waring, McElrath, Lefcoe, & Weisz, 1981; Wood, Barnes, & Waring, 1988) formulated a definition that suggests that intimate relationships are defined by more than the domains of intimate contact between partners. Drawing from clinical experience and research with married couples, they suggested eight characteristics of intimate relationships: conflict resolution, affection, cohesion, sexuality, identity, compatibility, autonomy, and expressiveness. Reis and Shaver's (1988) approach was similar to Waring's. They included the following in their definition of an intimate relationship: a temporal perspective, commitment, mutuality, common assumptions about the relationship, reciprocity, interdependence, and trust.

The authors of these conceptions often explicitly acknowledge that intimacy in a relationship is a process. They recognize that the partners in an intimate relationship engage in intimate interactions (whether these are summarized as "expressiveness," "verbal intimacy," or "communicativeness"). Moreover, they assume that intimate contact in a relationship fluctuates and is dependent on what the partners are doing and have been doing in the context of the relationship. Despite these claims, relational definitions may fail to describe the processes within intimate relationships that these trait-like descriptions purportedly summarize.

The strength of these comprehensive conceptions may also be their drawback. On the strength side, relational definitions, and the measures that emerge from them (see below), provide models for testing hypotheses about interconnections among components of intimate relationships. In addition, these conceptions acknowledge, as Reis and Shaver (1988) pointed out, that there is much that goes on in an intimate relationship that does not involve intimate interactions per se. Relational definitions can be unwieldy, however, because of their multidimensionality and their abstractness. They may include components of intimate relationships that do not necessarily define them as intimate. These components may not be unique to intimate relationships and may not be necessary for their inclusion in the category of intimate relationships.

Some relational conceptions have avoided abstractness and complexity by identifying as intimate a small number of relationship compo-

nents. These components are then used to distinguish intimate relationships from those that are not. These more parsimonious conceptions do
not attempt to fully describe intimate relationships. For example, Tolstedt and Stokes (1983) identified three dimensions of relational intimacy: verbal, emotional, and physical. Verbal intimacy is self-disclosure,
while physical intimacy "encompasses sex and other physical expressions
of love" (p. 574). Emotional intimacy "reflects feelings of closeness and
emotional bonding, including intensity of liking, moral support and ability to tolerate flaws in the significant other" (p. 574). Dahms's (1972) definition also identifies three dimensions—emotional, physical, and intellectual—that he claims capture intimacy within relationships. However,
one definition's weakness is another's strength. These definitions lack the
comprehensiveness of the broader relational definitions. Clinicians, for
example, might find couple assessment methods based on more comprehensive definitions of intimacy more useful.

Sample Measures

Comprehensive measures of relational intimacy tend to be multifactorial,
like the definitions of intimacy that spawn them. The content of
Maxwell's (1985) measure of *closeness* in relationships suggests that it
could be measuring a relational notion of intimacy. According to
Maxwell, this inventory measures "(1) separation distress, (2) naturalness
(disclosure of intense feelings), (3) touching (both general and in taboo
areas), (4) following (seeking out, gazing), (5) imitation, (6) reciprocity
and synchrony of behaviour, (7) help and gifts (given and received; not
normally from or offered to others), (8) similarity (in attitudes and values), and (9) disclosure (of intimate details)" (p. 217). The Waring Intimacy Questionnaire (WIQ; Waring & Reddon, 1983) has eight subscales
corresponding to their eight dimensions of intimacy indentified by Waring et al., along with a scale to detect desirability responding. Waring,
McElrath, Mitchell, and Derry (1981) also developed the Victoria Hospital Intimacy Interview (VHI) to assess the same dimensions. Sharabany
(1974; Sharabany & Wiseman, 1993) created an Intimate Friendship
Scale that assesses eight components of intimate relationships: frankness
and spontaneity, sensitivity and knowing, attachment, exclusiveness, giving and sharing, imposition, common activities, and trust and loyalty.
Schaefer and Olson's (1981) Personal Assessment of Intimacy in Relationships (PAIR) measures differences between each relationship partner's perceived and expected degree of intimacy in five areas of intimacy:
emotional, social, sexual, intellectual, and recreational. It also measures
differences between two relationship partners in their perceptions and

expectations about intimacy. Holt (1977) designed her Intimacy Development Inventory to assess Dahms's less comprehensive three-dimensional definition of relationship intimacy. The IDI has three subscales, that correspond to Dahms's dimensions: emotional, physical, and intellectual intimacy.

Perhaps in dramatic contrast to the multidimensional measures mentioned above, Aron, Aron, and Smollan (1992) developed a single-item measure of relational closeness called the Inclusion of Other in the Self Scale (IOS), which is based on their definition of closeness as an overlap of selves. Out of seven pictures of two circles with differing degrees of overlap, subjects are asked to pick the one that best describes their relationship. Scores on the IOS are moderately to highly correlated with other measures of intimacy and closeness.

Affective Conceptions

Conceptions of intimate relationships sometimes focus primarily on the feelings partners have for one another and about the relationship as a whole. They are centered on the positive emotions that people feel in their interactions and relationships. Definitions that emphasize the affective aspects of intimacy include Sternberg's (1988), Miller and Lefcourt's (1982), and Sexton and Sexton's (1982). These highlight warmth, affection, involvement, love, and deep feelings of acceptance between partners (Gilbert, 1976; Hatfield, 1988). The importance of the feeling aspect of intimate relationships was supported by O'Connor's (1992) research. In her sample of adult women she found that there was a difference between the feeling that one could confide in a friend and the actual practice of confiding (p. 62). For many women in her study, having such a feeling was sufficient reason to define the relationship as intimate.

Not surprisingly, affectively oriented definitions tend to draw from theories of emotion, such as Mandler's (1980). Berscheid (1983) identified two major components of emotion in Mandler's theory: autonomic nervous system (ANS) arousal and the cognitive-interpretive system. Theoretically, the ANS is innately primed to respond to an interruption in ongoing activity, particularly unexpected interruptions of practiced behavioral sequences. ANS arousal activates the cognitive-interpretive system to undertake a meaning analysis of the interruption. Berscheid argued further that people in close relationships are especially likely to experience strong emotions toward one another because they so frequently encounter opportunities for interruptions of familiar behavioral sequences. These opportunities to interrupt come about, in part, because people in close relationships make plans that include each other. The more important the other person is to those plans, the more intense the emotion the person is likely to experience when those plans are interrupted (whether those plans are to go to the movies Saturday night or to raise children together). The only way to prevent emotional arousal within a close relationship is to eliminate what Berscheid calls the partners' "interchain causal connections." These are sequences of behavior that are especially open to partner interruptions and therefore especially likely to generate emotion. Eliminating them, however, may result in peace and harmony at the expense of intimate interaction.

Drawing on Berscheid's notion that emotional intensity is an important aspect of intimate relationships, Hatfield and Rapson (1987) argued that this emotional intensity arises from the behavioral and cognitive aspects of intimate interaction. Behaviorally, intimates confide extensively in one another and maintain close physical proximity. Cognitively, in part because they confide, they come to acquire large amounts of intensely personal information about one another. These behavioral and cognitive aspects of intimate interaction create the emotional intensity central to intimate experience, which in turn affects each partner's confiding behavior and the information that each comes to acquire about the other. Partners can use this information to hurt and humiliate as well as to soothe, comfort, and give pleasure—hence, the emotional intensity of intimate relationships.

Sternberg (1988) argued that intimate relationships are bound to wane in emotional intensity over time. His argument states that because intimacy in a relationship is primarily an affective experience, the novelty and uncertainty of a relationship at the beginning will enhance partners' awareness of their intimate experiences together. As familiarity and predictability come to increasingly characterize the relationship, the intensity of emotion within the relationship decreases, causing the partners, at times, to be less aware of their level of intimacy.

Affective conceptions, then, have emphasized the experience of emotion in intimate relationships. Some of these conceptions suggest that intimate experience is intense experience. To the extent that theorists emphasize intimacy's emotional intensity, they are likely to argue that intimacy will wane over time as partners habituate and become predictable to one another. In contrast, affective conceptions also view the primary emotions of intimacy as deep caring, tenderness, and love. From this perspective, intimacy could easily remain stable or even increase as relationships endure over time.

Sample Measures

Measures that emphasize affective aspects of intimate relationships are not difficult to find. Most measures of intimacy seem to rest on the assumption that positive emotional experience of some kind is an important aspect of an intimate relationship. The intimacy subscale of Sternberg's (1988) Triangular Love Scale includes items such as "I have a warm and comfortable relationship with my partner," "I strongly desire to promote the well-being of my partner," "My relationship with my partner is very romantic," and "I feel emotionally close to my partner." The Passionate Love Scale (Hatfield & Sprecher, 1986) measures affective aspects of love relationships, asking participants to rate themselves on statements such as "I would feel despair if _____ left me," "I take delight in studying the movements and angles of _____'s body," and "I feel happy when I am doing something to make _____ happy." Moss and Schwebel's (1993) Relationship Intimacy Styles Questionnaire asks participants to rate things like "How much I can tell what my partner is feeling," "How much I wish I was with someone else," and "How much I enjoy being physically affectionate with my partner" according to the contribution each makes to their feelings about their relationship. Doi and Thelen's (1992) Fear of Intimacy Scale asks partners to rate how they would feel telling about things from the past, confiding their innermost thoughts, being spontaneous, and taking the risk of being hurt in the context of a close relationship. Tolstedt and Stokes's (1983) 10-item measure of affective intimacy assesses the degree to which individuals feel intimate with their spouses, the degree to which they felt important to their spouses, and their willingness to tolerate the less pleasant aspects of the relationship. Miller and Lefcourt's (1982) Miller Social Intimacy Scale (MSIS) includes two sets of items, 6 assessing the frequency of certain behaviors and the other 11 primarily assessing affect through such questions as "How much do you like to spend time alone with him/her?" and "How much do you feel like being encouraging and supportive of him/her when he/she is unhappy?" and "How affectionate do you feel towards him/her?" Walker and Thompson's (1983) measure asks participants to rate statements like "We love each other" and "We want to spend time together" according to how well the statements describe their feelings in their relationship.

Some paper-and-pencil intimacy inventories combine affectively oriented items with items measuring cognitions (such as expectations, perceptions, or knowledge of partner). The intimacy subscale in the Davis–Todd Relationship Rating Scale (Davis & Todd; 1985), for example, combines cognitive items such as "Do you know what kind of person he/she is?" and "Do you know this person's faults and shortcomings?" and

"Is this person's behaviour surprising or puzzling to you?" with affective items such as "Do you feel there are things about you that this person just would not understand?" and "Do you feel some things about yourself are none of this person's business?" The intimacy subscale of Burgoon and Hale's (1988) Relational Communication Scale only assesses cognitive/perceptual aspects of intimacy, as in "He/she didn't care if I liked him/her," "He/she considered us equals," and "He/she wanted me to trust him/her" (p. 22). These measures seem to imply a definition of intimate relationships in which affective and cognitive experiences are enmeshed. They leave open theoretical questions about how these aspects of intimate experiences relate to each other in the context of intimate relationships.

Behavioral Conceptions

Clinical behaviorists have viewed intimacy as synonymous with and resulting from the rewarding exchanges of relationship partners (Margolin, 1982). This view has traditionally arisen from operant and social exchange theories. According to operant theory, the important determinants of behavior can be found in the environment, which, in the case of intimate relationships, is the other partner. To the extent that relationship partners engage in behaviors they know to be pleasing to one another, they create a rewarding (or intimate) environment for each other. Thibaut and Kelley's (1959) social exchange theory has also been influential in shaping more behaviorally oriented views of relationships. This theory states that relationship partners are satisfied when the rewards of their relationship are proportionate to the costs. If the partners' rewards from the relationship sufficiently exceed the costs, the relationship should be satisfying. If the costs of ending the relationship exceed the costs of staying in it and/or the rewards of ending the relationship do not appear to exceed those of staying in, the relationship should endure (Margolin, 1982).

Perhaps because of their frequent exposure to destructive marital conflict in their consulting rooms, clinical researchers have emphasized the importance of effective conflict resolution as a prerequisite to intimate relating (Fruzzetti & Jacobson, 1990; L'Abate & L'Abate, 1979; Margolin, 1982). One reason effective conflict resolution is so important is that unresolved conflict leaves a residue of anger and resentment that interferes with the performance of rewarding behaviors (Christensen & Shenk, 1991; Fitzpatrick, 1988; Gottman & Levenson, 1986; Levinger & Huston, 1990; Raush, Barry, Hertel, & Swain, 1974). Further, as L'Abate and L'Abate noted, couples who can express the feelings of hurt and fear that often underlie their anger can have potent experiences of intimacy.

The traditional behavioral approach to understanding intimate relationships has not, until recently, been especially concerned with defining intimacy itself. Proponents of the behavioral approach have argued that the specific nature of relationship rewards—whether intimate, companionable, sexual, or supportive—was less important than the consequences of that rewarding behavior. The important task for psychologists, from the behavioral perspective, is to define behaviors that tend to have a positive impact on relationship satisfaction and stability, rather than develop distinct definitions of different kinds of rewarding behavior.

More recently, behavioral theorists have become more interested in defining intimacy specifically. For example, Fruzzetti and Jacobson (1990) constructed a definition of intimacy when marital interaction research revealed a destructive interaction pattern that arose specifically from conflicts about intimacy (Christensen, 1988; Fruzzetti & Jacobson, 1990). Behaviorally oriented writers have defined intimacy as a type of interaction occurring within a relationship, thus combining interactional and relationship conceptions (e.g., Hatfield, 1988). Fruzzetti and Jacobson's definition in Table 2.1 is a good example.

While not intended to describe intimate interaction per se, Acitelli's (1988, 1993) notion of "relationship talk" may prove to be an effective operational definition of intimate behavior in adults' intimate relationships. Acitelli defined relationship talk as the verbal expression of "a person's thinking about interaction patterns, or contrasts between himself or herself and the other partner in the relationship . . . [it] requires both self-awareness and a knowledge of the other, yet it encompasses more . . . the partner must have a metaperspective of the relationship" (Acitelli, 1993, p. 186). Acitelli described highly immediate disclosure, which could not exist outside of a relationship context. For this reason, her "relationship talk" effectively described one type of intimate verbal behavior within relationships.

Sample Measures

The hallmark of the behavioral approach to measurement is observational assessment of behavior (e.g., see Gottman, 1979; Markman & Notarius, 1987; Montgomery & Duck, 1991; Weiss & Heyman, 1990). Perhaps because of behavioral theorists' relatively recent interest in intimacy, there are few observational measures of intimate behavior in intimate relationships. In a 1987 review Markman and Notarius listed the six dimensions most commonly found in observational coding schemes for marital and family interaction and did not mention intimacy or any related behavior (such as self-disclosure). Even when intimate interaction behavior is assessed directly, few observational coding schemes attempt to code both for self-disclosure and for sensitive responding. One exception is a behavioral assessment of confiding communication, developed by Kobak and Hazan (1991). Kobak and Hazan asked one partner to disclose personally distressing information while instructing the other to "listen carefully and try to understand how the spouse [feels]" (p. 863). In this study, couples engaged in two sessions, so that each partner had a chance to be in each role. Couples were rated on two global scales: Disclosing (for the speaker) and Acceptance of Distress (for the listener). Kobak and Hazan achieved high levels of interrater reliability with these global scales ($r > .90$). A second observational coding scheme by Stover, Guerney, Ginsberg, and Schlein (1977a, 1977b), is a behavioral measure of speaking effectiveness and responder acceptance, recently used by Walsh, Baucom, Tyler, and Sayers (1993) in a study of intimate interaction in maritally distressed couples. In this paradigm, raters code response units (one partner's statements made in between two statements by the other) according to (1) the speaker's ability to share her or his feelings and thoughts in clear, specific, and subjective terms through the use of "I statements" and emotional labeling and (2) the responder's ability to verbally convey understanding and acceptance of the speaker's message.

Idiomatic communication may be a behavioral indicator of intimacy in relationships. Idiomatic communication contains patterns of symbolism, vocabulary, metaphor, and private gestural meanings that are unique to dyads and groups that have frequent close contact. Romantic partners, for example, might tug an ear to indicate they want to leave a party or might "propose sexual intercourse by saying, 'Let's go home and watch some TV'" (Bell, Buerkel-Rothfuss, & Gore, 1987). The use of idiomatic communication has been assessed with structured interviews (Hopper, Knapp, & Scot, 1981). Hopper et al. classified the idiomatic communication of young (mostly college student) couples into eight categories (in order of frequency): expressions of affection, teasing insults, partner nicknames, confrontations, requests and routines, sexual invitations, names for others, and sexual references and euphemisms. Interest in idiomatic communication stems from interest in how specific it is to communication in intimate relationships (Hopper et al., 1981).

Holt's (1977) Intimacy Development Inventory combines behavioral and cognitive/perceptual items. Examples of the former include "I encourage my partner to be his/her own person," "I put aside my personal needs when important problems arise for my partner," and "I express my true feelings toward my partner to him/her personally." Examples of cognitive/perceptual items include "My partner accepts me for what I am," "There is a close emotional tie between my partner and myself," and "I trust my partner not to take unfair advantage of me."

CONCEPTIONS EMPHASIZING INDIVIDUAL DIFFERENCES

Some very influential conceptions of intimacy have been most concerned with individual differences in people's approaches to intimate interactions and relationships. Two prominent individual difference approaches have arisen, one from psychodynamically oriented developmental theories, and the other from theories of motivation.

Developmental Conceptions

In developmental conceptions the emphasis has been on the psychological maturity required to sustain an intimate relationship. Psychoanalytic theorists were the first to take this approach. Freud (1933) proposed that children's resolutions of emotional conflicts in their preschool years are carried forward within the structure of their personalities and thereby determine the quality of their sexual relationships in adulthood.

Object relations theorists (e.g., Fairbairn, 1954; Klein, 1935; Winnicott, 1953) proposed that the foundation for adult intimacy capacity is the infant's internalization of its experiences with its mother in the first weeks and months of life. Bowlby (1969) followed the object relations school closely with his notion that "working models" of oneself and one's relationship partners are formed as a result of infants' experiences with their close relationships. Sullivan (1953) suggested that children acquire the competencies crucial for intimate relating from the close friendships of preadolescence. Erikson (1963) suggested that a true capacity for intimacy is not possible until young adulthood because the development of a secure and stable identity in adolescence is a prerequisite to developing such a capacity.

What these psychodynamically oriented theorists had in common was the belief that the capacity to form and maintain intimate relationships in adulthood is predicated upon the fulfillment of important needs at a critical point earlier in development. For example, in object relations theory the development of a capacity to be alone paradoxically provides the individual with the capacity to be intimate (Winnicott, 1953). This capacity to be alone does not develop fully unless the mother fulfills her infant's needs for holding, safety, and attention. If she does fulfill these needs appropriately, the child internalizes her nurturing image and becomes able to soothe, nurture, and comfort herself or himself (Winnicott, 1953). Without this capacity to be alone the pursuit of intimate relationships in adulthood may take on a desperate quality, and the maintenance of those relationships may be tainted with overwhelming fears of abandonment by the loved one. In the psychodynamic view, then, the fulfillment of needs in early life results in individual capacities that become the building blocks of, and sometimes the prerequisites for, a capacity for intimacy.

In Erikson's (1963) theory the capacity for intimacy requires the ability to commit to the endurance of relational bonds; it also requires the ability to temporarily fuse with another person during intense, close contact without fear of engulfment. Erikson proposed that to tolerate the close contact and commitment of self that intimacy requires the young adult must have the secure sense of self that can only come from the development of an adult identity.

Two more recently developed conceptions of intimacy capacity have grown out of Erikson's theory. Orlofsky and his colleagues (Orlofsky, 1978, 1988; Orlofsky et al., 1973) have suggested that the capacity for intimacy includes capacities for depth and involvement in relationships, for making commitments to relationships, and for maintaining self-definition or identity within relationships. White and her colleagues (e.g., Paul & White, 1990; White, Speisman, & Costos, 1983) have defined three components of intimacy capacity: (1) the cognitive component, which is perspective taking, or the ability to see the world through the eyes of another; (2) the affective component, which is empathy or the ability to experience vicariously the emotions and experiences of another; and (3) the behavioral component, which involves trustworthy behavior, sensitivity and responsiveness, and effective communication.

Sample Measures

Measures of the capacity for intimacy have been drawn largely from Erikson's theory of intimacy development. Included among these are the intimacy status interview (Orlofsky et al., 1973), the intimacy maturity interview (White et al., 1986), and two paper-and-pencil measures that assess the first six stages of development, as defined by Erikson: the Inventory of Psychosocial Development (Constantinople, 1969) and the Erikson Psychosocial Stage Inventory (Rosenthal et al., 1981). The intimacy status interview of Orlofsky et al. (1973) categorizes persons according to their style of coping with the intimacy crisis of young adulthood, a style that should reflect their capacity for intimacy (Prager, 1991). Ratings are made on the basis of subjects' levels of commitment, depth, and individuation in their closest romantic relationship and friendship (Orlofsky et al., 1973; Tesch & Whitbourne, 1982). The intimacy maturity interview by White et al. assesses five components of intimacy maturity: orientation (to the relationship), communication, caring, commitment, and sexuality. The intimacy scales of the two paper-and-pencil measures described here are similar in that each contains items that reflect both the successful and unsuccessful resolution of Erikson's intimacy crisis. Constantinople developed her inventory for college students, while Rosenthal et al. validated their measure on an adolescent sample.

Motivational Conceptions

Motivational definitions also strive to explain individual differences in intimate behavior. These definitions suggest that individuals differ in the extent to which they will attend to, respond to, and attempt to elicit intimacy-related interactions from others in their daily social interactions. McAdams's conception of intimacy motivation (1980, 1982a, 1988a) focuses on internal individual drives to share with others "openness, contact, reciprocal dialogue, joy and conviviality, caring and concern" (McClelland, 1985, p. 359). Motivational theorists, beginning with Freud, believe that motives energize behavior, including behavior necessary for survival. Intimacy motivation is a particular kind of motive: It is a stable disposition that organizes or explains behavior in many situations (McAdams & Constantian, 1983). The higher one's level of intimacy motivation, the more likely one is to engage in intimate behavior in the presence of motive-arousing conditions.

The need for intimacy may also be a disposition on which individuals differ. In a recent formulation, Prager and Buhrmester (1992) conceived of intimacy as one of a set of communal needs that all people experience to a greater or lesser degree. As a need, intimacy represents a "very generalized and broad-based wish or want" (Cantor & Malley, 1991). By definition intimacy needs are motivating. Fulfillment of intimacy needs results in satisfaction and good adjustment, while nonfulfillment should result in distress and loneliness (Wilson, 1967).

Sample Measures

The challenge of measuring intimacy motivation, needs for intimacy, and individual capacities for intimacy lies in the likelihood that none may be immediately accessible to conscious awareness. Drawing from a long tradition in the measurement of motivation, McAdams's (1982a, 1982b) measure of intimacy motivation uses thematic coding of imaginative stories written under potentially intimacy-arousing conditions, namely, the presentation of pictures from the Thematic Apperception Test (TAT; Murray, 1943). The TAT, which has been used in the formalized assessment of several other individual motives (McClelland, 1985), consists of a series of pictorial depictions of ambiguous situations involving one or more persons. People are asked to write stories about what they believe is going on in the pictures. The idea behind the test is that because the pictures are ambiguous, people will fill in the missing information with thematic content that is either explicitly or symbolically related to their own concerns, needs, and desires. Scoring the intimacy motive requires that a story contain at least one of two "prime-test" themes: (1) the notion that a relationship produces positive affect (i.e., the characters in the story must have an interaction that leads to positive feelings or sentiment) and (2) a dialogue in which characters engage in two-way communication that is noninstrumental. The strength of the intimacy motive is determined by adding scores on these two categories plus eight additional ones: psychological growth and coping, commitment or concern, time–space transcendence, union, harmony, surrender of control, escape to intimacy, and connection with the outside world (McAdams, 1984). McAdams and his colleagues have demonstrated the usefulness of his measure for predicting individual behavior in a variety of interpersonal situations (e.g., McAdams, Healy, & Krause, 1984). It predicts behavior within interactions and within groups, and it predicts certain characteristics of relationships over time.

Prager and Buhrmester's (1992) Plano Inventory of Need Satisfaction (PINS) asks people to rate how important a particular need is to them (by rating how much it would cause distress if it were unfulfilled) and how satisfied they are with its fulfillment. The inventory measures people's perceptions of intimacy need fulfillment in conjunction with their perceptions of the fulfillment of other important needs.

SUMMARY AND CONCLUSIONS

In this chapter I have distinguished two types of intimacy conceptions in the literature on the basis of their primary emphases: intimate interactions—behavior or experience—and intimate relationships—comprehensive, affective, or behavioral. I have also identified several distinct theoretical frameworks from which authors have drawn useful definitions of intimacy: humanistic, cognitive social learning, interpersonal (Sullivan), emotion, operant, and social exchange theories. Conceptions emphasizing individual differences in intimacy capacity are also important to understanding intimacy, and have emerged from their own frameworks—psychodynamic and motivational theories.

Intimate Interactions

Interactional conceptions that emphasize intimate behavior arose initially from humanistic theory. These conceptions have two important strengths: They recognize self-disclosure as a central and salient component of intimate interactions, and they are concerned with the important contribution that self-disclosing interactions can make to developmental adaptation and self-actualization.

The difficulty with interactional conceptions has been that intimacy can become overidentified with a few behaviors. Intimacy should not, for example, be equated with self-disclosure. People can use disclosure to confront and criticize, which tends to create distance rather than intimacy (Derlega & Chaikin, 1975; Helgeson, Shaver, & Dyer, 1987).

Interactional definitions that emphasize intimate experience along with intimate behavior began with Sullivan's (1953) interpersonal theory. Sullivan's emphasis on validation as a key component of intimate experience continues to be influential. Sullivan's proposition that children's intimate relationships have both immediate and long-term effects on their personalities and their mental health inspired a large body of work on children's development in the context of their relationships with parents and friends (see Chapter 5).

Since Sullivan, others have attempted to give detailed descriptions of the cognitive and affective components of intimacy. For example, Chelune et al. associated intimate experience with partners' expectations, making their conception reminiscent of cognitive social learning theory. Most conceptions of intimate experience emphasize both cognitive and affective aspects of that experience. Single concepts like validation or acceptance seem to capture cognitive and affective experience combined.

In truth, none of the conceptions reviewed here focuses solely on intimate experience to the exclusion of behavior. The differences among these conceptions lies in the degree to which some aspects of experience are emphasized over others. Conceptions of intimate interaction that most influenced the definition in this book are those that place relatively equal emphasis on behavior, affect, and cognition in intimate interactions (Hatfield, 1988; Reis & Shaver, 1988).

Intimate Relationships

Three types of conceptions of intimate relationships emerged from this review. The first type, what I call relational conceptions, are comprehensive, multi- dimensional categorizations of the types of intimate contact partners (usually couples) can have. From a researcher's viewpoint, their greatest strength may be their potential to generate hypotheses about how different aspects of intimate relationships influence one another. Measures that reflect relational conceptions, such as the PAIR, have considerable clinical utility because of the in-depth assessment they provide. If these conceptions have a weakness, it lies in the trait-like (and therefore potentially static) nature of their intimacy definitions. Moreoever, some of them include all aspects of relationships in their definitions, and therefore risk equating "intimate relationship" with "good relationship."

The second type of conception I discussed emphasizes the affective aspects of intimate relationships. Affective conceptions draw from emotion theories such as Mandler's. Berscheid's (1983) conception, for example, underscored the emotional impact that partners can have on one another as a result of their interdependence. Other conceptions, such as Sternberg's (1988) were more concerned with the positive feelings that partners have for one another, such as love, affection, warmth, and so forth. Still others placed emotional intensity at the center of intimate experience.

Affective definitions have intuitive appeal. Laypersons have equated intimacy with emotionally intense, transcendant experiences (Roscoe, Kennedy, & Pope, 1987). Further, it is difficult to imagine a definition of intimate relationship that does not acknowledge the positive feelings partners have for one another. However, these conceptions risk implying that low-key, (e.g., long-lived) relationships lack intimacy. They may therefore exclude relationships that many would regard as intimate.

Finally, conceptions of intimate relationships sometimes emphasize intimate behavior within relationships. Operant and social exchange theories have inspired work on the rewards and costs of partners' relationship behaviors, particularly their communication. Researchers with an interest in intimate partners' behavior have gone beyond operant theory's traditional concern with the positive versus punishing consequences of behavior to define intimacy explicitly (e.g., Fruzzetti & Jacobson, 1990).

Behaviorally oriented research has resulted in a substantial body of knowledge about couple interaction. Contented and distressed couples can be distinguised by the frequency of certain interaction behaviors, and by their contingent responses to one another (e.g., Margolin & Wampold, 1981). Though few studies of intimacy have emerged from this tradition, intimacy research would nevertheless benefit from its emphasis on conceptual specificity and behavioral observation.

Individual Differences

Conceptions emphasizing individual differences have been concerned with the capacities, motivations, and needs that partners bring to their interactions with others. Psychodynamic theorists have argued that people have differeing capacities to form, enjoy, and maintain intimate relationships as a result of their own individual history. Motivational theorists, such as that of McAdams (1988a), are more concerned with stable dispositions of individuals that predispose them to respond to intimacy-relevant cues in particular ways. McAdams may be less concerned with individual differences in people's capacities for intimacy than with individual differences in their preference and desire for intimate contact.

These conceptions bring rich descriptions of individuals in relationships. These descriptions can be useful for clinicians who wish to assess individual contributions to relationship problems. Some of these conceptions, such as Erikson's (1963), have also generated testable research hypotheses (e.g., Prager, 1989; White et al., 1986). Individual approaches have been criticized, however, for neglecting the important information that is gained from observing relationships versus individuals. Research has suggested that it may be necessary to assess both partners in order to understand their relationship (Acitelli & Duck, 1987).

A NEW MULTITIERED CONCEPT OF INTIMACY

I have sought, with my definition of intimacy (Chapter 1), to systematize existing conceptions without unnecessarily excluding behaviors, experiences, and relationships commonly considered intimate. As the review in this chapter demonstrates, existing conceptions of intimacy have emphasized a wide variety of phenomena: nonverbal behavior and self-disclosure, expectations of the other and intense emotions, passionate uncertainty and long-enduring affection. If my definition errs, it is because it risks encompassing peripheral cases of intimacy that most people would not regard as intimate.[3]

Despite its widely set boundaries, my definition of an intimate interaction nevertheless successfully excludes types of interactions that have not been considered intimate by scholars in the past. Specifically, by insisting that intimate interactions include experiences of positive affect, it excludes interactions that result in one or both partners feeling badly about themselves or their interaction partner. It could happen, for example, that Maya might disclose a personal belief to Gail which would make Gail feel put down or diminished. However personal the disclosure, this interaction is not intimate by the present definition.

By insisting that perceptions of understanding are part of an intimate interaction, my definition also excludes interactions in which one or both partners feel "opaque" or misunderstood. For example, if Les expresses sympathy and support to Pat in such a way that Pat doesn't believe he understands why she is distressed, then their interaction is not intimate, however much warmth and love they might both feel. Conceptions crafted by Beach and Tesser (1988), Chelune et al. (1984), Duck (1994a), Hatfield (1988), Jourard (1968), and Reis and Shaver (1988) all mention the importance of shared understanding and meaning as an outcome of intimate interaction. The exclusion of interactions that do not yield this outcome, then, is consistent with conceptions of intimacy in the research literature.

Finally, my definition excludes interactions that do not involve sharing something personal. For example, two people who interact so that they both feel warmth and understanding are not having an intimate interaction if they are discussing superficial or impersonal topics. The notion that intimate interactions involve sharing something personal may be closest to the core meaning of intimacy. This meaning emerges most clearly from intimacy's etymological origins. The word derives from the Latin word *intimus*, meaning "inner" or "innermost." Variations on the Latin word have survived in several languages, and all refer to the "most deeply internal or inmost" qualities of a person (Sexton & Sexton, 1982). The conceptions discussed in this chapter converge in their emphasis on the role that sharing or knowing a person's innermost aspects as central to intimate interactions.

With my definition of intimate relationships, I strove to specify components of relationships which, because they are necessarily associated with relational intimacy, can distinguish intimate relationships from other personal relationships. With an exception or two, existing conceptions have not approached defining intimacy in this way. They are more likely to list domains of intimate relating, or to define intimate relationships by the affect within those relationships. Many of these conceptions reflect the typical or desirable characteristics of intimate relationships instead of the distinguishing ones.

I first distinguish intimate relationships by the presence of frequent intimate interactions between the partners. I further define them by the partners' affection, trust, and cohesiveness. This suggestion is based on the premise that these relationship characteristics are necessary to sustain relational intimacy. As this review shows, however, the inclusion of these characteristics does not clearly emerge from any existing conception of intimacy. While some definitions mention affection, trust, and cohesiveness (e.g., Reis & Shaver, 1988; Sexton & Sexton, 1982; Sternberg, 1988; Waring et al., 1981), they also mention other relationship characteristics, such as commitment (Reis & Shaver, 1988), compatibility (Waring et al., 1981), interdependence (Perlman & Fehr, 1987), and mutual need-satisfaction (Clinebell & Clinebell, 1970). I have omitted the latter characteristics because existing empirical evidence suggests that commitment (Orlofsky, Marcia, & Lesser, 1973; Prager, 1989), interdependence (Kelley et al., 1983; Berscheid, Snyder, & Omoto, 1989) and compatibility (Fitzpatrick, 1988) are not necessarily linked with the sustenance of relational intimacy. Whether affection, trust, and cohesiveness are so linked remains to be tested empirically.

My selection of affection, trust, and cohesiveness does not rule out the likely possibility that other components of intimate relationships play a role in fostering relational intimacy. Furthermore, affection, trust, and cohesiveness can characterize relationships that involve little relational intimacy. What I am theorizing is that there are few (if any) intimate relationships that are not also characterized by these three characteristics.

My definition of an intimate interaction is designed to encourage conceptual clarity in measurement. The current definition encourages researchers to decide, before developing measures, whether they are measuring intimate interactions or relationships. It offers a framework for deciding further whether they wish to measure behavior, experience, or (most likely) both.

Each component of intimacy is best measured by a different combination of assessment methodologies. The strengths and weaknesses of methods commonly used to measure intimacy—self-report questionnaires, semi-structured interviews, and behavioral observations—depend upon which component the researcher seeks to measure. Self-report measures—questionnaires and interviews—may be optimum when the goal is to assess intimate experience. People's reports on themselves may work best for gathering information on feelings, perceptions, and expectations.

Behavioral observation, in combination with self-reports, may be the most effective way to assess intimate behavior. When interactions are videotaped, researchers can take advantage of the relative objectivity of third-party assessments. Since third-party raters are not themselves involved in the interaction or the relationship, their perceptions are not affected by expectations of, feelings about, or memories of either partner. Schemes for coding intimate behavior directly are few, however. This paucity is likely due, in part, to the contradiction that researchers present to participants when they ask them to engage in intimate conversation while being videotaped by total strangers. Participants might censure these "intimate revelations" under the circumstances.

Self-reports have also been used to gather information about behavior. Interaction record forms, which ask people to describe very specific behaviors and experiences at the time of their occurrence, likely reduce problems due to memory failure or motivated distortion. Some inventories are written with items that ask participants to describe themselves in very specific terms, which might also reduce distortion. Self-report inventories cannot ever completely correct for people's distorted perceptions of themselves, however.

The measurement of intimate relationships can benefit from all the methods discussed above. Behavioral observation cannot reveal how prevalent intimate interaction is between two particular relationship partners, but it can reveal whether intimate interactions are within the partners' repertoires. Self-reports can tap partners' perceptions of the modal characteristics of the relationship over time. Finally, daily records and participant observation checklists can provide estimates of how commonly partners engage in intimate interactions. Further, in interviews, well-placed probes can help detect whether the interviewee's notions of what intimate interaction is match preestablished criteria (e.g., as in the intimacy status interview [Orlofsky, Marcia, & Lesser, 1973]). Further, asking participants to generalize about their relationships for a specific time period can reduce error that come from broader inferences (Wheeler, Reis, & Nezlek, 1983).

The conceptions of intimacy reviewed here, and introduced in Chapter 1, converge on a definition of the superordinate concept 'intimacy:' intimacy is a positively cathected psychological relation between two or more people in which partners share that which is private and personal with one another. Like any superordinate concept, this one is broad and abstract, making it difficult to operationalize.

Unlike the superordinate concept, the basic intimacy concepts (intimate interaction and intimate relationship) fulfill the four functions of an intimacy conception listed in Chapter 1. First, these intimacy concepts have helped to organize a literature on intimacy that spans several disciplines and traditions. For example, they have allowed conceptions of intimacy that emphasize self-disclosure (Jourard, 1971) and sensitive responding (Berg, 1987) to be distinguished from conceptions that primarily address intimate relationships and their characteristics (Shaefer & Olson, 1981). Second, these basic concepts have clarified the dyadic nature of intimacy. They include conceptions which emphasize interactions or relationships (e.g., Reis & Shaver, 1988), while excluding those that emphasize capacities and motives (e.g., McAdams, 1984). Capacities and motives may contribute to people's effectiveness in intimate interactions and relationships, but are not synonymous with intimacy. Third, these intimacy concepts extend traditional social psychological definitions of intimacy (i.e., self-disclosure and sensitive responding) and include other experiences and interactions that laypersons commonly call intimate. They purposely include a variety of intimate experiences while still differentiating between intimacy and related concepts, such as love and closeness. Finally, the current intimacy concepts allow for boundary cases of intimacy, thus acknowledging the fuzziness of the concept. Just as there may always be "boundary cases" for concepts such as furniture (is a rug a piece of furniture?) so also will there always be boundary cases for intimacy.

INTIMACY THROUGH THE LIFE SPAN

Individual Development
and Intimacy

All the factors entering into the vicissitudes of self-esteem . . . are
wholly a matter of past experience with people . . . if experience is
definitely unsuited to providing competence for living with
others, at [a] particular level of development, the probabilities of
future adequate interpersonal relations are . . . reduced.
—HARRY STACK SULLIVAN, *The Interpersonal Theory of Psychiatry*

For several decades theorists have acknowledged the influence of interpersonal relationships on the development of personality. Adler (1964)
argued that parents' behavior toward children could predispose children
to feelings of inferiority and a lack of self-sufficiency. Sullivan (1953) suggested that children's personalities are shaped by their efforts to avoid interpersonal anxiety, which arises primarily from experiences of rejection,
punishment, or ridicule from others. Horney (1950) believed that a child
must have warm and affectionate relationships with others in order to develop a sense of basic security in a potentially hostile world. Fairbairn
(1954) argued that if children do not obtain satisfying experiences in important relationships, their ability to form successful relationships in
adulthood will be seriously compromised.

The next four chapters speak to three notions about the interrela-
tionship between individual development and intimacy. First, these
chapters propose that our intimate interactions and relationships affect,
for good or ill, our adaptations to the changing needs and stresses that
emerge with each stage of development. Underlying this proposition is
the assumption that we develop characteristic ways of behaving in the
context of our interactions and relationships with others and then generalize these patterns of behavior to other situations.

A second (and related) notion is that the character of intimate interactions and relationships is shaped by our adaptations to life-stage-related needs and stresses. The assumption here is that each stage of development is characterized by its own configuration of needs and stresses and that our behavior reflects in part our efforts to cope with those needs and stresses. These coping efforts affect interactions and relationships with others through our interpersonal behavior.

Third, these chapters propose that adaptations learned earlier in development may influence intimacy in later life stages. Adaptations to intimate interactions and relationships are not only generalized across situations within a single stage of development but may also generalize from earlier to later relationships. The expectations and associated behaviors from an early childhood relationship, for example, may in part shape how an adult approaches his or her relationships. Unlike traditional object relations theories, however, these chapters suggest that early childhood adaptations and intimate relationships are not the only ones that affect subsequent interpersonal behavior but that adaptations learned during any life stage can generalize to challenges faced later on (a perspective in line with Erikson, 1963).

I believe that neither intimacy nor individual development can be understood without considering the other (e.g., Bowlby, 1969, 1973; Erikson, 1959, 1963; Sullivan, 1953). I view the birth of a child as initiating a lifelong process of *mutual adaptation* between the child, his or her intimate relationship partners, and the broader social environment. Figure 3.1 depicts this mutual adaptation process, which serves as a framework for systematic study of individual development and intimacy across the life span.

The process depicted in Figure 3.1 rests on several assumptions about individual development. First, I assume that within any given set of circumstances some behaviors are more adaptive than others (Erikson, 1959; Loevinger, 1976; L. Sroufe, 1989). Notions about which behaviors are adaptive rely on theoretically derived characteristics of normative development (Erikson, 1959; Loevinger, 1976). They may also rely on findings from empirical studies of specific adaptations and their consequences (e.g., Elicker, Englund, & Sroufe, 1992).

Second, I assume that intimate relationships are most likely to have positive effects on individuals when they address their concerns or fulfill their needs (Buhrmester, in press; Rotter, 1982; Sullivan, 1953). The results of interactions that address concerns and fulfill needs can soothe, improve skills, expand knowledge, improve coping effectiveness, increase the clarity or complexity of thought, relieve symptoms, enhance mood, or facilitate goal attainment. The fulfillment of needs should be satisfying

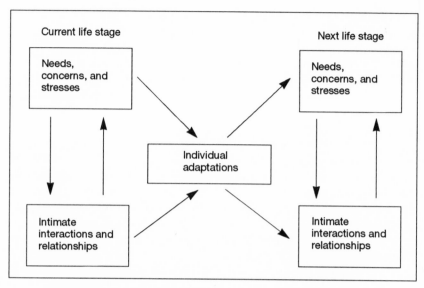

FIGURE 3.1. Individual development and intimate relationships.

and rewarding and should free up time and attention that would otherwise go into their pursuit (Maslow, 1968). Further, need deprivation leaves people in a negative state *specific* to the deprivation of that particular need (R. S. Weiss, 1986); for example, hunger is specific to food deprivation, and loneliness is specific to intimacy or companionship deprivation. States of deprivation, if they are sufficiently frequent, persistent, or severe, exert negative effects on development (Spitz, 1949).

The third assumption made here is that life stages carry with them particular needs, concerns, and stresses. The notion that life stages are marked by particular concerns has a long history in developmental psychology (Erikson, 1963; Freud, 1933; Gould, 1978; Levinson, 1978; Loevinger, 1976; Mahler, 1975). I will draw from theories that propose that life-stage-related changes in concerns, stresses, and needs mark development and that the ability to cope with later concerns and needs is based on the outcomes of prior coping attempts (Erikson, 1963, 1968; Freud, 1933; Havighurst, 1972; Sullivan, 1953).

A fourth assumption is that each life stage has the potential to add new skills, competencies, and coping styles to the individual's repertoire. As a result of engaging in life-stage-related activities, individuals develop new levels of breadth and depth in certain competencies. Limitations in competencies may similarly mark each life stage. In either case, individuals will bring age-related competencies to their interactions with significant others.

Figure 3.1 depicts the process by which intimate interactions and relationships may shape and be shaped by individual psychological development. It is an outgrowth of a model developed by Duane Buhrmester and me to describe the interplay between individual development and self-disclosing interactions (Buhrmester & Prager, 1995). This account proposes that intimate interactions and relationships can help people understand, think more clearly about, approach more skillfully, or resolve preoccupations of their current life stage (Elicker et al., 1992; R. Lerner, 1989). Depending on the kinds of individual adaptations they make within their relationships, people may be more or less prepared to tackle the problems of the next stage (Belsky & Nezworski, 1988). A detailed description of the three theoretical propositions in this account follows.

INDIVIDUAL DEVELOPMENT AND INTIMATE RELATIONSHIPS

Proposition 1: Interactions with others will affect how individuals adapt to developmentally related needs, concerns, and stresses. The account depicted in Figure 3.1 proposes that some of the most important environmental contingencies to which individuals must adapt come from intimate interactions and relationships. It further proposes that they therefore play a profoundly important role in shaping individual personality and coping style. In the course of daily interactions, intimate relationship partners likely make dozens of adjustments in their behavior in order to adapt to each other's styles of relating and other idiosyncracies. Theoretically, the most important relationships elicit adaptations from the partners that they generalize to other situations. These adaptations will either enhance or interfere with individual efforts to address life-stage-related needs and concerns.

Proposition 2: Whether a need or concern is voiced or not, it will affect the individual's interactions with others. The amount of interaction, the personalness of interaction, and the level of relational intimacy people seek with intimate partners may vary systematically with life-stage-related needs and concerns. For example, infants who need to be fed are less likely to seek social interaction than well-fed infants. Awareness of hunger will disrupt an infant's playful interaction. Older children and adults can more actively pursue gratification of their needs, perhaps verbalizing them directly, perhaps disclosing their concerns in hopes of receiving a helpful response (Buhrmester & Prager, 1995). The content and emotional tenor of verbal interaction may shift as intimate partners grow and their concerns change.

Proposition 3: Experiences in intimate interactions and relationships from earlier in life can affect a person's intimate interactions and relationships later on. Experiences with others can influence how we perceive others, what we expect and hope to find in relationships, and our styles of interpreting various interpersonal situations (Baldwin, 1992). These earlier experiences create what have been called object relations schemata (Rausch, Barry, Hertel, & Swain, 1974), working models of self-and-other (Bowlby, 1969), or, more simply, schemas. Schemas are sets of expectations about current interpersonal situations that are based on generalizations from previous experiences. They affect the way we think, feel, and behave in any given interpersonal situation. Furthermore, they guide our perceptions. What we attend to and perceive about others and our relationships is selected through our schemas (Mischel, 1993).

The chapters in Part II of this book address a fourth proposition as well. In them I presume that the availability of intimate others to address concerns or needs is affected by the context in which individual development occurs. There are several different levels of context (which will be discussed in detail in Part III). The immediate context affects the availability of intimate partners through the pressures and opportunities people confront in their day-to-day lives. At this level, individuals must determine which, if any, intimate partners are available (physically or psychologically) with whom to share certain concerns. One's close relationship partners have their own concerns and preoccupations that affect their responsiveness and sensitivity, for example. Contextual factors can also refer to personal individual factors such as genetic endowment, personality characteristics, competencies and skills, values and beliefs, and so on. At this level are the individual's own comfort level with intimate interaction and the individual's skillfulness in marshaling support and advice from others. Finally, context can refer to the sociocultural values, social roles, and standards for behavior available in the discourses of society. Gendered sociocultural norms may determine the availability of intimate partners, for example; specifically, American boys may be less likely to find friends to confide in than American girls.

In sum, the account depicted in Figure 3.1 suggests that each developmental stage or period in life carries with it certain needs, concerns, and stresses. These exert an influence on intimate interactions via their impact on individual behavior within those interactions. Interactions with intimate others will, more or less, fulfill needs or address concerns, and individuals will adapt or learn accordingly. These adaptations will be more or less useful when the individual addresses the needs and concerns of the next life stage and will undoubtedly be further modified or expanded as new sets of concerns are confronted.

For the remainder of the chapters in Part II, I use the model in Figure 3.1 to construct a life span account of individual development in the context of intimate interactions and relationships. My main purpose is to reveal patterns of mutual influence between individual development and intimacy through a selective review of the literature.

I have divided the life span into eight periods. Chapter 4 discusses the first two: infancy (birth to 18 months) and preschool age (18 months to 5 years). Chapter 5 discusses early childhood (5 to 9 years) and middle childhood and preadolescence (9 to 12 years). Chapter 5 addresses adolescence (12 to 18 years) and young adulthood (18 to 35 years), while Chapter 7 presents middle (35 to 65 years) and late (65+ years) adulthood.

Each chapter begins with a descriptive review of research on age- and life-stage-related characteristics of intimate relationships for that developmental phase. These reviews identify the major intimate partners of individuals in that life stage and the changes in those relationships both within the life stage itself and since the last life stage. Following the review, each section addresses hypothesized links between life-stage-related needs and intimacy. I introduce each of these subsections with a brief description of the specific need or concern in question. These introductory sections explain why developmental theorists and researchers believe that the concern might be ascendant during the current life stage.

Each section then considers how intimate interactions and relationships affect individual development by creating demands for individual adaptation. These discussions also examine how individual development (specifically, life-stage-related needs and stresses) affects intimacy via its impact on individual behavior within interactions and relationships. Finally, each section considers how adaptations to needs and stresses in earlier stages of development may generalize to intimate interactions and relationships in later stages.

CAN YOUNG CHILDREN BE INTIMATE?

Because the social psychological literature often confines discussions of intimate relationships to verbal interactions between adolescents and adults (e.g., see M. S. Davis, 1973; Reis & Shaver, 1988), the kinds of intimate interactions infants and young children can have merit discussion. Work on intimacy has often excluded children. Children's relationships with parents have been excluded because they are not egalitarian (M. S.

Davis, 1973). Definitions that equate intimacy with self-disclosing inter-actions, in which the private self is verbally revealed to another (e.g., Derlega, 1984), may exclude children who lack abstract reasoning abili-ties. Children's relationships may also be excluded when the expression *intimate relationship* denotes a sexual relationship. In this chapter, I will take advantage of the fuzzy boundaries around the concept of intimate in-teraction to include children's interactions and relationships.

The set of intimacy concepts defined in Chapter 1 can be used to clarify what kinds of intimate interactions young children can have. Re-call that intimate interactions have two components: (1) the sharing of personal and private things (intimate behavior) and (2) positive involve-ment and affect, accompanied by perceptions of understanding (intimate experience). Infants and young children engage in intimate behavior by this definition. Initially, most of these interactions are *nonverbal*. The younger the child, the more likely it is that intimate experience will be confined to touching, holding, caressing, and the gratification of basic bodily needs. Children gradually incorporate verbal intimacy as their abilities to understand and later produce speech increase with age. In-fants and young children can also have intimate experiences. Even before they can smile and laugh, infants can show positive affect in response to interactions (e.g., by relaxing and cooing when held). It is more difficult to argue that infants and young children have perceptions of understand-ing, however. The term *understanding* can imply an ability to take the per-spective of another, an ability not possessed by young children.

Children's perceptions of understanding in intimate interactions may be best defined in terms of their cognitive capabilities during any given life stage. In infants, for example, perceptions of understanding might best be confined to children's experiences of *attunement*. That is, infants may feel understood when they sense their intimate partners are attuned to their moods and needs. In the youngest children, then, posi-tive affect and perceptions of understanding may be one and the same.

Rather than asserting that children's immaturity precludes their par-ticipation in intimate interactions, I argue in this chapter that their changing cognitive capacities allow them to participate in *increasingly so-phisticated intimate interactions*. That is, as children gain cognitive capabil-ities, their perceptions of understanding can expand beyond feeling grati-fied in response to another's behavior and can incorporate an increasingly differentiated picture of the other person.

Finally, infants and young children also have intimate relationships. Chapter 1 defines intimate relationships according to the affection, trust, cohesiveness, and relational intimacy[1] that characterize them. From the outset most children's relationships include affection from people who love them. Adaptations children make to their early relationships with parents may reveal a level of trust appropriate to the typical pattern of interaction between child and parent. There is also evidence that children enjoy cohesiveness in their earliest relationships with parents, which ultimately extends to friends and other peers. Finally, the reviews that follow provide a picture of relational intimacy that increases in complexity as children broaden their repertoire of interpersonal skills. From infancy through middle childhood, children add capacities for goal-directed communication, for the labeling and articulation of feelings, for empathy and perspective taking, and for cooperation and negotiation. Each of these capacities has the potential of adding complexity and depth to children's intimate relating.

SUMMARY AND CONCLUSIONS

This chapter provides a theoretical framework for understanding how our evolving networks of personal relationships might shape, and be shaped by, our life-stage-related needs, concerns, and preoccupations. This framework, which sets the stage for all four chapters in Part II, was derived from one developed by Duane Buhrmester and me (Buhrmester & Prager, 1995). Its first purpose is to provide a unifying perspective on individual development and intimacy for the entire life span. Its second purpose is to generate meaningful hypotheses about links between life-stage-related changes in intimate interactions and relationships and individual development. The following four chapters use the framework to organize the literature on personal relationships through the life span and to integrate that literature with existing knowledge on normative developmental change.

⁓

Intimacy in Infancy and the Preschool Years

Links between individual developmental needs and intimate relationships are more extensively documented for infancy and the preschool years than for any other life stage. Thus far, considerable evidence exists for links between characteristics of parent–child interaction, the quality of children's peer relationships, and children's developing autonomy and social skills (e.g., see review by Eliker, Englund, & Sroufe, 1992).

Since the literature on children's relationships has not been explicitly concerned with intimacy, I confronted two important challenges while writing this and the following chapter. The first was to make some a priori decisions about which aspects of children's relating are intimate. For example, in this chapter I discuss attachment because, as I explain later, babies' attachment relationships may be their first intimate relationships. The second challenge was to identify life-stage-related concerns and competencies that are likely to affect intimate relating over time, and to generate hypotheses about how these affect and are affected by children's relationships. For example, a growing sense of autonomy, a developing gender identity, and an ability to share and communicate awareness are all likely to shape children's interactions with intimate partners. At the same time, each of these aspects of children's development are being shaped by those same interactions.

In this and the next chapter, I review the literature on children's relationships with their parents and peers and how these change over time. Following the reviews, I consider individual concerns and needs that are likely to influence and be influenced by children's relationships. As this discussion progresses from infancy and the preschool years to middle childhood and preadolescence, my notions about links between individual development and intimate relationships become more speculative, reflecting the state of our knowledge at this time.

INFANCY (BIRTH–18 MONTHS): LIFE-STAGE-RELATED DEVELOPMENTS IN INFANTS' RELATIONSHIPS

Relationships with Parents

Parents and other caregivers are the principal sources of intimate contact for infants in the first year of life. Rapid developmental changes are observable in interactions between infants and their parents during the first year. Infants become visibly more responsive to their parents over time (Blehar, Lieberman, & Ainsworth, 1977; Greenspan & Lourie, 1981). At around 8 or 9 months of age infants begin to use affective, vocal, and gestural communication to direct their parents' attention to events of interest (L. Sroufe, 1989). At this point, interaction in a functional parent–infant dyad takes on a "dancelike quality" (L. Sroufe, 1989), in that it consists of coordinated give-and-take responding (Brazelton, Koslowski, & Main, 1974). By the end of the first year infants' behavior toward their parents seems goal-directed, with infants' signals clearly expressing to parents the response they wish to receive (e.g., lifted arms communicating a desire to be picked up) (L. Sroufe, 1989).

Infants are readily comforted by any adult until somewhere around 7 months, at which age they will cry when their parents disappear and resist comforting by other adults (Shaffer, 1988). These early relationships with those who care for infants become what Bowlby (1969) called attachment relationships. Bowlby argued that attachment relationships ensure physical proximity between infants and caregivers. In so doing, they provide a safe and secure environment for infants to begin exploring themselves and their world.

Our attachment relationships in infancy may be our first intimate relationships. That is, these relationships are the first in the life span that can be characterized by the features of intimacy described in Chapter 1. Within these relationships infants have their first experiences of being understood (when they express needs and get them met) and of sharing positive affect with another human being. They also have their first experiences of physical closeness and tenderness, of being loved and loving.

Interactions with Peers

Developmental changes in infants' interactions with peers are observable during the first year of life. Newborns show responsiveness to age-mates in "contagion" crying (Saarni, 1988), and by 3 or 4 months, infants are more responsive to social than to nonsocial stimuli. They respond to peers with smiles, vocalizations, and touches and will offer toys and other objects (Nash, 1988). These kinds of sociable behaviors become more pronounced as the infant gets older and are well established by the end of the first year (Nash, 1988; Vandell, Wilson, & Henderson, 1980).

Over the course of the first year of life, then, infants become increasingly responsive and active shapers of their interactions with their parents. Toward the end of the year they have normally established one or more distinct attachment relationships, the quality of which tends to be stable over time (Sroufe, Egeland, & Kreutzer, 1990). Infants are responsive to peers but show little sign of developing specific relationships with peers during their first year.

NEEDS, STRESSES, AND INTIMATE RELATIONSHIPS IN INFANCY

In the following section I argue that babies' needs for (1) security and comfort and (2) sharing and communicating awareness play a role in shaping their interactions and relationships with parents. This review considers attachment styles as the primary indicator of infants' adaptations to needs for security and comfort within relationships with parents and other caregivers. Attachment styles may be important to the study of intimacy because they are an early indicator of the quality of infants' first intimate interactions. Expectations from these early intimate interactions may generalize to other relationships, thus affecting children's behavior.

Infants' adaptations to needs for sharing and communicating awareness may also be most apparent in their interactions with parents. Infants' increasingly deliberate efforts to engage their parents with whatever has captured their attention are intimate because they involve sharing and positive affect. The earliest sign of infants' ability to understand others' meanings may be seen in their capacity to read and respond appropriately to parents' facial expressions of emotion.

Security and Comfort

The Concern in Context

Infants' helplessness ensures that safety, security, and comfort are their paramount needs (Bowlby, 1969). The helplessness of the newborn human infant is its most overriding characteristic. Infants are unable to protect themselves and ensure their own survival. Their very life depends on a sustained and constant adult presence and attention.

Maturing psychomotor and cognitive abilities may ensure that infants' needs for security and safety are expressed with increasing directness within their intimate relationships with caregivers. Specifically, at age 6 weeks, refinements in the infant's depth perception are apparent. These refinements allow infants to perceive caregivers from a distance (Hartup, 1989a; L. Sroufe, 1989) and thereby detect their caregiver's whereabouts. Perhaps as a result, 6-week-old infants cry when they believe they have been left alone by their caregivers. This separation anxiety of the baby's first year may arise in part from increases in cognitive understanding that accompany these perceptual abilities.

Relationships with Parents

Most likely, infants' adaptive efforts to fulfill needs for security and comfort are shaped primarily within their intimate interactions and relationships with their parents (or other caregivers). These adaptive efforts are theoretically observable in the characteristic attachment style an infant demonstrates in interactions with each parent. Attachment styles are patterns of behavior children manifest following separation from and reunion with caregivers[1]. The experimental paradigm called the "strange situation" has been the primary setting in which researchers have observed these attachment styles. In the "strange situation," infants participate in a series of eight episodes designed to escalate the amount of stress they experience. Episodes in which babies are separated from and then reunited with a close companion (usually a parent) are specifically designed to elicit attachment-related behavior (Ainsworth, Blehar, Waters, & Wall, 1978; Bowlby, 1982).

The quality of parents' interactions with their infants may exert a significant influence on infants' patterns of attachment-related behavior

(Crittenden, 1990). The caregiver's sensitive and appropriate responding to the infant during feeding, crying, and face-to-face play (Ainsworth, 1967; Ainsworth et al., 1978) predicts a *secure* attachment pattern in both mother–infant and father–infant interactions (Cox, Owen, Henderson, & Margand, 1992; Main & Weston, 1981). A lighthearted parenting style (i.e., one characterized by fast tempo of speech and rapid changes in voice volume and pitch) is more likely to be associated with insecure attachment classifications than is a more tender (marked by nondramatic, soothing, even attentiveness) or more sober (marked by slow, uneven, delayed responding) parenting style. Secure infants are more likely to have eye contact and responsive facial expression with their mothers than are insecure infants (Grossmann, Grossmann, & Schwan, 1986) and are less likely to be ignored (Bretherton, 1988).

Parents' ability to attune to their infant's emotional expressions, or affect, is associated with more secure attachments between infant and parent (Grossmann, & Grossmann, 1991). Affective attunement refers to the caregiver's ability to respond promptly and appropriately to a young infant's emotional expressions (Ainsworth et al., 1978). With older infants, it refers to the caregiver's ability to reflect emotions back at the same valence and intensity with which the infant initially expressed them (Bretherton, 1988). Secure infants and their mothers display an ease of emotional access not apparent between insecure infants and their mothers. The mothers of a secure infant is equally responsive to all kinds of affect, makes herself available when her infant seems to need her, and is able to remain attentive when her infant is playing or exploring happily (Main, Kaplan, & Cassidy, 1985; Matas, Arend, & Sroufe, 1978).

Security of attachment may therefore be best interpreted as an assessment of the relationship rather than of the infant (Bretherton, 1988). In support of this, security of attachment classification was found to be stable for several years *within* relationships (Main et al., 1985) but not *across* relationships, that is from mother–infant to father–infant relationships (Cox et al., 1992). Moreover, stresses, social support, and other factors external to the dyad may affect an infant's attachment classification through their effects on the mother's responsiveness (Sroufe & Fleeson, 1986). Finally, maternal responsiveness early in infancy is more predictive of later attachment classification than is the young infant's behavior (Blehar et al., 1977). The infant's response to the "strange situation" and the resulting attachment classification, then, can be best understood as an assessment of the infant's first intimate relationships (Sroufe & Fleeson, 1986).

According to Bowlby's (1969) attachment theory, babies' adaptations to their early attachment relationships create a foundation on which later experiences with potentially intimate partners will be built. Cross-sectional and longitudinal research has supported Bowlby's theory. Classifications of attachment-related behavior patterns in infant–parent relationships predict other indicators of infant adjustment, maternal behavior, and infant–mother relationship characteristics, both concurrently and over time (see reviews by Bartholomew, 1993; Bretherton, 1988; Sroufe & Fleeson, 1986). This research is presented in more detail in the discussions of the relevant life stages.

Sharing and Communicating Awareness

The Concern in Context

During the first year, infants show evidence of an increasing interest in sharing and communicating their awareness of their surroundings with others. Manifesting this interest (and capacity) are interactions in which infants follow their mother's gaze[2] (Scaife & Bruner, 1975) or her pointing gestures (Murphy & Messer, 1977). Infants appear to experience pleasure as they discover their abilities to actively engage their parents' attention and to direct it to something of interest to them (L. Sroufe, 1989).

Infants' apparent desire to share and communicate their awareness may be a manifestation of two developing capacities. First, infants develop a capacity for goal-directed behavior during the second half of the first year; by 10 months of age they acquire the capacity to direct their gestures and vocalizations (J. Sroufe, 1991). Second, infants acquire what Stern (1985) described as an increasing awareness of intersubjectivity (i.e., an awareness of the distinctiveness and separateness of other minds besides their own). Theorists inferred this increasing awareness of intersubjectivity from the rapid and dramatic increase in infant behavior directed toward communicating whatever has aroused them or come into their awareness (Saarni, 1988). Also supporting the notion of an increasing awareness of intersubjectivity are infants' increasing use of facial cues to assess others' emotions and to direct their behavior accordingly. For example, Campos, Barrett, Lamb, Goldsmith, and Sternberg (1983) placed mothers of 10-month old infants on one side of a visual cliff, which consisted of a sturdy, transparent board placed over a substantial drop from the surface on which the baby was sitting. Infants, who were placed on the other side, would crawl across the board when mothers signaled to them with a joyful face but would not when mothers signaled with a fearful or angry face.

Relationships with Parents

When sharing awareness the infant seems to be seeking a reciprocal exchange in which both parent and infant can experience delight and mutual understanding. The infant's behavior is highly engaging to adults and draws them into interactions with the infant. (Imagine an infant pointing out the window at a cat, crying with delight, and then turning around to make eye contact after Mom or Dad witnesses the animal's presence.) Through their expressions of shared delight, adult and child may be providing one another with a rewarding experience of shared positive affect and understanding—in short, with an intimate experience. Because these kinds of interactions potentially provide infants with intimate experiences, their contribution to children's adjustment should be studied more thoroughly.

TODDLERS AND PRESCHOOLERS (18 MONTHS– 4 YEARS): LIFE-STAGE-RELATED DEVELOPMENTS IN INTIMATE RELATIONSHIPS

Relationships with Parents

During the preschool period parents and other adult caregivers continue to be the child's most important relationships. The quality of parent–child attachments is quite stable from infancy through the preschool years (Matas et al., 1978) with both fathers and mothers (Egeland & Farber, 1984; Main et al., 1985).

In their relationships with parents preschool children show more tolerance of separateness than they did earlier. Because of their broader range of experience and increased cognitive processing skills, preschoolers are less likely than infants to be alarmed in new situations (R. S. Weiss, 1986) and are more tolerant of their parents' temporary inaccessibility.

Toddlers also actively *seek* more separateness than do younger children in the context of relating to their parents. There is evidence that toddlers can comfort themselves with visual contact with their parents whereas physical contact is necessary for an infant's comfort (Sroufe & Cooper, 1988). Further, the more easily accessible mothers are, the less frequently toddlers seem to avail themselves of the opportunity to visually contact them (Carr, Dabbs, & Carr, 1975). As toddlers develop language skills, these seem to allow them even more distal contact with parents, further reducing their efforts to seek physical or visual contact.

Interactions with Peers

By the end of the second year toddlers can sustain interactions with their peers (Hartup, 1989b). Children of this age show a capacity for reciprocity and an ability to engage in cooperative play (Hartup, 1989a). Much of toddlers' play together involves creating a shared fantasy, in which "two friends do not simply *act* like tigers or dragons or ghosts—they *become* tigers or dragons or ghosts" (Parker & Gottman, 1989, p. 105). Children of this age demonstrate the ability to resolve conflicts with nonlinguistic vocalizations; later they will use verbal negotiations (Nash, 1988).

While increased smiling and other signs of delight suggest that coordinating play with an age-mate enhances children's enjoyment of play, their primary focus seems to be on the game at hand rather than on the friend. The sustained interactions of toddlers appear to be coordinated and reciprocal interactions rather than friendships. For this reason, Selman (1980) called these toddler pairs "momentary physical playmates." The friendships seem to be based on a shared momentary interest in a game or toy.

The momentary quality of toddlers' peer relationships begins to change by age 4. There is evidence that 4-year-olds can sustain a relationship with their age-mates over time. Four-year-old children greet one another joyfully upon reunion and talk about their friends in their absence (Levinger & Levinger, 1986). Some peer associations between nursery school children are clearly stronger than others, indicating companion preference in children of this age (Hartup, 1989b; Rotenberg & Sliz, 1988). Four-year-olds have been found to interact more frequently with peers they designate as friends than with those not designated as such (Hartup, 1989a).

Toward the end of the preschool years children begin to show a marked tendency to prefer play with same-sex playmates (Maccoby, 1990a). Same-sex playmate preferences seem to be associated with children's acquisition of the concept of gender and a growing preference for "gender-appropriate" toys and games (Fagot, 1978). This preference for same-sex playmates begins a process by which children form their closest friendships with same-sex peers, a process that will last through adolescence and into adulthood.

NEEDS, CONCERNS, AND INTIMATE RELATIONSHIPS DURING THE PRESCHOOL YEARS

During the preschool years children's needs for (1) autonomy and individuation, (2) sharing and communicating awareness, (3) enjoyable interactions with peers, and (4) consolidating gender identity may each influence (and be influenced by) their intimate interactions and relationships. Developmental theory (e.g., Mahler, 1975) argues that through their interactions with intimate others, children learn whether they can be autonomous beings and still retain the love and intimacy they experienced with their parents during infancy. Cross-sectional research (e.g., Matas et al., 1978) suggests that the quality of parent–child interactions predicts children's functioning in situations that demand autonomy and self-control.

The sharing and communicating of experience by preschool children involves the acquisition of a variety of competencies that are likely to affect their concurrent and later functioning in intimate interactions and relationships. In particular sensitive, attuned interactions with parents foster skills in children such as verbalizing emotions and expressing empathic concern (Bretherton, 1988).

Children also learn much about intimate relating through their interactions and relationships with peers (Sullivan, 1953). An understanding of the processes by which children learn to relate to peers is therefore important to the study of intimacy. First, children who interact sensitively and skillfully with peers during the preschool years seem more likely to form intimate friendships later on (Eliker et al., 1992). Second, the need for enjoyable interactions with peers may itself be related to life stage. The efficacy of children's adaptations to peer interaction seems to be affected by characteristics of parent–child interaction. Possibly, children acquire competencies through interactions with parents that may result in more effective behavior with peers.

Preschool-age children are just beginning to demonstrate concerns with consolidating a gender identity. The effect of this concern on preschoolers' interactions with others is currently most evident in peer relationships, where children increasingly avoid social contact with the opposite sex (Maccoby, 1990a). This exclusively same-sex social contact may result in gender-related styles of behaving in intimate interactions and relationships

Autonomy and Individuation

The Concern in Context

Toddlers' apparently decreasing efforts to maintain physical contact with their parents during the late infancy and preschool periods may be due in part to increasingly salient needs for autonomy and individuation (Erikson, 1963; Mahler, 1975). Psychodynamic theorists have proposed that

individuation needs in toddlers emerge when they discover that the plea-
sures of pursuing inner aims are at times more rewarding than those found
in pursuing coordinated aims with parents and other caregivers (Mahler,
1975; L. Sroufe, 1989). As Mahler (1975) noted, this "practicing period,"
during which children become preoccupied with exercising and proving
their developing competencies, can be a period of joyous self-discovery.

Needs for individuation may be inferred from children's demonstrated pleasure in controlling their own movements. Children show dramatic
increases in motor coordination and cognitive skills from the second to
the fifth year and happily experiment with walking toward and away from
objects and people of interest, as if to test their newfound abilities
(Mahler & McDevitt, 1980).

Perhaps as a reflection of their evolving interest in autonomy, toddlers play for longer and longer time periods without companionship and
direction from their parents. Their greater attention span and increasing
capacity to think consciously about sequences of events may allow them
to be more entertaining to themselves. After the second year, children
can lose themselves in fantasy play complete with imaginary plots and
characters (Bretherton, 1988; Parker & Gottman, 1989).

Relationships with Parents

In their interactions with parents toddlers purportedly have the opportunity to learn how intimate experiences may happily coexist with their capacities for separateness, distinctiveness, and independence. Developmental theorists have emphasized the importance to children of having
positive early relationship experiences in conjunction with their developing autonomy and individuation (e.g., Erikson, 1963; Mahler, 1975).
Theorists like Chodorow (1979) have suggested that we generalize to our
adult intimate relationships what we learned from our parents during
childhood about the coexistence of autonomy and intimacy. (I will discuss these long-term effects in conjunction with the relevant life stages.)

The quality of children's intimate interactions with parents may enhance their ability to function autonomously. Specifically, there is evidence that the security of toddlers' attachments to their parents, particularly to their mothers, predicts the persistence and affective quality of
their independent play and exploration (L. Sroufe, 1989). Securely attached 18-month-old children show more tolerance for frustration, more
persistence in a difficult task, and more effective use of their mothers for
assistance than insecurely attached children (Matas et al., 1978; Sroufe
& Fleeson, 1986). In one study, when mothers were inattentive, most of
the participating youngsters (regardless of attachment classification)
showed less pleasure and persistence when exploring a new environment

and sought proximity with the mother less often. Children's autonomous play is more thematic when their parents are more attentive(Sorce & Emde, 1981).

Interactions with parents may encourage toddlers' independent exploratory play when parents use a teaching process referred to as "scaffolding." This involves a balance between direct assistance on the one hand and verbal instructions encouraging children to "fix things" themselves on the other (Hartup, 1989a). Research suggests that mothers' skillfulness at encouraging children when they are frustrated and their ability to use scaffolding play a role in promoting children's exploration and problem solving (Maslin, Bretherton, & Morgan, 1986). A parent's scaffolding efforts, then, appear to have beneficial effects on a child's problem-solving abilities independent of the pair's attachment classification (Maslin et al., 1986; Nash, 1988).

Finally, preschool-age children's autonomy and self-control are higher when their parents use an *authoritative* rather than an authoritarian or permissive parenting style (Baumrind, 1967, 1971). In laboratory studies, children who showed more self-reliance had parents who were nurturing, and who reasoned with them, listened carefully to their point of view, and resisted their attempts at coercion. Parents of less autonomous children were either permissive (i.e., they were nurturing but did not make demands or exercise any control) or authoritarian (i.e., they were highly controlling and sometimes punitive, and failed to listen or encourage verbal give-and-take).

Parents' interaction styles may be a response to, as well as a cause of, children's efforts to fulfill autonomy needs. For example, parents' use of scaffolding rather than direct intervention may increase in response to their child's evolving autonomy. Parents seem to increase their use of verbal instruction in response to improvements in child's verbal skills (L. Sroufe, 1989).

Sharing and Communicating Experiences

The Concern in Context

Children develop a host of competencies during the preschool period that are likely to make ongoing contributions to their intimate interactions and relationships (e.g., Derlega & Chaikin, 1975). Children's capacities for communicating about feelings and emotions increase substantially during the preschool period. Preschool children also reveal an increase in their ability to read and understand emotions (Dunn, Bretherton, & Munn, 1987). Although children can display a range of emotions by the end of the first year (Izard, 1990; Izard, Huebner, Risser, Mc-Ginnes, & Dougherty, 1980), their ability to *interpret* others' emotional signals greatly increases in the second year (Saarni, 1988). It is then that their capacity for intersubjectivity (i.e., for sharing emotions) becomes more apparent, probably because they are now able to verbalize their feeling states (Stern, 1985). As a result, preschoolers engage in shared interpretations of events and the motives behind actions, and are able to clarify misunderstandings (Dunn et al., 1987; Saarni, 1988). Later, around age 4, children develop the ability to "grasp that their truth is not necessarily another's truth" (Bretherton, 1988, p. 92). At this time they understand more clearly than before that someone may be experiencing a different emotion than the one they are feeling, perhaps even about the same event.

Coinciding with the development of emotional understanding and expressiveness is an emerging capacity for empathy (i.e., for resonating emotionally to the emotions of another). By age 2, toddlers show a capacity to anticipate their own emotions (Saarni, 1988). By age 4 they can anticipate the emotions of another. Kestenbaum, Farber, and Sroufe (1989) found that 4-year-olds vocalized their concern for and attempted to approach another child who was in distress.

Relationships with Parents

Preschool children's abilities to express their feelings may be cultivated in the parent–child relationship (Bretherton, 1988). When mothers display more skill at affective attunement, their young children seem more inclined to verbalize their own feeling states (Dunn et al., 1987). Bretherton (1988) reported that parents often match their own emotional expressions to their child's. Appropriate matching is believed to affirm the very young child's experience and to provide older children with language to represent their feeling states to themselves and to others. Conversely, there is evidence suggesting that when parents ignore or misread their child's signals for attachment and autonomy, there is disturbance in the communication between parent and child (Bretherton, 1988).

Enjoyable Interactions with Peers

The Concern in Context

Scholars once believed that friendship was relatively unimportant to preschoolers because young children were unable to articulate the meaning of their friendships in interview studies (Dunn, 1993). More recent work indicates, however, that young children demonstrate loneliness and unhappiness when they do not have friends (Cassidy & Asher, 1992).

Developmental theorists have proposed that exposure to interactions with peers during the preschool years may be an important facilitator of children's social skills (Buhrmester, in press; Hartup & Moore, 1990) and success in making friends later on (Lewis & Feiring, 1989; Parker & Asher, 1987). This premise has been supported by work with nonhuman primates (Suomi & Harlow, 1972, 1978) that showed that monkeys raised in isolation were less competent when given the opportunity to interact with peers than those who had prior peer contact.

Preschool-age children enjoy joint play with peers and form somewhat stable friendships (Dunn, 1993; Lewis & Feiring, 1989). Children's interactional behavior differentiates friends from acquaintances. Preschoolers select as special friends children who are the most fun to play with and play with them for longer periods (Hartup, 1989a).

Relationships with Parents

Close associations have been found between preschool children's interactions with their parents and the quality of their interactions with peers (e.g., Kerns & Barth, 1995). Several aspects of the parent–child relationship may be associated with the quality of children's peer relationships. First, the development of preschool children's social skills with peers may be facilitated by a secure parent–child attachment (Cohn, Patterson, & Christopoulos, 1991; Elicker et al., 1992; Kerns & Barth, 1995; Putallaz & Heflin, 1990). Longitudinal research indicates that children who have secure attachment relationships with their mothers at 12, 15, or 18 months become more sociable, empathic, and capable of reciprocity, and are more frequently imitated by other children later on (Hartup, 1989b). It has also been found that secure children approach and respond to others with more positive and less negative affect (LaFreniere & Sroufe, 1985; Lamb & Nash, 1989; Lieberman, 1977; Sroufe & Fleeson, 1986; Waters, Wippman, & Sroufe, 1979).

The concurrent attachment relationship between parent and child also covaries in predictable ways with the quality of toddlers' peer interactions. Park and Waters (1989) studied pairs of 4-year-old friends who were rated as secure–secure or secure–insecure on the basis of their current attachment relationships with their mothers. Their results indicate that the interaction between secure–secure pairs is more harmonious, less controlling, more responsive, and happier than that between the secure–insecure pairs. Children with insecure (particularly avoidant) attachment to their mothers are more likely to be involved in peer interactions in which one child is victimized by derogation, sarcasm, and hostility (Egeland & Sroufe, 1981). Further, insecurely attached children appear more dependent than securely attached children on nursery school teachers (Hartup, 1989a) and are rated by their teachers as being less empathic with peers (L. Sroufe, 1983). Although the data are correlational, this body of research supports the notion that relationships with parents shape toddlers' interactions with peers (Sroufe & Fleeson, 1986).

Children's expectations about relationships with other children may arise from parent–child relationships. These expectations theoretically affect children's behavior in those relationships (Arend, Gove, & Sroufe, 1979; Erickson, Sroufe, & Egeland, 1985; Sroufe, 1983). Children's expectations (also called working models, schemas, or emotional templates) combine and integrate antecedent emotional states (e.g., fear), goal-directed behaviors (e.g., reaching for a parent), and emotional outcomes (e.g., reassurance and comfort) (Bowlby, 1973; Leventhal & Scherer, 1987). Working models were initially believed to be evident in the pattern of infants' behavior within their attachment relationships (Ainsworth et al., 1978; Bowlby, 1973; Bretherton, 1991). Patterned interactions between infants and their caregivers theoretically reflected sets of expectations, or working models, about the relationship. Attachment theorists later proposed that these working models affected children's behavior with their peers as well.

Children's ability to read and respond skillfully to emotional expression in others may account for the positive correlations found between the quality of the parent–child relationship and the child's relationships with peers (Cohn, Patterson, & Christopoulos, 1991). Parke, MacDonald, Beitel, and Bhavnagri (1988) found that children rejected by peers are less able than popular children to recognize and correctly label the emotional expressions of unfamiliar others. In turn, rejected children spend less time playing with their parents (Parke et al., 1988). Their fathers are more controlling during physical play (MacDonald, 1987), their mothers are more likely to endorse aggressive parenting strategies (Pettit, Dodge, & Brown, 1988), and both parents ignore or neglect them more frequently (Attili, 1989). Children who have certain kinds of interactions with their parents, then, may be less likely to become skillful at reading and decoding others' emotional expressions. As Cohn et al. (1991) suggest, "the child's ability to recognize others' emotional expressions may play a mediating role in the connection between parent–child relations and peer social acceptance" (pp. 326–327).

Finally, children's interactions with peers may be more person-centered and prosocial when they have learned to be reflective in their interactions with parents (Applegate, Burleson, & Delia, 1992). Applegate et al. proposed that parents' social knowledge is reflected in the complexity of their discourse with their children, which in turn influences children's cognitive complexity. Children's cognitive complexity then appears to shape their interactions with their peers.

Parents' influence on children's social competencies may *not* be limited to the parent–child interaction itself. Parents may help augment children's social skills when they actively seek opportunities for them to interact with peers (Hartup & Moore, 1990; Lamb & Nash, 1989; Parke et al., 1988). Parents can organize social activities, ensure children's access to other children, and plan or supervise children's play activities with age-mates (Ladd, Profilet, & Hart, 1992). For example, children who spend time in extra familial child care have more extensive opportunities for interaction with other children than those raised at home and sometimes show superior social skills (Howes, 1988; Mueller & Brenner, 1977; Vandell, Henderson, & Wilson, 1988).

Another way parents may affect children's social competence is by serving as models of effective social interaction. Children may learn prosocial interaction skills by observing their mother's interactions with others (Hartup & Moore, 1990). For example, Nash and Lamb (1987) found that 14-month-old children who best tolerated being left alone in a playroom with a peer and the peer's mother had observed their mother in a previous interaction with the peer's mother. The mothers of those toddlers who were distressed in this situation had not interacted much with the peer's mothers. Thus parents may serve as models and create bridges between their children and others.

Gender Identity

The Concern in Context

Preschool children may be actively concerned with establishing a sense of gender identity and an understanding of gender constancy (Kohlberg, 1966). Gender identity is a feeling of confidence in one's femaleness or maleness, whereas gender constancy is an understanding that one always will be the gender one is now. By the age of 4, children understand the concept of gender and know whether they are boys or girls (P. Smith, 1987). Simultaneously, they may become aware of the importance of gender in their social world (Bem, 1993; Liben & Signorella, 1993) and may avoid disapproval for cross-sex-typed behavior.

Relationships with Peers

There is clear evidence that children's concerns with gender identity affect their interactions with others, principally with peers. Late in the toddler period children show a strong preference for play with same-sex age-mates and become increasingly resistant to including opposite-sex peers in their play. This preference for same-sex play groups coincides with children's ability to identify their own gender and to understand the importance of gender as a category of persons and activities in their surrounding milieu (Maccoby, 1990a). This confinement to same-sex play groups itself may have an impact on development (see discussion in Chapter 5).

SUMMARY AND CONCLUSIONS

This chapter's review demonstrates dramatic life-stage-related changes in intimate relationships during infancy and the preschool years. Infants' responsiveness to others increases with each month that passes (e.g., L. Sroufe, 1989). Babies' ability to form specific attachments to one or more adults by the 6th month or so may have special significance for their individual development and for their future relationships with others (Bowlby, 1969, 1982; Crittenden, 1990). Their protests when their caregiver goes out of sight indicate that an attachment relationship has probably formed (Bowlby, 1969). Attachments are directed toward parents and other adults,[3] although infants are responsive to peers as well (Nash, 1988).

Toddlers enjoy togetherness and contact with parents but, compared to infants, seek more time to play alone (R. S. Weiss, 1986). Toddlers become increasingly entertaining to themselves and seem less concerned as time passes with maintaining constant contact with parents (Hartup, 1989a, 1989b). Toddlers, compared to infants, are more able to engage in sustained play with age-mates (Dunn, 1993). Preschool children characteristically create games of fantasy in which all can become immersed (Parker & Gottman, 1989). As children's communication with parents and peers during these years becomes increasingly verbal, their ability to resolve conficts and express their feelings expands greatly (Saarni, 1988). The quality of parent–child attachments, in contrast, tends to be stable from infancy through the preschool years (Matas, Arend, & Sroufe, 1978).

This chapter's review reveals established links between life-stage-related competencies, concerns, and needs and observed changes in infants' and preschoolers' relationships. For example, there is evidence that as infants demonstrate more interest in sharing and communicating their awareness with others (e.g., Scaife & Bruner, 1975), their parents' expressiveness and sharing seem to intensify (L. Sroufe, 1989).

Scholars have also made progress toward understanding how children's relationships might influence their competencies, concerns, and needs. Most of this work has investigated influences exerted by the parent–child relationship on the child's development and peer relationships. Toddlers' ability to enjoy independent play, for example, seems to be facilitated by parents who are attentive and available (Sroufe & Fleeson, 1986). Relationships with parents also seem to affect the quality of children's peer relationships. Cooperative and enjoyable interactions between preschoolers and their peers are associated with the quality of the parent–child attachment (Cohn, Patterson, & Christopoulos, 1991), the amount of time children and parents spend playing together (Parke et al., 1988), and parents' parenting strategies (Pettit et al., 1988).

Evidence is also accumulating that peer relationships themselves may exert an important influence on children's development. Peers, for example, may be primary socializing agents for children's gender-typed social styles (Maccoby, 1990b). The best recipe around for learning gender-typed social behavior may be just what children do: confine social interactions to same-sex peers, most of whom are intensely concerned with "proper" boy- or girl-like behavior while limited to concrete thinking. Children assist each other, then, to incorporate socially sanctioned roles and identities by rewarding conforming behavior and punishing deviance.

Research has already extensively explored links between infants' and preschoolers' life-stage-related needs and the quality of their relationships, particularly with parents. A large proportion of this work explores the implications of parent–child attachment relationships for preschoolers' concurrent psychosocial functioning. Intimacy researchers may wish to study, in addition, the concurrent and long-term effects of interactions involving sharing and communicating awareness. These interactions, in which infants and their relationship partners together experience delight and other positive emotions, may create (or fail to create) expectations in the infant that people can experience positive feelings together. These expectations could, reasonably, provide an important foundation for later intimate relating.

In sum, a developmental approach to studying intimacy should focus attention on the interplay between life-stage-related concerns, needs, and stresses and intimate interactions and relationships. This approach promises to deepen our understanding of life-stage-related changes in people's intimate relationships. It may also suggest ways that people are especially resilient, and especially vulnerable, with respect to particular kinds of relationships at particular times in life. For infants and preschoolers, attachment relationships with parents seem especially important. The quality of the parent–infant attachment predicts the quality of a preschooler's peer interactions and autonomous play. Children's experiences with sharing and communicating awareness, however, may be as important in shaping their expectations for intimate contact and deserve more attention.

Intimacy in Early and Middle Childhood

Perhaps less is known about intimate relating during the elementary school years than during any other period in the life cycle. Some evidence suggests that school-age children's most important and frequent intimate partners are their parents (Furman & Buhrmester, 1985). Unfortunately, little information is available about the kinds of intimate contact that parents and children share or about the impact of this contact on either the child's or the parent's development.

While a few studies have addressed intimacy in children's friendships (e.g., Furman & Buhrmester, 1992), information in this area is also sparse. What can be seen in the review that follows is that friendships take on increasing importance in children's lives during the elementary school years.

It is evident that children acquire a substantial number of cognitive and social competencies during the early and middle childhood years that seem likely to contribute to the quality of their intimate relationships, both concurrently and in the future. A capacity for taking another's perspective, for example, which becomes quite sophisticated by the end of the elementary school years, has been postulated to be a necessary ingredient for intimate relating (e.g., Paul & White, 1990). Further, positive relationship experiences during the school years may compensate for adaptation deficits from earlier development (Skolnick, 1986).

Developmental theorists since Freud (1933) have assumed that during the latency period children are less interested in intimacy than at other times. The lack of research on intimate interaction during this period may be due in part to the legacy of Freud's ideas. It is possible, of course, that information on children's needs, concerns, and stresses during the latency years may prove Freud correct. Until more research specifically addresses intimacy during this period, however, we cannot conclude definitively that school-age children are either interested or uninterested in intimacy.

Because research on intimate interaction and relationships in early and middle childhood is still in its infancy, this chapter takes a somewhat different tack than the others in Part II. It focuses on the same propositions as the previous and following ones but draws from the wider literature on children's relationships to generate hypotheses about children's intimacy.

EARLY CHILDHOOD (4–9 YEARS): LIFE-STAGE-RELATED DEVELOPMENTS IN INTIMATE RELATIONSHIPS

Relationships with Parents

By children's own reports, parents continue to be primary intimate partners in the early school years (Furman & Buhrmester, 1985). They are rated as the most important sources of companionship (Buhrmester & Furman, 1987) and support (Furman & Buhrmester, 1992) among children younger than 10 years of age.

Some studies have shown continuity in the parent-child relationship from infancy to the early childhood years. The longitudinal work of Main et al. (1985) indicates that the quality of interactions between 6-year-olds and their mothers can be predicted from assessments of attachment quality in infancy. In this study mother–child dyads classified as secure in infancy were, when the child was 6 years of age, fluent in their conversations with one another and able to discuss a broad range of topics. In contrast, dyads classified as avoidant in infancy spoke of impersonal matters, asked mainly yes/no questions of one another, and were unable to elaborate on conversation topics. In the same study children who were securely attached to their mothers at 12 months appeared to have freer access to their feelings and memories about family life at the age of 6 whereas 6-year-olds classified as avoidant with their mothers at 12 months had difficulty discussing their feelings about their family. This research indicates that significant individual differences exist in the kinds of interactions children have with their parents and in the feelings children may have about those interactions. The kinds of observational studies of intimate parent–child interaction commonly found in the literature on preschoolers' relationships are much harder to find in the research on young school-age children, however.

The frequent negotiations of parents and children regarding the enforcement of household rules may take on added significance in early childhood (R. S. Weiss, 1986). Parents' styles of negotiating and cooperating with their children around household rules may shape the development of children's own communication skills, not only within the parent–child relationship but with peers as well. These effects are discussed in more depth below.

Relationships with Friends

Children readily differentiate friends from acquaintances by the early elementary school years. Five-year-old children reserve very personal disclosures for friends but not for acquaintances (Rotenberg & Sliz, 1988). Children spend more of their discretionary time with friends (Hartup, 1989a) and describe friends as more supportive than casual acquaintances (Berndt & Perry, 1986), particularly toward the end of this period (i.e., in fourth grade). School-age friends, compared to nonfriends, smile and laugh with each other more, pay closer attention to equity rules, and direct their conversations toward mutual ends rather than toward each other as individuals (Newcomb & Brady, 1982). Little is known, however, about intimate interactions between school-age friends.

Gender-related patterns in children's friendships are quite distinct during the early school years. It is during this period that the commonly observed pattern of same-sex affiliation stabilizes and becomes nearly universal (Maccoby, 1990b). Even though boys and girls play quite separately, however, there are few sex differences in attitudes toward friendship or in the provisions of children's friendships. Both boys and girls see parents rather than friends as the major providers of intimacy (Buhrmester & Furman, 1987). Boys and girls rate their friendships as comparably supportive (Berndt & Perry, 1986), although girls do report liking their friends more than boys do (Berndt & Perry, 1986). There is little or no evidence of sex differences in friendship intimacy (Buhrmester & Furman, 1987).

There is limited evidence from observational studies of white, middle class friendship dyads that gender-distinct communication styles emerge as early as second grade (Tannen, 1990a). By age 7, girls sit closer to one another when they converse, meet one another's gaze more frequently, and seem more absorbed and entertained by talk than boys. Boys show mutual affection with mock insults and teasing while girls show support through agreeing with one another and augmenting one another's conversation. During early childhood, then, gender differences in communication styles may be emerging, but there are few differences in the benefits boys and girls report gaining from their friendships.

NEEDS, CONCERNS, STRESSES, AND INTIMATE RELATIONSHIPS DURING EARLY CHILDHOOD

Several life-stage-related needs, concerns, and stresses seem likely to affect and be affected by school-age children's intimate interactions and relationships. To be discussed here are (1) needs for fun and cooperation, (2) concerns with developing competencies and making social comparisons, and (3) concerns with gender-role conformity. Needs to have fun and cooperate with others may emerge from and propel children toward spending time with friends. This chapter proposes that children's increasing ability to enjoy interactions with age-mates may in part be a function of their own (and their peers') developing social competencies (e.g., for perspective taking and empathy) (Strayer & Eisenberg, 1987). Enjoyable interactions with peers may be the arena in which these competencies are first practiced. In turn, these skills are likely to provide a foundation for intimate relating later on.

Children's concerns with developing competencies, comparing themselves to their peers, and gender-role conformity are discussed together in this section because each concern seems likely to influence (and be influenced by) children's peer relationships in tandem with the other concerns. Each may emerge from children's voluntary confinement to same-sex friendships, and they may also result in children being less interested in intimacy than in conformity and making good impressions on others.

Fun and Cooperation

The Concern in Context

Elementary school children potentially have the most fun when they play cooperatively with other children. A concern with learning how to cooperate with others may emerge as a function of children's desires to have fun.[1]

During the early childhood years children show significant increases in prosocial behavior with their peers (i.e., behavior that is altruistic, cooperative, and/or collaborative) (Sroufe & Cooper, 1988). They also show increases in empathy and perspective-taking abilities. Empathy involves "feeling into" another's emotional experience (Strayer & Eisenberg, 1987). Perspective taking, which accompanies the development of affective empathy, is the cognitive ability to project oneself into another's viewpoint. Most 6-year-olds can comprehend that others may interpret situations differently than they do (Selman & Byrne, 1974).

Empathy and perspective-taking skills may thereby set the stage for children's developing capacities for collaboration and fair play. An ability to simultaneously hold in mind their own and another's point of view may augment children's capacity to "give a little and take a little" in their interactions with others. Ultimately, these skills are likely to contribute to an adult capacity for maintaining intimate relationships.

Relationships with Parents

Children's skills with cooperation and negotiation may be learned in part from their interactions with their parents (e.g., Cole, Baldwin, Baldwin, & Fisher, 1982). To the extent that parents are warm and collaborative—for example, by combining firm limits with respect for children's feelings and ideas—children seem more likely to learn negotiating skills (Maccoby & Martin, 1983). In contrast, when parents use power-assertive means of setting limits with their children, children often respond with noncompliance and resistance (Stafford & Bayer, 1993).

Parenting styles can affect children's relationships with their friends. A review by Cohn et al. (1991) indicates that when parents express less warmth to their children and behave more punitively, their children are more likely to be rejected by peers. Fathers' attentiveness, warmth, and companionship are especially potent predictors of peer acceptance (Patterson, Kupersmidt, & Vaden, 1990). Children's antisocial behavior may mediate the relationship between parents' punitive and neglectful behavior and children's peer relationships (Cohn et al., 1991).

Finally, evidence is accumulating that the quality of the attachment relationship between parents and infants is predictive of elementary school children's relationships with peers. Sroufe et al. (1990) found that an assessment of parent–child attachment quality in infancy is predictive of emotional health and peer competence in early childhood, despite intervening periods of poorer adjustment during the preschool years. Cohn (1990), using concurrent assessments of parent–child attachment and peer competence, found that insecurely attached first-grade boys are "less well-liked by peers. Further, peers perceived them as more aggressive and disruptive than their more secure counterparts" (Cohn et al., 1991, p. 322).

Individual differences in children's cooperative behavior should in turn exert an influence on relationships with parents and peers. When children practice their own persuasive skills with parents, for example, they may do so in the form of refusals to comply with parental requests (A. Eisenberg, 1992). A parent may behave more coercively when the child is less cooperative, even if the uncooperative behavior is serving some constructive end for the child, for example, helping the child understand why the parent is seeking his or her cooperation (Stafford & Bayer, 1993). There is little work on parent–child interaction, however, that explores the effect of a child's behavior on the parent.

Relationships with Friends

Children's preoccupation with having fun may encourage them to develop friendships and to master the skills of collaboration and fair play. As mentioned above, research findings indicate that young children view friends primarily as people with whom they share enjoyable activities (Berndt & Perry, 1986; Buhrmester & Furman, 1986; Furman & Buhrmester, 1985). Perhaps because the games they play with friends are more fun when everyone plays cooperatively, children make the effort to learn cooperation.

Young children's friendships can in turn promote gains in social skills necessary for cooperation and collaboration. Children provide one another with assistance (and insistence) to ensure that play is equitable, and therefore fun, for all involved. Children's desire to make and maintain friendships, then, may serve to activate their desire to learn how to cooperate, the friendship interactions themselves being the context in which new skills are acquired and practiced (Hartup, 1989a).

Developing Competencies and Social Comparisons

The Concern in Context

Concerns with developing competencies and making social comparisons may shape school-aged children's peer interactions. Erikson (1963) proposed that elementary school children are preoccupied with "industry vs. inferiority," that is, with acquiring and maintaining skills that are publicly observable and have real-world significance. When they are unable to excel in one way or another, children may become preoccupied with a sense of inferiority (Erikson, 1963).

Elementary school children's tendency to become preoccupied with how they measure up to their peers may be an outgrowth of their concern with developing competencies. Children in this age group use social comparisons as a basis for self-evaluations (Damon & Hart, 1982). On those competencies and skills that count in school and the peer group (e.g., school and athletic performance, leadership skills, accomplishments in extracurricular activities), the performance of peers becomes the standard against which children judge their own abilities and themselves (Harter, 1990).

Gender Role Conformity

The Concern in Context

Research suggests that school-age children are concerned with conforming to gender stereotypes (Thorne & Luria, 1986) and may actually distort or forget information that is inconsistent with those stereotypes (Liben & Signorella, 1993). Both developmental and contextual factors are likely contributors to their concern with gender stereotypes. Developmentally, the strengths and limitations of children's intellectual capacities may ensure that they will be concerned with gender role conformity. On the one hand, school-age children demonstrate an increased ability to apply various categories to themselves, including gender (Thompson, 1975). On the other hand, because children of this age do not think abstractly, gender role prescriptions can take on the character of physical laws or moral imperatives rather than conventional social rules (Bem, 1989). Further, young school-age children (ages 5–7) are just acquiring an understanding of gender constancy (Bem, 1989, 1993; Slabey & Frey, 1975).[2] Children may be concerned with following the "gender rules" because they fear they will cease being male or female if they neglect to do so.

Contextual factors probably contribute to children's concerns with gender conformity as well. Children are aware from an early age how important gender conformity is in their families and their peer groups (Bem, 1983; Thorne & Luria, 1986). Between the ages of 4 and 6, children's gendered behavior may be a product of concerted efforts to reconcile budding gender identities with cultural conceptions of gender (Kohlberg, 1966). School-age children must either conform to socially sanctioned gender roles or face negative social consequences among peers (Thorne & Luria, 1986).

Relationships with Peers

Concerns with establishing a sense of individual competence and industry, combined with concerns about gender role conformity, may together exert an influence on children's relationships with friends. In particular, these combined concerns may explain the emerging preference for play with same-sex peers (Bukowski, Gauze, Hoza, & Newcomb, 1993) and the consequent development of gender-distinct interaction styles (Tannen, 1990b).

Children are concerned with excelling in spelling, arithmetic, athletics, and artistic endeavors; perhaps they are also concerned with excellence in "doing gender." West and Zimmerman (1991) described performing the complex set of interpersonal behaviors that come to distinguish male and female social styles as "doing gender." Surely, children must learn the skills of their respective gendered social styles just as they must learn other skills. If this is so, children's increasingly gendered interpersonal behavior in the elementary school years might best be understood as the product of age-related efforts to achieve competence in culturally valued (and therefore peer-valued) tasks.

These concerns could also explain a lack of interest in intimacy with peers among children in this age group. Intimate interaction may not serve children's needs to conform, compete, and impress one another. As long as the latter set of needs is predominant, it is possible children will either be indifferent to or resist intimate interaction. This is because intimate interactions reveal that which is private, whereas concerns with social comparison and conformity seem squarely focused on presenting an impressive and/or acceptable public persona. More research is needed to determine whether young school-age children are uninterested in intimate peer interactions and whether concerns with conformity contribute to a lack of interest in intimate interaction.

MIDDLE CHILDHOOD AND PREADOLESCENCE (9–12 YEARS): LIFE-STAGE-RELATED PATTERNS IN INTIMATE RELATIONSHIPS

Relationships with Friends

There is disagreement in the literature about whether childhood friendships begin to show signs of adult-like intimacy during the middle childhood and preadolescent phases. It was Harry Stack Sullivan who first hypothesized that adult-like intimacy initially becomes possible between children and their friends at around age 10. Sullivan (1953) believed that children of this age could form "chum relationships" characterized by verbal self-disclosure. Research examining children's conceptions of friendship has tended to support Sullivan's view, suggesting that sixth graders are more likely than younger children to refer to intimacy, support, and empathy as important features of friendship (Bigelow & LaGaipa, 1975).

Research on children's descriptions of actual friendships, however, suggests that there is no clearly discernible increase in intimacy among friends of this age, especially for boys (Buhrmester & Prager, 1995).

The preadolescent years may be a transitional time in the development of intimacy between childhood friends. Although a few studies indicate that preadolescent (i.e., 11-year-old) children are more open, frank, and likely to discuss private concerns with their friends than are younger (8- or 9-year-old) children (DeRosier & Kupersmidt, 1991; Jones & Dembo, 1989), there is more evidence showing few changes from early to middle childhood (see review by Buhrmester & Prager, 1995). The most reliable increases in intimacy occur after puberty. When results do suggest change, it is nearly always girls rather than boys who show evidence of some increase in intimate interaction with friends (e.g., Buhrmester & Furman, 1987).

In contrast to the early childhood period, however, sex differences are discernible in the quality of preadolescents' friendships. Some studies show that girls are already beginning to spend more time talking with their friends than boys are, both on the phone (Crocket, Losoff, & Peterson, 1984) and face-to-face (Raffaelli & Duckett, 1989; Sharabany, Gershoni, & Hofman, 1981). Studies indicating sex differences at this age, however, coexist with those showing no differences (Berndt & Perry, 1986; DeRosier & Kupersmidt, 1991). When differences are found, they are often notably less dramatic than the sex differences of adolescence (Sharabany et al., 1981). It is possible that when sex differences are found at this age, they are due in part to the increasing significance of intimate conversation among girls, an increased significance that has not been found for boys (Buhrmester & Furman, 1987). In self-reports, girls may therefore emphasize intimate interactions more than boys do, although the frequency of such conversation may not vary significantly between boys and girls. Because of this mix of findings, preadolescence is best conceived of as a transitional period during which changes in depth of self-disclosure between friends occur for some children.

For both girls and boys negative gossip in conversations between friends is prevalent during this life stage (Parker & Gottman, 1989). There is evidence that middle childhood friends are more likely to devote time to talking about other children than are younger or older pairs of friends or than children and their parents (Gottman & Mettetal, 1986; Rafaelli & Duckett, 1989). Typically, such gossip identifies offensive behavior committed by a child known to all. When children tell one another about behavior they find offensive, they may be revealing their values and standards for proper conduct, for example, that one shouldn't "rat" on others, or that one must play fair at games (Buhrmester & Prager, 1995).

Relationships with Parents

There is evidence that parents continue to be children's most frequent conversation partners and that parents serve as important sources of companionship (Buhrmester & Furman, 1987). One study found that parents (particularly mothers) were chosen as "first comfort figures" by over half of a group of fifth graders (Marcoen & Brumagne, 1985). As is the case with young school-age children, however, little is known about the nature of intimate interaction between preadolescent children and their parents. Similarly, little is known about life-stage-related concerns and needs that might emerge from, or shape, intimacy between children and parents during this period.

NEEDS, CONCERNS, STRESSES, AND INTIMATE RELATIONSHIPS DURING MIDDLE CHILDHOOD AND PREADOLESCENCE

Life-stage-related needs, concerns, and stresses likely to affect and be affected by intimate interactions and relationships during middle childhood and preadolescence include (1) needs for approval from peers, (2) concerns with conformity to peer group standards, and (3) a concern with friendship. Once again, this review considers the impact of two life-stage-related concerns in tandem: needs for approval and concerns with conformity. The effect of these concerns on children's interactions with friends may be revealed in the prevalence of negative gossip. Negative gossip in turn may exacerbate children's needs for approval and conformity. Needs for approval and conformity may encourage socially desirable public behavior while discouraging intimate interaction. Perhaps in contrast to concerns with approval and conformity are preadolescent children's concerns with genuine friendship. Children's tendency to seek exclusiveness in friendship may reflect an increasing awareness of their own vulnerability to hurt and disappointment in close relationships.

Approval from Peers

The Concern in Context

Concerns with approval, in combination with concerns about peer group standards, may exert considerable influence on the nature of children's friendships during middle childhood. While children are known to seek approval from parents from very early in life, preadolescents' needs for approval may be focused as much on peer group as on parental acceptance (Berndt, 1979). The extended time periods that children spend with peers once they enter school may create a context in which approval from peers is bound to become a concern (Buhrmester & Prager, 1995). Spending more time with peers may also intensify another concern: enjoyable and entertaining social activity. The more acceptance and approval they gain from peers, the more likely children are to be included in exciting and pleasurable games and activities. There is also evidence that children who are not included may experience painful feelings of loneliness and depression (McGiboney, 1993), an indication of how important peer approval is at this age. Finally, children are aware that others have thoughts and feelings about them—and may even be talking about them! Gaining peer acceptance may be a way of reassuring oneself that others' thoughts and talk will be benign.

Conformity to Peer Group Standards

The Concern in Context

A concern with peer group norms may logically accompany a concern with being liked. Adherence to peer group norms may be the means by which peer approval and acceptance is gained (Brown & Gilligan, 1992). Perhaps because preadolescent children lack the cognitive sophistication (i.e., formal operations) required to understand that social norms are conventional and subject to interpretation, they follow these standards rigidly (Sroufe & Cooper, 1988). Further, because others in the peer group are also rigid adherents, it becomes important for children to be aware of and follow these rules if they want others to like them (Brown & Gilligan, 1992; Thorne & Luria, 1986). During middle childhood, then, children may be preoccupied with knowing and following peer group standards, even if they have participated in creating them.

Relationships with Peers

Children's concerns with approval and conformity likely affect and are affected by their relationships with their peers. The negative gossip about others commonly heard in conversations between friends of this age could easily emerge from and intensify children's concerns with social approval. Negative gossip may provide children with the opportunity to both set the norms that result in social approval and to become informed of the norms that concern their friends and other peers (Mettetal, 1983).

Sharing negative attitudes about others may also serve as an indirect source of approval for the children who participate: Implicit in the disparaging remarks about others is the unspoken premise that "present company" is excepted from the criticism (Buhrmester & Prager, 1995). "Present company" is actually getting advance warning about behavior that is sure to result in social disapproval.

Participation in negative gossip may also serve to intensify children's concerns about peer approval. Children can become witnesses to their peers' rejection of others based on violations of peer group social norms and at times may experience that rejection firsthand (i.e., may themselves become the objects of negative gossip). Participation in the disparagement of others, then, may have the effect of making children more vigilant about their own social behavior.

Children's strict adherence to peer group norms may represent their best effort to avoid disapproval. Continued acceptance by peers seems to require sticking to the rules of interaction as closely as possible. For example, adherence to peer group norms is observable in children's continued efforts to conform to sex-typed standards of behavior during middle childhood (Brown & Gilligan, 1992; Katz & Ksansnak, 1994). Within their sex-segregated social groups children's interactions with their friends appear to sustain and even intensify their efforts to conform (Brown & Gilligan, 1992; Maccoby, 1990b; Tannen, 1990b).

Differences in the way boys and girls conduct their friendships surely reflect in part children's efforts to conform to gender role standards. Negative gossip and sex-segregated play groups may each contribute to differences in female and male friendship styles, while at the same time reflecting children's efforts to conform. Through negative gossip children can impart to one another the rules for gendered behavior and the consequences of violating those rules. Through their sex-segrated play groups they practice gendered behavior and essentially guarantee that they will overlearn same-sex-typed interaction styles and underlearn opposite-sex-typed styles (Tannen, 1990b). It would be surprising if friendship patterns did not reflect this gendered behavior to some extent.

Relationships with Parents

A history of secure attachment to parents may ease preadolescent children's efforts to gain approval, acceptance, and enjoyment in relationships with age-mates. Elicker et al., (1992) observed the interaction of 10- and 11-year-old children who had been tested in Ainsworth's "strange situation" (Sroufe, 1983) at 12 and 18 months of age. They found that children who had been securely attached to their mothers as infants were rated as much more socially effective at preadolescence than were children who had been insecurely attached. Secure children were more involved and talkative with their peers during a 2–3 week summer camp program than were insecurely attached children, spent less time alone, and were less dependent on adults. Secure children were also more successful at conforming to peer group standards for gendered behavior (Eliker et al., 1992). They spent less time with opposite-sex children, sought them out less frequently, and, according to observer ratings, "follow[ed] explicit and implicit rules regarding gender boundary relations and behavior" (p. 97).

Friendship

The Concern in Context

During preadolescence children show an increased concern about friendship for its own sake (Bigelow & LaGaipa, 1975; Selman, 1980). Although, as mentioned previously, parents are still primary companions for children of this age, the amount of time children spend socializing with friends is increasing during this life stage (Rawlins, 1992).

Preadolescent children's emerging concern with friendship is perhaps nowhere more evident than in their emphasis on exclusiveness in friendships. Preadolescents are openly loath to share their friends with other peers, are jealous of the possibility that a friend may prefer someone else, and need to feel confident that their feelings of friendship are reciprocated (Rawlins, 1992). Perhaps this concern with exclusiveness emerges because children after age 10 seem more conscious of friendship as a relationship that persists over time. Children have, according to Rawlins (1992), "an emerging expectation of permanence and the simultaneous awareness that friendships are difficult to establish and preserve" (p. 34).

Because children explicitly value friendship and understand that it can persevere or not, they may become preoccupied with threats to its continuance. Girls in particular verbalize a desire for frequent contact with their friends and a desire to limit their friends' contact with others (Rawlins, 1992). Children's increased emotional involvement in their friendships may also contribute to their interest in exclusiveness. More emotional involvement means friends have more reward value (Gottman, 1983) and can cause emotional hurt. By protecting their friendships, then, children may be protecting their own vulnerability.

Children's increasing ability to enjoy and appreciate close friendship may stem from their more advanced understanding of the psychological aspects of self and others (Selman, 1980). Preadolescents' notions of self include traits and abilities and rely less on the physical attributes that made up the self-concept in earlier years. Simultaneously, they are beginning to understand that others have an internal world that affects their perspective. By age 10, children not only comprehend that others have a different perspective from theirs but also understand that different motives, goals, and feelings about situations prompt these different perspectives (Selman & Byrne, 1974).

Relationships with Parents

Individual differences in the quality of the parent–child relationship in preadolescence may account for differences in children's levels of interpersonal understanding. These differences in understanding may in turn predict children's ability to make friends during middle childhood and preadolescence. The longitudinal study by Elicker et al. (1992) indicates that deficits in social skills shown by children with anxious attachment histories are accompanied by a tendency for these children to make fewer friends at summer camp than other children. Pair nominations showed that 76% of children with secure histories, but only 50% of children with anxious histories, had made at least one friend during 4 weeks of summer camp. Independent observations suggested that children with secure histories spent more time in free play with their friends than did children with insecure histories. Similar results were reported by Grossmann and Grossmann (1991).

Parent–child interactions other than attachment may also predict the quality of children's peer relationships in middle childhood. Dishion (1990) sampled 9- and 10-year-old children and their parents to learn whether parenting practices predicted the development of antisocial behavior and peer rejection. Results indicated that parents who upon observation "displayed inconsistent, negative and punitive behaviors were more likely to have sons who engaged in antisocial behaviors . . . [and who were] actively disliked and rejected by peers" (Cohn et al., 1991, p. 330).

SUMMARY AND CONCLUSIONS

The present chapter attempts to draw conclusions about school-age children's intimate interactions and relationships in the absence of a significant body of empirical work in the area. In response to this challenge, it reviews literature on changes (and stability) in peer and parent–child relationships that have implications for understanding intimacy. Also reviewed is literature on those life-stage-related needs, concerns, and stresses faced by school-age children that might affect or be affected by intimate interactions and relationships during this period.

Research indicates that friendships become increasingly important when children reach school age. Change is evident in the clear distinctions children now make between peers who are friends and those who are merely acquaintances (Berndt & Perry, 1986). Preferences for same-sex friends and companions are overwhelmingly evident in early childhood (Maccoby, 1990a). Tannen (1990a) observed distinct gender-related styles of interaction as early as second grade.

While some sophisticated children, particularly girls, may engage in intimate self-disclosing conversation for its own sake during preadolescence (Buhrmester & Furman, 1987), most evidence indicates that there are few dramatic changes from early to middle childhood (Buhrmester & Prager, 1995). That girls spend more time just talking to their friends than boys do has been documented (Raffaelli & Duckett, 1989).

Preadolescence may provide children with psychological preparation for the substantial increases in friendship intimacy they are likely to experience during adolescence and young adulthood. On the one hand, preadolescents are newly vulnerable in their friendships; they prize friendship highly and are prone to feelings of jealousy and possessiveness in relation to their friends. On the other hand, preadolescents' vulnerability is protected because the level of intimacy in their friendships is limited. If they had to cope simultaneously with the combined effects of increased significance and increased intimacy in their friendships, they might become overwhelmed. To the extent that intimacy is limited during a time when friendships are rapidly increasing in importance, children may avoid coping simultaneously with two sources of increased vulnerability.

Middle childhood friends are more likely to engage in negative gossip about other peers than are younger children (Parker & Gottman, 1989). Buhrmester and Prager (1995) suggested that negative gossip gives children the opportunity to discuss and explore the standards for proper behavior in the peer group. Should more research be devoted to children's life-stage-related needs and concerns, the psychological and social functions of gossip during middle childhood may become more apparent.

There is a notable absence of research on parent–child intimacy during the elementary school years. Available evidence suggests that parent–child relationships demonstrate stability through these years (e.g., Main et al., 1985) and that parents are children's most intimate partners (Buhrmester & Furman, 1987; Marcoen & Brumagne, 1985). Research aimed at increasing understanding of intimacy in these relationships seems warranted. Perhaps children who are able to be intimate with parents during middle childhood will find it easier to establish intimate relationships with peers in adolescence. A growing body of evidence indicates that parent–child relationships are critically important arenas in which children learn social behavior (e.g., Parke & Ladd, 1992). It seems likely that parents serve as models and teach children about enjoying and competently handling intimate interactions.

Chapter 3 hypothesized links between children's adaptations to life-stage-related needs and concerns and the kinds of interactions and relationships they have with parents and peers. That account has been used here to generate a number of specific hypotheses about intimacy and individual development. It seems reasonable to propose, for example, that as children's interest in having fun expands to include shared play, they will seek one another out more as playmates (Maccoby & Martin, 1983). One might predict, therefore, that the more interested children are in having fun, the more time they would spend will friends. Perhaps the more children play together, the more aware they are that cooperation enhances joint play and the more likely they are to be concerned with learning how to cooperate effectively (e.g., Hartup, 1989a). In turn, children who are more concerned with cooperation may have more opportunities to participate in joint play because other children enjoy their company more. Thus, children's concerns with having fun and cooperation could encourage them to adapt by learning more effective cooperation skills, which in turn should enhance their concurrent and future opportunities for enjoyable friendships. More opportunities for friendship should mean more opportunities to engage in intimate interaction, as Chapter 6 will indicate.

Some of elementary school children's life-stage-related concerns, and the contexts that spawn them, may actually discourage them from pursuing intimate interactions and relationships with peers. Children who are primarily concerned with acceptance and conformity, for example, may reasonably believe that the risks of sharing personal material with a friend are too high. Such disclosures increase the risk of rejection by the friend, who is also concerned with conformity, and by others if the friend "spills the beans." These concerns may also lead children to cherish the friendships they have, however, because of the relief intimate friendships offer from pressures to conform (see Chapter 6). Further, they may prompt children to look more to parents as confidants. Interactions with parents, and perhaps siblings, may provide the lion's share of school-age children's intimate contact. More empirical work is needed to evaluate these hypotheses.

Additional advances in our understanding of the links between children's development and personal relationships may come when we assess children's needs, concerns, and preoccupations more directly. With older children and adults, self-reported concerns and needs can be assessed separately from behavior in interactions, allowing for direct tests to be made of the relationship between conscious preoccupations and intimate interactions. For example, individual differences may exist among children's concerns with gender role conformity (Eagly & Wood, 1991), with some children being more resistant to conformity than others. If concern with gender role conformity is in fact shaping children's relationships with peers, then children who are more concerned with conformity should be most loath to play with members of the opposite sex and to stray from the behavior associated with their own gender.

The challenge for intimacy researchers may be to identify behaviors throughout childhood that serve as age-appropriate indicators of intimate interaction and experience. Little is known about age-related patterns in how frequently or easily children talk to parents about things that bother them, for example. Similarly, scholars know little about the normal range of affectionate physical contact between parents and children and what, if any, implications there are for different amounts and types of parent–child affection at different life stages. Without knowledge of normal age-related changes, it is difficult to generate meaningful hypotheses about variations from normal patterns and any long-term implications these variations might have for children's later adaptations.

Intimacy in Adolescence
and Young Adulthood

To Carthage I came [in my youth], where there sang all
around me . . . a cauldron of unholy loves. I loved not yet, yet
I loved to love, and out of a deep-seated want . . . I sought
what I might love.

—St. Augustine, *Confessions*

Adolescence and young adulthood bring dramatic increases in capacities
and opportunities for intimate relating in Western culture. These increased capacities and opportunities are closely linked to developmental
changes in concerns, needs, and stresses. Perhaps it is not surprising that
most intimacy research has addressed these life stages.

First, the cognitive advances of adolescence allow perceptions of understanding, identified in Chapter 1 as critical intimate experiences, to
be abstractly symbolized in the course of intimate interaction. Adolescents, more than younger children, can reflect on and verbalize their experiences with intimacy. Because of their advanced cognitive skills, adolescents can engage in a new type of verbal intimacy. Extensive
self-disclosure between friends is first widely observed in adolescence.
Perhaps underlining the significance of the cognitive achievements of
adolescence, conceptions of what intimacy is and what one seeks in an
intimate friend remain remarkably stable from adolescence through the
adult years (Lowenthal, Thurnher, & Chiriboga, 1977).

Second, sexual maturity ushers in new possibilities for intimacy. Most (if not all) Americans have their first experiences of sexual intimacy (if not sexual intercourse) during adolescence (Janus & Janus, 1993). Sexual interactions are not automatically intimate interactions, however; they are only intimate if the participants experience intimacy while engaging in sexual behavior. In other words, sexual behavior is intimate if it generates positive emotions about self and partner and results in partners feeling understood. Coerced sex, for example, is never intimate.

Finally, peers, instead of parents, become preferred intimate partners. Adolescence is the first time that peer relationships consistently appear to be as intimate as parent–child relationships. By the end of adolescence (or early in the young adult years) peer relationships supersede parent–child relationships in their level of relational intimacy.

This chapter addresses the next two stages of the life span: adolescence (12–19 years) and young adulthood (19–35). It explores the three propositions introduced in Chapter 3 with regard to these life stages:

1. Intimate interactions and relationships may enhance (or obstruct) individual efforts to adapt to life-stage-related needs and stresses;
2. Adaptations to life-stage-related needs and stresses shape intimate interactions and relationships through their impact on people's behavior within them.
3. Expectations and adaptations from earlier life stages can affect behavior, and therefore relationships, in later stages.

This chapter, like the previous ones, organizes the literature and illuminates areas where further research is needed. The organization in this and the following chapter parallels that used in the chapters on children's intimacy. I begin my discussion of each stage with a review of research on life-stage-related changes in intimate relationships. Next, for each life stage, I propose possible linkages between the needs, concerns, and stresses associated with that life stage and developmental changes in intimate relationships. Each section discusses how concerns and needs affect people's choice of intimate partners and the kinds of interactions they have with those partners. Potential influences of intimate relationships on how individuals adapt to and resolve their concerns and preoccupations are also explored. Finally, possible effects of earlier adaptations are considered.

ADOLESCENCE (12–19 YEARS): LIFE-STAGE-RELATED DEVELOPMENTS IN INTIMATE RELATIONSHIPS

Friendships

While research results on preadolescents are equivocal regarding age-related changes in friendship intimacy, available evidence indicates that there are significant increases in the prevalence and depth of adolescent intimate friendships (Savin-Williams & Berndt, 1990). Adolescents explicitly value opportunities to share their thoughts and feelings with their friends (Buhrmester, 1990; Townsend, McCracken, & Wilton, 1981), and consider this a top priority in choosing a friend (Berndt, 1982; Kon, Losenkov, de Lissovoy, & de Lissovoy, 1978). Increases in frequency and personalness of self-disclosure to same-sex friends have been documented from the preadolescent to adolescent period for girls (Buhrmester, 1990) and from the early to midadolescent period for boys (Sharabany et al., 1981). The intimate exchanges of adolescent friends result in better knowledge of friends' personalities and preferences (Diaz & Berndt, 1982). While children of younger ages sporadically describe their friendships as intimate, adolescents (particularly girls) do so with much greater consistency. Intimate friendship, then, becomes much more common in adolescence.

Differences between girls' and boys' friendships become more pronounced during the teen years (Buhrmester & Prager, 1995). Girls' friendships become intimate earlier in development (e.g., Blyth & Traeger, 1988), achieve greater amounts of intimacy (e.g., Diaz & Berndt, 1982; Tannen, 1990a), and remain more intimate throughout adolescence (e.g., Smollar & Youniss, 1982). Girls are more likely than boys to rate their same-sex best friends as the ones in whom they confide most frequently. Boys may confide as often to parents, particularly mothers, as to friends (Richardson, Galambos, & Petersen, 1984).

Romantic Relationships

While increases in intimacy between same-sex friends begin early in adolescence, there are also increases in intimacy between opposite-sex peers that begin a bit later (Buhrmester, 1990; Sharabany et al., 1981). The few studies that address opposite-sex relationships during adolescence focus on verbal intimacy, and indicate a rapid and pervasive increase that begins earlier for girls (Buhrmester & Prager, 1995). Research on opposite-sex verbal intimacy does not reveal gender differences as consistently as does research on intimacy between same-sex friends. When boys and girls get together, they sometimes seem to split the difference, disclosing at moderate levels of intimacy (Buhrmester & Carbery, 1992; Papini, Farmer, Clark, & Snell, 1988). When sex differences are found, however, they nearly always show females disclosing more within these relationships (Furman & Buhrmester, 1992; Sharabany et al., 1981).

Little is known about adolescent experiences of sexual intimacy. It is nevertheless well documented that most American adolescents are sexually active by the age of 19. Further, a larger percentage of adolescents are having their first (consensual) sexual experience by age 17 (Janus & Janus, 1993); this is particularly true of gay male youths (Savin-Williams, 1995). First heterosexual experiences most often occur within intimate, committed dating relationships (Christopher & Roosa, 1991). Couples who are satisfied with their dating relationship are more likely to become sexually active. Girls who have frequent sexual intercourse with their boyfriends, however, may feel more powerless in those relationships than do girls who are less active (Jorgensen, King, & Torrey, 1980). Many factors affect teens' decisions to be sexually active, but the quality of the dating relationship appears to be the single most influential factor (Christopher & Roosa, 1991). Despite the possibly important role played by relationship factors in teen sexual decision making, little is known about the relationship between sexual intimacy and other aspects of intimacy in adolescent dating relationships. In fact, we need more information about intimacy of all types in teenagers' dating relationships.

Parent–Adolescent Relationships

There is little or no evidence of an increase in intimacy with parents during adolescence; some studies suggest that self-disclosure to parents decreases during the adolescent period (Hunter & Youniss, 1982). On the one hand, feelings of warmth between adolescents and their parents (particularly mothers) remain high (Youniss & Ketterlinus, 1987), although these feelings coexist with explicit adolescent concerns about "getting away" (White et al., 1983). The bulk of available evidence suggests that parent–adolescent relationships remain important attachment relationships for teens (e.g., Greenberg, Siegel, & Leitch, 1983), and parents are important consultants regarding certain kinds of adolescent decisions, such as whether and where to go to college (Wilks, 1986). On the other hand, there is evidence that adolescents keep secrets from their parents (Spencer, 1994). Parents, therefore, are no longer primary confidants.

Sex differences pervade the findings on adolescent relationships with their parents. On the basis of their review of the literature on parent–child self-disclosure, Buhrmester and Prager (1995) concluded that daughters self-disclose to their mothers more than sons do, while sons disclose more to fathers than do daughters. Both sons and daughters, however, disclose more to their mothers than to their fathers. The general picture that emerges is one of considerable intimacy between mothers and daughters, of moderate levels of intimacy between sons and both their parents, and of distance in father–daughter relationships.

NEEDS, STRESSES, AND INTIMATE RELATIONSHIPS DURING ADOLESCENCE

This section suggests that adolescents' intimate interactions and relationships are shaped by the following needs, concerns, and stresses: (1) the dramatic bodily (and cognitive) changes that accompany puberty, (2) needs for approval and acceptance, (3) concerns with gender role conformity, (4) needs for individuation, (5) needs for autonomy, and (6) an increasing interest in intimacy. In turn, adolescents' intimate interactions and relationships with others should affect their adaptations to these needs and stresses. This long list of concerns reflects the many changes developmental theorists and researchers attribute to adolescence. It also reflects the many areas of developmental change that likely affect and are affected by intimate interactions and relationships.

While adolescents, like their younger peers, address their life-stage-related concerns with parents and with friends they also have romantic relationships. It seems indisputable that adolescents' changing bodies, needs for acceptance, concerns with gender role conformity, and increasing concerns with intimacy would have a profound effect on their interest in and capacity to form romantic relationships. Further, it seems likely that adolescent experiences in romantic relationships could shape the expectations and adaptations they carry with them into young adulthood. Despite their likely importance, however, work on adolescent romantic relationships is still in its infancy.

Bodily Changes

The Concern in Context

Perhaps the first preoccupation of adolescence is the one that marks the beginning of this developmental period: the emotional and bodily changes of puberty. Pubertal changes occur rapidly and carry with them preoccupations with bodily appearance and physical attractiveness, with sexual feelings and impulses, and with concerns about future reproductive roles (Adams & Gullota, 1989; A. C. Peterson, 1983). An additional pre-occupation of adolescents—romance and sexuality—is undoubtedly an outgrowth of pubertal maturity.

There is evidence that the onset of puberty is a more stressful preoccupation for girls than for boys (Ruble & Brooks-Gunn, 1982). For example, the cultural valorization of thinness prompts American girls to become disproportionately dissatisfied with their body weight as they mature physically (Crockett & Peterson, 1987; Dornbusch et al., 1984; Striegel-Moore, Silberstein, & Rodin, 1986). In addition, menarche may arouse ambivalence by signifying the onset of maturity while carrying the weight of negative social attitudes toward menstruation (Brooks-Gunn & Ruble, 1983; Ernster, 1975). Finally, girls may anticipate the joys and pains of childbearing and/or childrearing with ambivalence. Perhaps they are aware of the conflicts that societal gender and work roles create between mothering and individual achievement (Bardwick & Douvan, 1971).

Puberty may also be more stressful for gay and lesbian youth (C. Patterson, 1995). Like their heterosexual counterparts, gay and lesbian youth must learn to accommodate to sexual feelings of increasing salience and intensity. Same-sex attractions, however, can alter teens' expected course of identity development. Further, it puts them at risk for denigration, harassment, and violent assault from peers (Hershberger & D'Augelli, 1995).

Relationships with Friends

The onset of puberty may facilitate increases in intimate interaction between friends. From an adolescent's perspective puberty may be a stressful process. Because their peers are going through the same changes, teens may seek each other out and confide in one another about what they are experiencing, or waiting to experience (Buhrmester & Prager, 1995).

That puberty occurs earlier for girls than boys, and is more stressful for girls, may contribute to the earlier growth of intimacy in girls' friendships. Intimate interactions can provide adolescents with support, encouragement, and advice when they face difficulties (Derlega & Grzelak, 1979). To the extent that pubertal changes create more stress for girls, they may be more motivated than boys to seek support and nurturance in intimate interactions with same-sex friends. Female friends may make the ideal targets for confidences. For one, discussing menstruation with a male is generally considered taboo (Brooks-Gunn & Ruble, 1983). Secondly, friends who are going through similar changes can help each other feel less alone in their concerns (Buhrmester & Prager, 1995). Finally, it is common for mothers and daughters to experience conflict around the time of daughters' puberty (Hill & Holmbeck, 1986; Paikoff & Brooks-Gunn, 1991; Steinberg, 1988), further arguing for girlfriends as the ideal confidantes for girls' concerns about their changing bodies.

Because gay youth are unlikely to find commiseration with peers, they may wait several years before confiding in anyone about their same-sex attractions (Savin-Williams, 1995). A homophobic social context, particularly evident among adolescents (Hershberger & D'Augelli, 1995), may result in a lack of intimacy between gay youth and their same-sex friends.

Relationships with Parents

Children's pubertal changes may elicit changes in parent–child relationships as well. The increasingly adult-like appearance of post pubertal adolescents may prompt parents to think of their adolescent children as older and more responsible. Parents may expect more of their children and make more demands (Douvan & Adelson, 1966). Similarly, some parents may come to tolerate more independent thinking and disagreement from an adolescent than from a younger offspring. By altering parents' perceptions of the adolescent, puberty may initiate a new level of egalitarianism in adolescents' relationships with their parents.

Approval and Acceptance

The Concern in Context

Concerns with approval and acceptance within the peer group may continue into adolescence for both boys and girls, particularly during the early years. Young adolescents become concerned with self-presentation, that is with the image of themselves they convey to their peers (Buhrmester, Goldfarb, & Cantrell, 1992; Parker & Gottman, 1989). Advances in cognitive functioning that occur during adolescence contribute to adolescents' concerns with their self-images. Adolescents' matured perspective-taking ability allows them to view themselves from the perspective of a "generalized other" (Selman, 1981), a development that sets the stage for intense concerns that others are evaluating their every word and action (Harter, 1990). As noted by Buhrmester and Prager (1995), the immediate context of the peer group creates these concerns in part, because many conversations among peers are in fact devoted to scrutinizing and evaluating other peers (Gottman & Mettetal, 1986; Rafaelli & Duckett, 1989). Pressures to conform to peer group standards continue during early adolescence, and teenagers may be painfully aware that this conformity is necessary if they want to have status and acceptance among their peers.

Relationships with Friends

As same-sex friends become intimate, their relationship may become a haven from concerns with self-image within the broader peer group (Buhrmester & Prager, 1995). Teenagers are less likely to "act phony" with their intimate friends than with anyone else (Harter & Lee, 1989). By teens' own reports, friends are people who are trustworthy, who can keep secrets, and who will not talk behind one's back (Rawlins & Holl, 1987). With friends, teens have more freedom to violate peer group standards without risking humiliation and rejection than they would with more casual acquaintances (Rawlins & Holl, 1987).

Gender Role Conformity

The Concern in Context

There is evidence that most adolescents are concerned with maintaining the gender-related behaviors that will gain them acceptance and status in their peer group. During early adolescence there is an observable increase in boys' and girls' gender-role-conforming behavior (Douvan & Adelson, 1966; Hill & Lynch, 1983). Further, peers are actively rejecting and punishing of others who do not conform to gender role standards. Adolescent boys may engage in brutal teasing of their nonconforming peers, which can escalate to violent assault (Buhrmester & Prager, 1995; Thorne & Luria, 1986). Girls will exclude and isolate those who do not conform to the "nice and kind" feminine stereotype (Brown & Gilligan, 1992).

Later in adolescence, however, the flexibility of teens' gender-related conceptions increases. Katz and Ksansnak (1994) found that flexibility of self-perceptions and tolerance of nonconforming behavior in agemates increases from early to late adolescence, especially for girls. By the college years teens can be more selective about which aspects of those stereotypes they incorporate for themselves and require of others (Thorbecke & Grotevant, 1982). Little work has been done thus far, however, documenting changes in intimate relationships that might be sequelae to increasingly flexible gender role conceptions.

Relationships with Romantic Partners

There is reason to believe participation in heterosexual romantic relationships is more stressful for girls than for boys because of gender-related pressures on girls (Hill & Lynch, 1983). Although adolescent girls may generally have lower self-esteem than boys (Tobin-Richards, Boxer, & Peterson, 1983; Unger & Crawford, 1992), girls who date earlier appear to be particularly vulnerable to problems with self-image. Girls have traditionally been consigned to a passive role in adolescent courtship, which may contribute to feelings of powerlessness and a lack of control over their fate. Further, girls continue to cope with a double standard of behavior, which imposes stricter and narrower standards on girls' behavior than on boys'. The repercussions for violating these norms for girls may include peer rejection, which itself is associated with lower self-esteem and poor adjustment during adolescence (Unger & Crawford, 1992).

Relationships with Friends

The lower levels of intimacy in boys' relationships with one another may stem from gender role norms. Acute concerns with self-image and gender role conformity (Hill & Holmbeck, 1986) may exert a more inhibiting effect on boys' intimate relationships than on girls'. Intimate conversation may violate the norms of male-to-male interaction while integrating more easily into female-to-female interaction. Males' interactions with friends have been characterized as status oriented, and frequently punctuated with interruptions, contradictions, boasting, and other forms of self-display (Maccoby, 1990a). Females' interactions, in contrast, are enabling and more often consist of agreement, encouragement to speak, and elaborations on one another's points (Maccoby, 1990a; Tannen, 1990b). The risks of sharing personal and private feelings may be higher for boys because disclosure requires that boys violate well-established communication norms (Buhrmester & Prager, 1995).

Stereotypic gender roles may affect boys' intimate relationships more than girls', but the difference may be more of degree than kind (Duck & Wright, 1993). Brown and Gilligan (1992) noted recently that the "nice and kind" requirement of feminine sex-typed behavior inhibits certain kinds of communication. Girls may be ostracized for acknowledging their strengths, for expressing self-confidence, or for displaying intelligence, since these acts may seem competitive and therefore inconsistent with the promotion of group harmony. Additional research is needed to learn how much intimate friendships are affected by these norms.

Relationships with Parents

Gender role norms are also likely to explain differences in intimacy between sons and daughters and mothers and fathers. First, gender roles in the family dictate that mothers will be the primary caretakers of children. Children's lifelong closeness with their mothers, relative to their fathers, should logically persist in adolescence (Buhrmester & Prager, 1995).[1] Second, mothers have most likely acquired the same gender-typed, enabling interaction style as their daughters have. They may therefore encourage more confiding from their adolescent children than fathers. Fathers' male socialization may result in a "constricting" interaction style that is unlikely to facilitate children's self-disclosures (Maccoby, 1990a). Third, fathers' "breadwinner" role usually takes them away from home, making them physically less available to form close relationships with their children.

Daughters in particular seem to lack opportunities to build close relationships with their fathers (Wright & Keple, 1981; Youniss & Smollar, 1985). Daughters are less likely to share masculine-sex-typed interests with their fathers than sons are and may have interaction styles (enabling vs. status-oriented) that are incompatible with each other (Buhrmester & Prager, 1995). Fathers may take an especially authoritarian and controlling role with their daughters during adolescence (Youniss & Smollar, 1985), creating more distance.

Individuation

The Concern in Context

As young adolescents get older, concerns with self-presentation and image may start to compete with needs to define the real self (individuation) and behave authentically (Harter, 1990). The achievement of formal operations allows adolescents to begin the process of resolving discrepancies between multiple possible selves. During late adolescence concerns with defining the self expand with teens' increasing awareness of and concern with impending adulthood. Now they must consider decisions about their occupational goals, religious and political beliefs, and standards for interpersonal behavior (Marcia, 1966; Schenkel & Marcia, 1972). Erikson (1968) viewed this period of preoccupation with defining a provisional adult self as an "identity moratorium" during which youth are actively preoccupied with questions regarding who they are and will become.

Relationships with Friends

Intimate interactions between friends may increase in adolescence because they provide teens with opportunities for self-clarification. Intimate interactions with friends can provide a forum for coconstructive dialogues (Youniss, 1980). Within these dialogues teens can participate together in exploring and constructing selves. The egalitarian authority structure of friendship (in contrast to the unilateral structure of adolescent-adult relationships) lends itself to such dialogues and relieves the pressure adolescents might feel to succumb to the views of adult authority (Youniss, 1980).

Relationships with Parents

Adolescents are more likely to engage in verbally intimate interactions with their parents if their parents support their efforts to individuate. In an observational study of parent–adolescent interactions, Spencer (1994) found that adolescent self-disclosure increased when parents acknowledged the teen's point of view and did not try to control his or her thinking. When parents "were willing to set aside their own prejudgments long enough to listen to the adolescent's explanations and attributions . . . [they] were most likely to elicit frequent and intimate self-disclosures from their adolescents" (Spencer, 1994, p. 84).

Autonomy

The Concern in Context

Related to their concerns about becoming adults are teenagers' preoccupations with self-reliance and independence from parents (Blos, 1967). Teens' changing physical appearance and their increasing capacities to make their own decisions and monitor their own behavior increase their awareness that they will soon need to be more independent (Douvan & Adelson, 1966). Teenagers are concerned with autonomy, or the freedom to regulate their own activities, and self-reliance, or the freedom to make their own decisions about matters that affect them (Hill & Holmbeck, 1986). Undoubtedly, the American cultural context, with its emphasis on agency and individualism (Ambert, 1992; Cooper & Cooper, 1992; Guisinger & Blatt, 1994), intensifies teenagers' desires to be independent.

Relationships with Parents

A preoccupation with autonomy and self-reliance may affect intimacy in adolescents' relationships with their parents (White, Speisman, & Costos, 1983). If adolescents decrease their self-disclosure to their parents, it may be to create arenas of privacy within which they are protected from unwanted parental supervision (Derlega & Chaikin, 1977; Hill & Holmbeck, 1986). Teenagers also engage in self-presentational efforts with parents (Harter & Lee, 1989), perhaps withholding confidences about forbidden behavior (e.g., alcohol use, sexual activity) to avoid parental reprimands and constraints (Buhrmester & Prager, 1995). Adolescents may create some distance in their relationships with their parents, then, in the interest of fostering their own independence (Douvan & Adelson, 1966).

Recent evidence does not support an earlier notion, however, that disengagement from parents is a necessary or desirable step toward meeting teenagers' needs for autonomy or individuation (Cooper, Baker, Polichar, & Welsh, 1993; Cooper & Cooper, 1992; Grotevant & Cooper, 1986). Adolescents whose interactions with their parents balance warmth on the one hand with free expression of differences on the other, are most likely to be engaged in identity exploration (Campbell, Adams & Dobson, 1984; Cooper, in press; Grotevant & Cooper, 1986). According to Cooper and Grotevant (1987), self-exploring adolescents, more than their nonexploring peers, express to their parents the ways in which they view the world differently from their parents while simultaneously expressing openness to their parents' ideas. Remaining close to and maintaining open communication with parents, then, may encourage developing individuation in adolescents.

Intimacy

The Concern in Context

Intimacy itself becomes a preoccupation during the adolescent years. The development of formal operational thinking in adolescence may allow teens to understand and articulate how valuable intimate friendship is to them. Further, adolescents are sexually mature and therefore prone to falling in love, which arouses yearnings for closeness and intimate contact.

Relationships with Friends and Romantic Partners

Adolescents' friendships may increase in intimacy for all of the reasons presented thus far in this section. An additional reason, however, may be that teens value intimacy increasingly as an end in itself. Adolescents' formal reasoning abilities should contribute to their skillfulness, and therefore their appeal, as intimate partners. Adolescent friends can not only provide a sympathetic ear but can consider, for one another's benefit, complex sets of alternative constructions to use when solving problems (Parker & Gottman, 1989; Tannen, 1990a). They can apply their abstract reasoning abilities to understanding emotions and emotional life (Selman, 1980).

Relationships with Parents

Adolescents' adaptations to relationships with parents may influence to some extent whether their efforts to form intimate relationships with peers are successful. Several cross-sectional studies suggest that there are linkages between parent–adolescent relationships and adolescent peer relationships. Girls who describe their relationships with their parents as intimate have more satisfying and more intimate relationships with their best girlfriends (Sharabany & Wiseman, 1993; Walker & Thompson, 1983). Cooper and Cooper (1992) reviewed research suggesting that children learn negotiation skills in interactions with parents and then apply those skills in interactions with friends. They noted, for example, that teenagers whose parents do not listen to them or who cut off their ideas are most likely to behave the same way with their friends.

A recent study by Venberg, Beery, Ewell, and Abwender (1993) suggests that parents can have a direct influence on adolescents' ability to make friends. These researchers found that adolescents whose parents took an active role in assisting them to make friends following a change in the family's residence later have more intimate friendships.

YOUNG ADULTHOOD (19–35 YEARS): LIFE-STAGE-RELATED PATTERNS IN INTIMATE RELATIONSHIPS

Friendships

Friends continue to be important intimate partners as adolescents become young adults. During the early years of the young adult phase, friends are likely to maintain high levels of contact with one another and to have relationships of considerable intimacy (Rawlins, 1992). Self-disclosure continues to be important in building intimacy between friends (Helgeson et al., 1987). College students who have more frequent intimate interactions with their friends report higher levels of well-being (Reis et al., 1985). Close friends are college students' first choice of confidant; the presence of a romantic partner often does not alter this primacy (Prager et al., 1989). Just as in adolescence, then, close friends have their most intimate relationships with one another and are the primary source of relational intimacy and companionship during the early years of young adulthood.

The transitions to marriage and parenthood bring change to young adult friendships (Rawlins, 1992). Friends have less contact after marriage (Milardo, Johnson, & Huston, 1983). Friendships that might threaten the couple's stability may be dropped, and contact with others diminishes (Rubin, 1985; Tschann, 1988). There may be decreases in friendship intimacy besides decreases in contact (Booth & Hess, 1974; Tschann, 1988). Spouses meet most young adults' needs for intimacy (Carbery, 1993), and the demands of new parenthood usurp time that was once available for friends (Oliker, 1989; Rawlins, 1992; Shulman, 1975).

Despite the obstacles that a couple- and family-oriented society throws in the way, friendships show considerable resilience and continued importance through the transitions of young adulthood, particularly for women (Lowenthal et al., 1977; Stein, Bush, Ross, & Ward, 1992; Tschann, 1988). Married women report that they disclose as much or more to close friends as to their husbands (Oliker, 1989; L. Rubin, 1983). Women's friends serve as important sources of support as women help one another cope with the stresses of the transitions to marriage and parenthood (Oliker, 1989; Rawlins, 1992).

Young Adults and Their Parents

While the overall intimacy in young adults' relationships with their parents remains low relative to the intimacy in their friendships, there are life-stage-related fluctuations in intimacy between parents and young adults (Frank, Avery, & Laman, 1988; Franz & White, 1985). There is, unfortunately, only a handful of studies documenting the nature of these changes.

Young adults' relationships with their parents seem to change because of transitions in young adults' lives. When young adults are anticipating their first move away from home, they may increase their aggressiveness and distancing toward their parents, perhaps to ease the separation (Kurash & Schaul, 1980)—it's easier to go away mad. Later, they may experience a kind of rapprochement, with a subsequent increase in visits home, exchanges of letters, and long-distance telephone calls (Kurash & Schaul, 1980; R. S. Weiss, 1986). The transitions to marriage and to parenthood may also have an impact on young adults' relationships with their parents. The most consistent finding is that daughters (but not sons) develop closer relationships with their mothers following these transitions (L. Fischer, 1981; Frank et al., 1988; White et al., 1983). A simultaneous increase in conflict and hostile feelings on the part of daughters has also been documented (L. Fischer, 1981). Moreover, both sons and daughters have reported increased feelings of estrangement from fathers following each transition (Frank et al., 1988; Lowenthal et al., 1977). A more recent study, however, found that contact between sons and fathers is higher when the son is also a father and that sons rely on fathers for advice and support with their parenting efforts (Carbery, 1993). Firm conclusions regarding normative changes in young adults' relationships with their parents await further research.

Romantic Relationships

At some point during the young adult period most people living in a Western cultural environment are ready to make a long-term commitment to a romantic relationship. Heterosexuals commonly formalize their commitment via marriage; in the United States at least 95% marry at some point in their lives (U.S. Bureau of the Census, 1989). By the end of the third decade of life 53% of men and 63% of women are married. For others, including lesbian and gay couples, this commitment is represented by a decision to cohabit (about 3% of the U.S. population).

The early years of cohabitation and marriage are characterized by frequent intimate contact. Research suggests that this transition marks a time of great personal happiness and stress for homosexual (Kurdek, 1994) and heterosexual couples (Fischer & Sollie, 1993; Huston, McHale, & Crouter, 1986). For most heterosexual couples the first year of marriage is a time of high levels of romantic feeling (Lowenthal et al., 1977) and verbal intimacy (Swensen, Eskew, & Kohlhepp, 1981). Compared to older couples, young marrieds are more emotionally expressive, intense, and direct in their communication, and use more humor, (Sillars, Weisberg, Burgraf, & Zietlow, 1990). They are also more affectionate and engage in more frequent sexual activity than their elders (Huston et al., 1986).

As evidenced by the exceptionally high divorce rate following the first year of marriage (National Center for Health Statistics, 1991), the first year can also be a time of dissatisfaction and conflict. Even relatively satisfied couples show a decline in positive relationship behaviors over the first year (Huston et al., 1986) that may continue for several years (Kurdek, 1991a). Kurdek's work suggests that this decline in romantic feelings is specific to marriage, since it does not occur with equal intensity in cohabiting couples. Without the security of marriage, partners in cohabiting couples may keep their guard up more, permitting their partners to sustain idealized notions of them for a longer period. For married couples, though, the first year may be a time of high hopes that are either dashed fairly quickly or attenuated to match an imperfect partner.

During young adulthood it is likely that romantic relationships become primary attachments, replacing relationships with parents in that function (Ainsworth & Bowlby, 1991; R. S. Weiss, 1986). Securely attached romantic relationships seem to provide participants with a sense of safety, comfort, and well-being (Ainsworth, 1989). Further, romantic partners can show evidence of separation distress when involuntarily parted from one another and often rejoice when reunited following a separation (Ainsworth, 1989).

Research on the quality of attachments between husbands and wives has begun recently. Preliminary findings indicate that married individuals are more likely to be classified as securely attached compared to those who are either not romantically involved or are in dating relationships (Hazan & Shaver, 1990; Kobak & Hazan, 1991). Security of attachment was found to remain relatively constant across the first year of marriage for one group of couples (Senchak & Leonard, 1992). Further, couples who reported higher levels of relational intimacy were more likely to have secure attachments, both when newly wed and after one year of marriage (Senchak & Leonard, 1992).

The most significant changes that occur in young adults' romantic relationships coincide with the transition to parenthood. Eighty percent of Americans become parents; they commonly view parenting as an important source of self-esteem and life satisfaction (Feldman, 1987). Following an initial honeymoon period, however, the birth of the first child heralds decreases in marital intimacy and satisfaction for both husbands and wives (Belsky, Lang, & Rovine, 1985). Perhaps because they take on the bulk of child care responsibilities, wives may experience more severe declines in satisfaction (Belsky et al., 1985). Exchanges of affection, sexual activity, and companionship between husbands and wives decline as time and energy, particularly the mother's, are taken up with infant care (Abbott & Brody, 1985; MacDermid, Huston, & McHale, 1990; Wilkie & Ames, 1986). Sex roles can become more stereotyped (McHale & Huston, 1985; Ruble, Fleming, Hackel, & Stangor, 1988), exerting a negative impact on wives' marital satisfaction if they had expected more equitable sharing of child care responsibilities (Belsky et al., 1985).

NEEDS, CONCERNS, STRESSES, AND INTIMATE RELATIONSHIPS DURING YOUNG ADULTHOOD

Young adults' intimate interactions and relationships are likely to shape and be shaped by (1) a concern with formulating and committing to an adult identity, (2) a need and increasing capacity for intimacy, and (3) concerns with young adult life transitions. My discussion of the first two concerns draws heavily from the personality theory of Erikson (1959, 1963), who suggested that the development of a clearly delineated adult identity facilitates young adults' efforts to participate in intimate relationships. According to Erikson, people without clearly delineated identities risk feeling engulfed in their intimate relationships. These fears of engulfment prevent them from enjoying the temporary state of fusion that intimate interaction provides. Once a secure identity is established, however, young adults can make important advances in their capacities for intimate relating. This section examines the impact of young adults' capacities for intimacy on their romantic relationships and friendships.

Concerns with life transitions also affect and are affected by young adults' intimate interactions and relationships. For many people in Western culture young adulthood is a time of important life transitions: moving out of the family home, becoming part of a couple, and becoming a parent. These transitions are in part defined by the changes in intimate relationships they represent. The intimate interactions and relationships young adults are involved with before, during, and after these transitions seem to shape their adaptations to them.

Identity

The Concern in Context

Young adults become preoccupied with the process of exploring, formulating, and committing to an adult identity. Provisional commitments to a life's work, to an ideological orientation, and to an orientation toward relationships with others are the building blocks of identity in Western culture (Erikson, 1963; Marcia, 1966; Thorbecke & Grotevant, 1982).

Contextual factors such as social class and gender can affect the timing of identity exploration and the salience of identity-related issues. Young adults who are attending college, for example, have the luxury of time to think about their identities before they take on adult roles (Munro & Adams, 1977). Working-class youth may not have this luxury and are more likely to emerge from high school with clear commitments to an adult identity (Keniston, 1982). Gender-related expectations about future adult roles may lead young women and men to place different amounts of emphasis on occupational versus interpersonal aspects of identity (Hodgson & Fischer, 1979; Maines & Hardesty, 1987; Marcia, 1980; Thorbecke & Grotevant, 1982). Finally, gender role prescriptions modify the relationship between identity development outcomes and adjustment. For example, making commitments to goals and beliefs without engaging in exploration seems to have adverse effects on men's, but not women's, adjustment (Josselson, 1987; Marcia & Friedman, 1970; Prager, 1983b).

Relationships with Romantic Partners and Friends

A substantial body of work based on Erikson's (1963) theory has supported his proposed link between exploration and commitment to an identity and the formation of intimate relationships in young adulthood (Hodgson & Fischer, 1979; Orlofsky et al., 1973; Tesch & Whitbourne, 1982). According to Erikson's theory, the links are there because young adults have more difficulty forming intimate relationships when they have not first committed to an adult identity. Erikson also suggested, however, that involvement in the identity exploration process itself may facilitate intimacy between romantic partners and friends. He said, "Such attachment is often devoted to an attempt at arriving at a definition of one's identity by talking things over endlessly, by confessing what one feels like and what the other seems like, and by discussing plans, wishes and expectations" (p. 95). In other words, the identity exploration process may encourage young adults to seek out verbally intimate interactions with romantic partners and friends.

There is evidence that both friends and romantic partners are likely to engage in self-clarifying dialogues with one another in young adulthood (Prager et al., 1989). Through intimate interactions young adults can get direct opinions about their ideas and plans. They can formulate their thoughts more clearly while clarifying them to their listener (Buhrmester & Prager, 1995). Moreover, young people can coconstruct one another's identities through reciprocal interactions in which they express, listen to, clarify, and ultimately formulate together their goals, beliefs, values, and attitudes (McNulty & Swann, 1994; Youniss, 1980). The importance of intimate friendship in young adulthood, then, may stem in part from the valuable contribution interactions with friends can make to young adults' identity development.

During the transition to college old and new friends may support young adult efforts toward identity clarification in different ways. Old friends from adolescence provide young adults with a sense of continuity with the past, an important foundation for identity development (Erikson, 1968). Adolescent friendships, however, may be viewed as anachronisms. They may create pressure toward sameness and foreclosure at a time when the young adult wants to explore fresh alternatives. New friends, in contrast, may be chosen precisely because they support and validate what one is becoming and have no memory of what one was (Rawlins, 1992; L. Rubin, 1985).

Becoming part of a couple and being recognized as such by others can also shape young adult identity (Troll, 1985). When dating partners begin to appear as a couple in their social and familial groups, both add something ("Greg's wife" or "Joan's husband") to their individual identities. In addition, young adults may identify vicariously with their partners' attributes or accomplishments (Beach, Mendolia, & Tesser, 1992) or with one another's affiliations, for example, by developing loyalty to the partner's favorite political cause (Josselson, 1987). Becoming a couple also carries with it the risk of losing certain parts of one's identity, however. For example, Bernard (1972) described a process called "dwindling" whereby women lose a sense of distinctiveness because they accommodate too much to their husbands' identities. Acquiring a couple identity, then, can paradoxically both contribute to and threaten identity.

The development of private self-consciousness may form another link between identity exploration and commitment and the formation of intimate relationships. The identity exploration process may aid in the development of private self-consciousness, which in turn augments the development of intimate relationships (Davis & Franzoi, 1987). Private self-consciousness refers to one's awareness of and ability to articulate one's inner life. As young adults explore their occupational and ideological options, both internally and in interactions with others, they may be simultaneously developing the skills for making their inner lives explicit. As their inner lives become explicit, they are more amenable to being shared with another, and this sharing is a crucial component of intimate interaction (Altman & Taylor, 1973; Jourard, 1971; see Chapter 1).

Intimacy

The Concern in Context

Erikson (1963) postulated that the need for intimacy becomes a conscious preoccupation during the young adult period. "Intimacy vs. isolation" purportedly becomes a crisis during this life stage since no one automatically emerges from the young adult years having successfully cultivated one or more intimate relationships. Rather, there is a risk of isolation, or the "avoidance of . . . experiences [of close affiliations] because of a fear of ego loss . . . lead[ing] to a deep sense of isolation and consequent self-absorption" (1963, p. 264). Young adults therefore actively seek trust and acceptance in their friendships (Tesch & Martin, 1983) and are preoccupied with finding a long-term intimate romantic partner (Cantor, Acker, & Cook-Flannagan, 1992). They are more attracted to potential friends and dating partners who disclose about themselves (Hill & Stull, 1987), and are more satisfied with relationships that are more intimate (Prager, 1989). Those who are unsuccessful in their efforts are some of the loneliest people around (Cutrona, 1982; Peplau, Bikson, Rook, & Goodchilds, 1982; Shaver, Furman, & Buhrmester, 1985). Young adults, then, are absorbed in the task of developing those friendships and romantic relationships that are potentially intimate.

Young adults, at least in Western culture, are uniquely situated to develop new levels of skill and competency relevant to intimate relating, particularly within romantic relationships (Erikson, 1963). They are free to live independently of their parents (and therefore to set up their own households with another person), they are old enough to earn their own living, they are sexually and reproductively mature, and they have reached the peak of their attractiveness to potential partners (Cross, 1971). A variety of contextual factors converge, then, to ensure that young adults will be preoccupied with establishing intimate romantic relationships and will be confronted with opportunities to develop the competencies they need to maintain those relationships.

Erikson (1963) proposed that forming and sustaining an intimate relationship in young adulthood required three capacities: (1) a capacity for commitment, or the ability to make a significant investment in a relationship "without fear of ego loss" (p. 264); (2) a capacity for depth, or an ability to reveal oneself, to involve oneself emotionally, to share oneself sexually, and to air one's differences with another; and (3) a capacity to maintain individuation (or a clear definition of self) in the context of pressures to fuse with another (see Chapter 10 for further discussion of this issue). Drawing from Erikson's theory, Orlofsky et al. (1973) developed a classification scheme for identifying individual differences in the capacities required to build intimate relationships in young adulthood. The scheme classifies young adults into "intimacy statuses" based on whether they have established relationships characterized by commitment, depth, and partner individuation (Orlofsky et al., 1973; Prager, 1991; Tesch & Whitbourne, 1982). Individual intimacy capacity and the scheme proposed by Orlofsky et al. are discussed in the following section.

Relationships with Friends and Romantic Partners

Since the intimacy status classification scheme of Orlofsky et al. stems from an effort to assess individual capacities for intimacy, the intimacy status should predict (1) successful, satisfying intimate relating on the part of young adults and (2) other characteristics of young adults that coincide with successful, satisfying intimate relating. Several studies have addressed the second point (see review by Orlofsky, 1988). Results from this research, which is primarily cross-sectional in design, indicate that young adults who have friendships and romantic relationships characterized by depth, commitment, and partner individuation have higher scores on measures of other Eriksonian psychosocial dilemmas (Orlofsky, 1978), particularly identity (Hodgson & Fischer, 1979; Orlofsky et al., 1973). They are psychologically androgynous rather than sex-typed (Schiedel & Marcia, 1985; Tesch, 1984), have a more internal locus of control, and have lower levels of anxiety (Prager, 1986) and depression (Basco, Prager, Pita, Tamir, & Stephens, 1992). The formation of intimate relationships in young adulthood, then, is associated with good adjustment and psychosocial maturity.

Young adults whose relationships are high in depth, commitment, and partner individuation also engage in more intimate behavior in those relationships. They are more disclosing with romantic partners (Prager, 1989), use more constructive conflict resolution strategies (Prager, 1991), and report higher levels of relationship satisfaction (Basco et al., 1992; Prager, 1989). They know and understand their friends better (Orlofksy, 1976) and are more competent at articulating their feelings (Orlofsky & Ginsburg, 1981). They are more selective with their confidences, saving their most private disclosures for close relationships (Prager, 1986).

Unfortunately, the intimacy status measure assesses intimate relationships from the point of view of only one partner. Additional research is needed to determine whether these findings can be replicated using more dyadic assessments of intimate relationships (for efforts in that direction, see Basco et al., 1992; Prager, 1991).

A second scheme for classifying young adults' capacities for intimate relating comes from attachment theory (Bowlby, 1969). Hazan and Shaver (1987) defined three adult attachment styles: secure, avoidant, and ambivalent (derived from the categories used by Ainsworth et al., 1978, to describe infant–parent attachment). Theoretically, young adult attachment styles reflect working models of self and others. Working models were defined by Bowlby (1969) as expectations that are shaped during childhood relationships with parents and that affect adult relationships for good or ill. Theoretically, a secure working model enables the young adult to enjoy intimate relationships with others without crippling fears of abandonment or engulfment.

Attachment style represents an aspect of individual intimacy capacity and, in that light, should predict the quality of a young adult's intimate relationships (Hazan & Shaver, 1987; Shaver & Hazan, 1988). Research has documented that securely attached young adults enjoy better communication, more self-disclosure, and less conflict in their romantic relationships. Compared to avoidant (and sometimes ambivalent) young adults, they feel more loving and describe their partners as more trustworthy (Collins & Read, 1990; Simpson, 1990). Securely attached young adults also behave more sensitively to their partner's emotions and appear more willing to both seek and provide support when needed (Simpson, Rholes, & Nelligan, 1992).

The work on attachment styles, together with the intimacy status research, suggests that young adults' intimacy capacities affect the kinds of intimate relationships they can establish and maintain. However, both intimacy status and attachment style studies leave open the question of whether individuals bring critical capacities into their relationships or whether good relationships elicit and nurture these capacities. It is likely that both processes occur. For example, there are reasons to believe that the romantic attachment relationships of young adults can have reparative (or damaging) effects on the working models the attachment styles theoretically reflect. Romantic relationships may precipitate accommodation processes in working models (or schemas) because, as R. S. Weiss (1986) noted, these relationships recapitulate and replace the parent–child attachment relationship, providing (or not) a source of security and comfort to the partners. Variations in how successfully romantic relationships provide security and comfort may therefore contribute as much to adult attachment styles as do variations in attachment quality with parents. The working models assessed in young adults may be reflections as much as architects of current romantic relationships (Bartholomew, 1993).

Relationships with Parents

As the review above indicates, there is little evidence that young adults' concerns with intimacy are focused on relationships with parents. Attachment theory, however, has postulated that relationships with parents influence young adults' expectations about intimate peer relationships (i.e., their attachment styles) via the working models carried forward from the earlier parent–child relationship (Hazan & Shaver, 1987).

Hazan and Shaver (1987) found support for this hypothesis using college students' recollections of childhood interactions with mothers and fathers. Young adults with secure attachment styles describe more positive memories of their childhood interactions with their parents than do insecure young adults. They also describe their current intimate relationships as more satisfying.

Research using the Adult Attachment Interview has explored a similar hypothesis, namely, that the quality of attachment in young adults' relationships with their own children is influenced by working models derived from their relationships with their own parents (Main & Goldwyn, 1984). The Adult Attachment Interview measures young adults' conceptions about attachment, intimacy, and their own upbringing, conceptions that are presumably reflective of their relational schemas. For example, mothers with autonomous working models openly valued attachment relationships and could provide plausible, coherent, and balanced descriptions of their parents and their own upbringing. Main and Goldwyn's results indicate that babies of autonomous mothers are more likely to be securely attached than babies of other mothers. Haft and Slade (1989) found that autonomous mothers could reflect their babies' affect back to them more effectively than could mothers (1) who seemed preoccupied with family-of-origin issues (the "preoccupied" group) or (2) whose descriptions of their parents and their upbringing were incoherent (the "disorganized" group) or (3) who dismissed the value of attachment relationships and claimed not to need them (the "dismissing" group). Further, dismissing mothers tended to reject their babies' bids for contact and reassurance and were not attuned to their babies' negative affect.

This research supports the notion that working models from earlier parent–child relationships may influence young adults' behavior in relationships with peers and with their own children. Conclusions must still be drawn with caution, however. Until the necessary longitudinal work has been completed, associations between adult attachment styles and early parent–child relationships are purely speculative. Further, a few studies have shown discontinuities between concurrent parent–child and peer relationships, and between earlier parent–child relationships and later adult relationships (Hightower, 1990; Hunter, 1985; Skolnick, 1986). Inconsistent findings may reflect environmental opportunities such as relationships with friends or nonparental adults (e.g., paid caregivers, grandparents, and teachers) that might mitigate the association between experiences with parents and adult intimate relationships.

Life Transitions

The Concern in Context

Some of the most exciting and potentially joyful life transitions that people experience in their lives may come during the young adult life stage. During these years most North Americans move out of their parental homes and set up housekeeping for themselves for the first time. Most begin their life's work, get married (or begin a cohabiting relationship), and begin having children. It is a time of beginnings, as they wade into the waters of adulthood for the first time in every area of life.

There is reason to believe that as young adults face these transitions in turn, they become preoccupied with the challenges that each transition places before them. Further, there is evidence that intimate relationships can shape people's experiences with each transition and provide them with the resources they need to meet the challenges of these transitions successfully. Finally, the concerns and preoccupations that the transitions of young adulthood bring with them affect behavior within intimate relationships and shape the course of those relationships in the process.

In this section I discuss the transitions to living on one's own, to marriage, and to parenthood as they affect and are affected by the important relationships in young adults' networks. As the review above indicates, many developmental changes that occur within the young adult period coincide with young adult life transitions. In the following sections I review some explanations for why this is so.

Relationships with Parents

Young adults' preoccupations with making it on their own once they have left home may explain any "rapprochement" they experience with their parents at this time. Young people living on their own for the first time may need validation from others that they have the maturity and means to make it successfully. Parents may be an important source of this validation for several reasons. First, young adults are aware that their parents "knew them when" they were younger and more helpless. Parents can therefore give feedback to young adults about how much they have matured and how much more capable they have become. Second, parents have had the role all along of guiding the young person toward greater independence. In addition, because they have been adults for years, parents know what it takes to make it as an adult and are therefore better judges than age-mates of whether the young adult has what it takes. For these reasons, validation from parents may be important to young adults making the transition to living on their own.

A series of studies by Lopez, Campbell, and Watkins (1988, 1989a, 1989b) explored several dimensions of the parent–young adult relationship that might predict students' adjustment to college. Their findings showed that parental overinvolvement, intensity of parental marital conflict, and parent–child role reversal all predicted a poor adjustment to college on the part of students. Students' needs for validation from their parents may be frustrated by parental overinvolvement and marital con-

flict, each in a different way. Parental overinvolvement may directly frus-
trate students' needs for validation by communicating to students that
they need to be closely supervised because they are not competent.
(Parental overinvolvement may also be elicited by young adults who lack
a sense of autonomy.). Marital conflict may make parents, who are caught
up in their own emotional turmoil, unavailable to the student their attention is needed. Finally, parent–child role reversal, by definition, results in students attending to their parents' needs instead of parents attending to the students'. Under any of these conditions students' needs
are less likely to be met and their adjustment to the transition to college
more likely to be compromised.

Also supporting the notion that parental support is an important
predictor of young adults' adjustment to college is a recent study by
Cutrona, Cole, Colangelo, Assouline, and Russell (1994). Cutrona, et al.
found that support from parents predicted college students' academic performance (assessed by cumulative grade point average), over and above
variance accounted for by American College Test (ACT) scores. In contrast, support from friends or romantic partners did not significantly predict students' academic performance.

Attachment and support from parents may be less predictive of
men's than women's transition to college. In a study of U.S. college students, women's, but not men's, social competence and well-being were
predicted by attachment to parents (Kenny & Donaldson, 1991), especially when parents explicitly supported daughters' individuation. It is
possible that young men are less affected by parental support because they
are under greater pressure to deny their needs for aid and assistance. In
trying to live up to the image of the American "self-reliant male" (Doyle,
1989), young men may refuse to avail themselves of the support parents
can provide. Data from the study by Frank et al. (1988) support this notion: Their findings suggest that young men more frequently than young
women are "pseudoautonomous," feigning indifference to conflicts with
parents, actively disengaging themselves from them, and openly displaying contempt for their efforts to help them. Parents may, however, sub-
scribe to the same masculinity myth and may therefore provide less support to their sons than to their daughters.

Some studies indicate that parents and their young adult offspring
become closer following the transition to parenthood (Carbery, 1993; L.
Fischer, 1981; White et al., 1983) while others indicate more distance or
conflict (Frank et al., 1988; Lowenthal, Thurnher, & Chiriboga, 1977).
Research may yield mixed results because contextual factors are mediating the effects of this transition on young adults' relationships with their
parents. Allan (1993) has suggested a number of possible mediating fac-

tors. First, parents and adult children may live too far apart to maintain intimate ties easily. Second, the history of the relationship between parent and young adult will mediate the impact of the transition to parenthood. If they were not intimate before, for example, parents and grown children may become closer after the birth of a grandchild. If they were intimate before, the time commitments of new parenthood may interfere with young adults' efforts to stay close to parents. Third, the health and vitality of the older generation will affect their level of involvement with their grandchild, which may in turn affect the parent–young adult relationship. Finally, the young parent's marital status may have an important impact on the needs he or she hopes a parent will fulfill. Unmarried young parents may be especially inclined to form closer bonds with parents, perhaps because they count on their parents' assistance with their own parenting efforts.

Relationships with Friends and Romantic Partners

Relationships with friends seem to be affected by all three of the important transitions of young adulthood. As young adults become preoccupied with adjusting to and enjoying their new life following the transition to college, they seek to make new friends. In one study (Cutrona, 1982), college students reported that their friendships were their most satisfying relationships. Perhaps this is because their friends shared their preoccupations and could therefore commiserate, advise, and support most effectively.

The formation of close and satisfying friendships is in turn, an important factor determining the quality of the student's adjustment to college (Rawlins, 1992). Cutrona (1982) found that the loneliest students are those who are unable to make good friends or who pursue a romantic relationship at the expense of friendships. The single most important reason for loneliness reported by first-year college students in Cutrona's study was that old friends and family had been left behind.

Whether relationships with romantic partners have much impact on young adults' adjustments to leaving home is unknown. One study (Shaver et al., 1985) indicates that romantic relationships, like many friendships, fail to withstand the changes young adults experience when they make the transition to college. Perhaps it is this tendency to end romantic relationships from high school, coupled with the fact that few students sustain romantic relationships early in their college career, that explains the relative dearth of information about this issue.

The transition to marriage, of course, is an important transition both for the young adult individually and for the romantic relationship.

(Whether the move to a cohabiting from a dating relationship is experienced as an equally important transition is unknown at present). Engagement and marriage precipitate a preoccupation with establishing and fostering the marital relationship. This preoccupation could explain, in part, why relational intimacy and satisfaction are so high in early marriage. The transition focuses the young adult's attention on the partner and the new marriage, and spouses may thoroughly enjoy being the object of one another's attention. Clearly, the nature of the attention is a mediating factor in this relationship, however. Spouses may also focus negative attention on each other and the marriage at this time, which may explain why dissatisfaction and (sometimes) divorce are also frequent following the transition to marriage.

The preoccupation with the romantic partner and the marriage may also explain the decline in contact with friends (Booth & Hess, 1974; Cohen, 1992; Milardo et al., 1983; Tschann, 1988). Young couples' concerns with establishing their marital relationship and building a home may overshadow their interest in maintaining contact with friends, at least temporarily. Further, young partners' concerns with forming a couple identity may explain why some friendships are viewed as threatening to their relationship (such as cross-sex friendships or drinking buddies from singles bars) and why newlyweds may abandon these friends.

The transition to parenthood seems to hasten a decline in adults' intimate contact with other adults, whether spouse, friends, or parents. Because of the 24-hour-per-day demands of new babies, parents may find themselves curtailing all activity except work and infant care, including sleep! Because they are consumed with the parenting task, young adults also devote less attention to the quality of their marital relationship and friendships (Cohen, 1992; C. Fischer, 1982). It is unlikely, however, that this decrease in contact with other adults reflects a declining need for the benefits that intimacy with other adults provides (Carbery, 1993). More likely, becoming a parent precipitates for some adults a willingness to put personal need fulfillment aside in favor of meeting the child's needs (Ambert, 1992; Lopata, 1971). Parents may tolerate less intimate contact with other adults because they are willing to forgo the satisfaction that such contact brings.

Conversely, supportive intimate relationships with others can ease the transitions to marriage and parenthood for young adults. The presence of committed and enduring friendships predicts spouses' well-being during and following the transition to marriage (Fischer & Sollie, 1993). Friends' approval of one's choice of romantic partner is likely to be important to young adults (Rawlins, 1992).

A satisfying intimate relationship between marital partners is predictive of each partner's adjustment to the transition to parenthood and of the quality of parenting as well. New mothers with supportive husbands have fewer problems with pregnancy and fewer postpartum depressions and are more competent and responsive with their infants (e.g., Biller, 1993; Gottlieb & Pancer, 1988). Work by Belsky (1979) indicates that the quality of the husband–wife relationship is associated with the extent of fathers' (but not mothers') involvement in infant care. Couples who are more happily married share more in parenting (also see Levi-Shiff & Israelashvili, 1988).

SUMMARY AND CONCLUSIONS

This chapter has organized the literature on intimate relationships through adolescence and young adulthood to emphasize the continuing interplay between individual development and intimate relationships. Needs, concerns, and stresses of these two stages have served as vantage points from which to view possible linkages between intimate interactions and relationships and individual development. These life stages are associated with richer bodies of knowledge about intimacy than any other. As with research on childhood, however, support for linkages between individual development and intimate relating has yet to be established for many of the issues people confront during these life stages.

Two important changes set adolescent intimate interactions and relationships apart from those of earlier life stages. First, early in adolescence friendships emerge as teenagers' most intimate relationships (Savin-Williams & Berndt, 1990). Young adolescents value intimacy in friendship highly (Buhrmester, 1990) and choose friends based on whether they can confide in them (Berndt, 1982). Second, later in adolescence romantic relationships become important. Middle to late adolescence marks significant increases in intimacy between teens and potential (or actual) romantic partners (Sharabany et al., 1981). Sexual activity becomes a preoccupation for teens of various sexual orientations (Janus & Janus, 1993; Savin-Williams, 1995).

Young adulthood is a time of transitions in intimate relationships. During the early (e.g., college) years of young adulthood, friends continue to be primary intimate companions and preferred confidants (Prager et al., 1989). Most people commit themselves to a romantic partnership before the end of the young adult period (U.S. Bureau of the Census, 1989), which often results in young adults having less time for friendships (Tschann, 1988). Less contact does not immediately mean less intimacy, however, especially for women (Oliker, 1989).

The early years of marriage and cohabitation are marked by frequent intimate interactions, both verbal and sexual (Kurdek, 1994). It is likely that romantic partners form an attachment-like relationship with one another, that provides some of the feelings of safety, security, and comfort that were once obtained from parents (Ainsworth & Bowlby, 1991).

Some of the work on adolescence and young adulthood has sought to identify links between life-stage-related concerns and intimate relationships in adolescence and young adulthood. For example, research conducted by Cooper, Grotevant, and their colleagues (e.g., Grotevant & Cooper, 1986) has established associations between teens' explorations of self and identity and their interactions with parents. Other research has suggested that there may be links between young adults' adjustment to the transition to college and their relationships with their parents (Lopez, Campbell, & Watkins, 1989a, 1989b). Connections between marital quality and young adults' life-stage-related concerns, such as the transition to parenthood, have also been reasonably well documented (e.g., C. Fischer, 1982).

A proposition deserving more attention is Erikson's notion that young adulthood is a critical period for augmenting skills and competencies for intimate relating. Work on attachment styles (Bartholomew, 1993; Hazan & Shaver, 1987), intimacy maturity (White et al., 1983) and intimacy status (Orlofsky, 1988; Prager, 1991) has drawn from Bowlby's and Erikson's theories to explore possible competencies required for effective intimate relating in adulthood. The multilevel conception of intimacy introduced in Chapter 1 may provide a blueprint for new conceptions of intimacy capacity. At the level of interaction, intimacy capacity may refer to the person's skills with intimate behavior (e.g., self-disclosure, verbal responsiveness, and nonverbal involvement [see Chapter 8]. The attachment style, intimacy maturity, and intimacy status conceptions do not refer to interaction skills, however, but to a person's capacity to maintain satisfying intimate relationships (e.g., Kobak & Hazan, 1994). The conception of intimate relationships introduced in Chapter 1 suggests that intimate relationship capacity may be assessed by a person's ability to sustain relational intimacy, affection, trust, and cohesiveness with another person over time. The measurement of intimacy capacity, therefore, might involve several independent assessments, which in combination would operationalize intimacy capacity.

Another potentially fruitful area of study is same-sex romantic relationships. Further work in this area can potentially illuminate the impact of both gender and sexual orientation on intimate interactions and relationships (see Part III of this book). The extent to which adolescents and young adults develop a gay or lesbian identity as a result of their same-sex erotic attractions seems to vary considerably among individuals (C. Patterson, 1995). It seems likely that an individual's resolution of such identity issues would affect his or her expectations of and commitment to same-sex romantic relationships. The integration of that individual into a gay community, and a gay network of friends, would also likely be affected. Research on sexual identity and its impact on intimate relationships, then, would likely shed light on processes by which individual development and intimate interactions and relationships interact during adolescence and young adulthood.

In sum, researchers have accumulated a rich database on intimacy in adolescence and young adulthood. These are times of increasing interest in and capacities for intimacy with friends and romantic partners. Intimacy increasingly becomes a conscious preoccupation as people actively seek intimate friendships and enduring romantic relationships. These are also times of concern with self. Adolescents become preoccupied with their changing bodies and their increasingly intense sexual feelings. They also become concerned with their developing autonomy and individuation while still seeking approval and acceptance from parents and peers. Young adults confront the challenge of formulating an adult identity. They must test themselves for the first time in the adult worlds of higher education, work, and parenting. Intimate interactions and relationships cannot help but be colored by these concerns. In turn, they provide the context in which adolescents and young adults explore and resolve these concerns. The ultimate goal of research on intimacy during these life stages is to illuminate the processes by which intimacy and these life-stage-related concerns and stresses transform one another.

Intimacy in Middle and Late Adulthood

And Naomi said: "Turn back, my daughters; why will ye go with
me? have I yet sons in my womb, that they may be your
husbands? . . . go your way; for I am too old to have a husband.
. . . but Ruth . . . said, "Entreat me not to leave thee; . . . wither
thou goest, I will go; where thou lodgest, I will lodge; thy people
shall be my people, and thy God my God."
—RUTH 1:11–16

Intimate interactions and relationships continue to have a profound impact on life-stage-related concerns and needs through the middle and late
years of adult life. There is also reason to believe that adults' adaptations
to these needs and concerns continue to shape their intimate interactions
and relationships through the last years of life.

There is a shift in our discussion of individual development and intimate relationships when we get to the middle years of adulthood. The association between age and the development of competence is less dramatic during the last half of life. The earlier in development we go, the
more precisely are gains in competence associated with age (e.g., change
during infancy can be charted in terms of months rather than years).

The correspondence between age and life stage is also not as strong
in adulthood as it is during childhood and adolescence. Life stage refers to
the age-related roles the individual has taken on, including but not confined to school/work, family, and community roles. Because age norms are
well understood within a given culture, high correlations nevertheless remain between life stage transitions and the broad age periods of adulthood (e.g., many adults retire around age 65). Adults are significantly
more likely to deviate from age-related norms than children are. For example, the percentage of adults in the United States who deviate from

middle-class age-related norms for college attendance (i.e., beginning at 18 and finishing at 22) is considerably higher than the percentage of 6-year-olds who deviate from the norm of starting first grade! Therefore, age periods and life stages are rougher approximations of one another in adulthood than in childhood (Blieszner & Adams, 1992).

This chapter explores the interrelationships between life-stage-related needs, concerns, and stresses and intimate relating in middle (35–65 years) and late (65+ years) adulthood. As before, each section begins with a review of life-stage-related changes in intimate relationships. The current chapter reviews changes in adults' relationships with romantic partners, parents, and friends. In addition, it examines parents' intimate relationships with their children as they mature and become adults.

MIDDLE ADULTHOOD (35–65 YEARS): LIFE-STAGE-RELATED DEVELOPMENTS IN INTIMATE RELATIONSHIPS

Romantic Relationships

Marriage is the centerpiece of most American adults' network of intimate relationships. Within Western culture the marital relationship is expected to meet most of an adult's intimacy needs (O'Connor, 1992).

Although intimacy is not synonymous with satisfaction, the extensive literature on marital satisfaction can provide some clues about the way intimacy changes over time in marital relationships. A well-documented decline in marital satisfaction often begins with the birth of the first child. This decline is observable in longitudinal (Ryder, 1973) and cross-sectional studies (Harriman, 1983). Lower levels of marital satisfaction persist while there are children in the home; childless couples, on average, report higher levels of marital satisfaction (Ambert, 1992).[1] There is, however, evidence of a "devitalization" of marriage over time that occurs whether children are in the home or not (Huston et al., 1986; Lowenthal et al., 1975). Both husbands and wives report a drop in the pleasing things their partners do for them and in the time they spend on joint leisure activities. Couples become less affectionate over time and less expressive of their positive feelings toward one another.

Spouses may find themselves out of synchrony because of life-stage-related fluctuations in gender roles. After the birth of the first child, gender roles are often more stereotypical and divided (England & Farkas, 1986; Ruble, et al., 1988). A few studies have suggested that during this period wives are more likely than husbands to feel that their intimacy needs are not being adequately met in the marriage (Christensen & Shenk, 1991; Hite, 1987; Oliker, 1989; L. Rubin, 1983).

By middle age (i.e., ages 40–55) a renegotiation of gender-specific roles sometimes occurs (Tamir, 1982). Wives who have devoted the bulk of their early adult years to childrearing are likely to renew their interest in agentic pursuits (Gutmann, 1980). Full-time homemakers may change careers and enter full-time employment (England & Farkas, 1986). Husbands, in contrast, have often spent their early adult years in pursuit of occupational success; in middle age they may become more family oriented and may hope for more affection and attention from their wives (Tamir, 1982). If a wife's attention has simultaneously shifted outside the family, her husband's needs for intimate contact with her may be frustrated. If a husband attempts to obstruct or thwart his wife's efforts to pursue extra familial interests, intense marital conflict can ensue (Roberts & Newton, 1987).

Adults and Their Parents

Little is known about developmental changes in intimacy between adults and their parents. There are few norms or expectations regarding adults' relationships with their parents, perhaps because of recent changes in longevity. Adults in the middle years today are much more likely to have living parents than were adults of previous generations. Between 1900 and 1976 the number of middle-age couples with two or more living parents increased from 10% to 47% (Huber, 1993).

It is possible that as parents age and become frail, they will depend more heavily on their adult children. Some have speculated that this dependency results in a role reversal in the relationship (Cicirelli, 1983). Little is currently known about how these changing roles affect intimacy in those relationships.

Relationships between adults and their parents may change when the adult becomes a parent. Women have reported that once they become a parent, their relationship with their own mother becomes more like a peer relationship (Bretherton, Biringen, Ridgeway, Maslin, & Sherman, 1989). Even after becoming parents, however, women will struggle to have good relationships with their mothers (Bretherton et al., 1989). Less is known about adults and their fathers.

Adults and Their Children

While little is known about parent–child relationships from the parents' perspective (Ambert, 1992; Bretherton et al., 1989; Hartup, 1986), a few studies indicate that these relationships are quite satisfying. Mothers of 2-year-olds recall feeling extreme joy and love at the time of their child's birth (Bretherton et al., 1989). They remember their children as having been happy and easy to take care of as young infants. In an observational study of fathers and their infants, Greenberg and Morris (1974) noticed expressions of elation and attachment in fathers, along with extensive touching and looking. In Lewis's (1986) interview study of 100 English fathers of infants, fathers described important changes in their lives and in their attitudes toward family and work as a result of their parenting experiences.

Parents also acknowledge how difficult baby care is on them. On the basis of her review of the literature on the effects of children on parents, Ambert (1992) concluded that mothers of infants are fatigued, and that they feel burdened, confined, and isolated by the unremitting responsibility of infant care. A focus on difficulties, however, did not preclude more positive descriptions of the child's good qualities, particularly when children were a little older (Whitbourne, 1986).

In Whitbourne's (1986) interview study of parents with children of all ages, parents' comments about their relationships with their children were dominated by themes of generativity. Parents expressed empathy and concern for their children's health, welfare, and well-being. They reported feeling a strong sense of responsibility to care for their children materially and emotionally. Some adults claimed that becoming a parent itself expanded their identity and kindled generativity needs.

Adults also mention inhibitions on autonomy, freedom, and time for self-care when describing their relationships with their children (LaRossa & LaRossa, 1989; Whitbourne, 1986). Most parents report that they were unprepared for how the parenting role took over their lives. This theme is most likely to predominate when the children are infants and preschoolers (Gottlieb & Pancer, 1988). Over time, however, children may take on household responsibilities and relieve parents (Ambert, 1992). Older girls are especially likely to be involved in helping parents take care of younger siblings (Benin & Edwards, 1990; Cicirelli, 1976).

The existing literature on parent–child relationships does not indicate how much a relationship with a child meets a parent's intimacy needs (Ambert, 1992). Two recent studies, both on young adult samples, suggest that parents do not commonly look to children to fulfill their needs for intimacy. Carbery (1993) asked parents to report on which interpersonal needs were fulfilled in their relationships with their children. Adults reported several needs that children met (e.g., companionship, attachment), but intimacy, notably, was not among them. Peterson and Stewart (1993) found that the strength of affiliation-intimacy motives among young adults was not correlated with the number of children they had, their professed interest in children, or their involvement and satisfaction with parenting. Were studies to investigate the impact of physical intimacy (i.e., touching and holding) with children on parents, more positive associations might be identified (Ambert, 1992). Similarly, studies conducted with adults who are older (and who therefore have older children) might show that children more frequently function as verbally intimate companions.

Friendships

Research explicitly examining friendship in middle adulthood, or comparing it to friendship in other age groups, is sparse (Blieszner & Adams, 1992). There is evidence that intimate friendships are beneficial to individuals during the middle adult years (Stein et al., 1992) but that adults lack the time to nurture and attend to them (Cohen, 1992). As in earlier stages of the life cycle, women's friendships tend to be more intimate than men's (O'Connor, 1992).

Age-related trends are quite similar for women and men regarding friendship. For both sexes, there is evidence of a decline in the number of friends people maintain during the middle adult years as compared to young adulthood (Fiske & Chiriboga, 1990; Lowenthal et al., 1977; Nardi, 1992b). There is also a decline in the frequency of contact with friends (Dickens & Perlman, 1981). The number of new friends people make decreases, and the friendships maintained are often those of longer duration (Lowenthal et al., 1977). Further, one study found that when they are compared to people at other stages of life (younger and older), both men and women in the middle adult years describe their friendships in highly simplistic terms (Lowenthal et al., 1977). While it is possible that intimacy between friends may also decline over the life cycle (M. Brown, 1989), some evidence indicates that intimacy declines less than frequency of contact (Dickens & Perlman, 1981). Intimacy seems to decline more in men's than in women's friendships (Nardi, 1992b; Rawlins, 1992; Tschann, 1988).

NEEDS, CONCERNS, STRESSES, AND INTIMACY IN MIDDLE ADULTHOOD

In middle adulthood, intimacy is likely to affect and be affected by needs and stresses related to work, generativity, and a changing time perspective. Because North American adults' concerns with work continue to be profoundly shaped by gender, this section devotes a separate discussion to work, gender, and intimate relationships.

Work

The Concern in Context

Because work is so important and consumes so much time for most adults in the United States, its impact must be considered in any discussion of adults' intimate relationships. Adults are clearly concerned with satisfaction and achievement with work (Levinson, 1978). Work is important in part because adults have many financial responsibilities during this period. The middle adult years are also a time of increasing satisfaction with work, however (Bee, 1992; Whitbourne, 1986). Older workers, particularly men, are more likely than younger ones to have been promoted into the job they wanted (Rosenbaum, 1984) or to have molded their jobs to their own specifications (Mortimer & Lorence, 1979).

Balancing work and intimate relationships is a primary preoccupation among American adults employed full-time (Snarey, 1993; Voydanoff, 1993). Because the structure of work in the United States is not changing as fast as are family role expectations (L. Gilbert, 1993; Snarey, 1993), both men and women struggle to integrate their work and family commitments.

Relationships with Romantic Partners

Adults' experiences with work and marriage seem heavily interdependent. Hazan and Shaver (1990) argued that work is the adult form of exploration and that persistence and balance with work should thrive when adults have a romantic partner who provides them with a secure base. In their sample of adults of all ages they found that a secure attachment style within the context of a marital relationship was predictive of work–play balance and satisfaction with work. A secure intimate relationship may encourage *and* result from a balance between work and play.

The marital relationship can also have a negative influence on adjustment to work. There is evidence that if one partner disapproves of the other partner's job, this disapproval can interfere with the working adult's satisfaction with both job and marriage (Friedman, 1991; J. Wilkie, 1988). Marital conflict seems worst when a husband's traditional gender role expectations conflict with his wife's expectation of more flexible roles (J. Wilkie, 1988).[2]

Work roles should in turn exert a decisive impact on romantic relationships. When people work long hours and/or weekends, have little autonomy or job security, have to change jobs or locations frequently, and/or have a negative social climate at work, their family relationships seem to suffer proportionately (Friedman, 1991).

Relationships with Children

Work can have a negative impact on parents' relationships with children. Friedman's (1991) review suggests that the greater the number of family responsibilities adults take on, the more likely they are to report that work negatively affects those relationships.

Research examining the impact of work on parent–child relationships has generally restricted itself to the mother–child relationship. This research indicates that children's development is neither helped nor harmed when mothers work in jobs other than full-time homemaking (Clarke-Stewart, 1989; Etaugh, 1980; Gilbert, 1993; Hoffman, 1979). One exception has been research on mother–child attachment quality. Some studies have indicated that infants of full-time homemakers are more likely to be securely attached than infants of mothers employed full-time outside the home (Clarke-Stewart, 1989; Etaugh, 1980). These results must be interpreted cautiously because most of this research uses Ainsworth's "strange situation" to assess mother–child attachment. That is, the "strange situation" may not be strange to infants who see their mothers come and go regularly and may not cause them distress. This lack of distress may make infants appear insecurely attached (e.g., they may not seek mothers out for comfort at reunion). Research conducted on samples living outside the United States, where all-day mother–child contact is less common, supports this interpretation. This research reveals a distribution of attachment classifications similar to that obtained in studies of employed mothers and their children in the United States (Clarke-Stewart, 1989). This research does not rule out the possibility, however, that an adult who happily parents full-time maximizes the likelihood of a secure attachment with his or her baby.

Full-time employment may have more impact on father–child than on mother–child relationships. A mother employed full-time will spend significantly more time caring for her children than a father who is comparably employed (Pleck, 1985; also, see review by Fox & Hesse-Biber, 1983). Perhaps mothers' relationships with their children are more intimate *because* employment has less impact on the time and effort they spend on parenting activities (see Chapters 5 and 6).

A lack of intimate contact with their children may take its toll on parents' well-being. While there is little research in this area, a couple of studies on fathers are suggestive. Greenberg and O'Neil (1990) found that worries about children contribute significantly to experiences of role strain among fathers employed full-time. Robinson and Barret (1986) found that even those fathers who believe their most important contribution to their children's lives is financial security express sadness about their lack of intimate contact with their children.

The impact of the parent–child relationship on adults' progress at work might also merit further study. A review by Snarey (1993) reports mixed results regarding the effect of family involvement on men's careers. While some research shows negative correlations between family involvement and either socioeconomic status or the status of men's positions in their organization, most show success with work and family to be positively correlated. Relationships with children, of course, have a profound effect on women's careers when women temporarily halt a career to care for children full-time (Moen, 1985).

Relationships with Friends

The heavy demands of the workplace may cut into friendships even more than into relationships with family members (Cohen, 1992). Adults often give what little free time they have to their families (Cohen, 1992; L. Rubin, 1985).

The workplace can also be a source of friends, however. On the basis of a recent review, Rawlins (1992) concluded that people who are very interested in their work often fill their personal relationship networks with people employed in similar occupations. The shop talk shared by these friends may be quite intimate when it involves self-expression and emotional catharsis around issues related to work. The presence of friendships at work has a positive impact on job satisfaction (Winstead, Derlega, & Montgomery, 1995).

Rawlins lists workplace factors that can determine whether a collegial relationship will take on "the person-qua-person orientation or depth of mutual concern of friendship" (p. 163). To the extent that workplace culture emphasizes cooperation and concern rather than competition among coworkers, friendships seem more likely to develop. The nature of the work itself may also be a factor. Jobs with "inherently self-serving, divisive, and/or highly competitive aims" (p. 162) may be less likely to engender friendships than those with more nurturing purposes. Workers' status relative to one another also seems to be a crucial factor. Workers who are equals are most likely to form friendships, even if they are competing for recognition. Supervisor–supervisee relationships, in contrast, contain an authority structure that inhibits genuine friendship.

Work, Gender Roles, and Intimate Relationships

The Concern in Context

The focus of women's and men's concerns with balancing work and family demands may be different. Men may place more emphasis on workplace success and achievement while women are more concerned with family relationships (Roberts & Newton, 1987).

Several factors may contribute to men and women having different preoccupations in middle adulthood. Men may emphasize work because work satisfaction and success are so highly correlated with their self-esteem at this age (Tamir, 1982). In addition, the earnings advantage of men can result in both spouses supporting the husband's career more than the wife's for economic reasons (England & Farkas, 1986). This support may further encourage men to concentrate on success at work. Moreover, when couples intensify their sex-typed behavior following the transition to parenthood (Belsky et al., 1985), fathers may shoulder most of the breadwinner role (Hawkins & Belsky, 1989). Their concerns for their family's financial security may translate into concerns with workplace success (Larson, Richards, & Perry-Jenkins, 1994).

Women's concerns with family relationships likely stem from and contribute to the primary responsibility they take for the care of children (Fox & Hesse-Biber, 1983; Gilbert, 1993; Maret & Finlay, 1984; Pleck, 1985). When people spend more time caring for children, they experience more conflict between family and work demands (Friedman, 1991). Further, as mentioned already, women are more likely than men to leave the workforce or cut back to part-time during their childrearing years (Moen, 1985). Reduced involvement in paid work and more involvement in family work may ensure that women are more concerned with family life.

Relationships with Romantic Partners

Different preoccupations among husbands and wives may contribute to decreases in marital satisfaction over time. Spouses' diverging concerns and interests may limit opportunities for intimate interaction. Further, men's concerns with workplace success may override concerns about family relationships. As a result, men may wish to avoid negotiating marital conflicts (Gottman, 1994) and devote their energy to other pursuits. Wives may resent husbands being less involved with family concerns (Belsky, Youngblade, Rovine, & Volling, 1991).

This divergence in husbands' and wives' preoccupations at midlife may contribute to the prevalence of the demand–withdraw pattern of marital interaction. Demand–withdraw describes a pattern in which one spouse (usually the husband) withdraws and the other spouse (usually the wife) tries to engage the withdrawn spouse (Christensen & Shenk, 1991; Fruzzetti & Jacobson, 1990; Napier, 1978). The disproportionate number of wives who demand and husbands who withdraw may result from sex differences in life-stage-related preoccupations. Perhaps wives make efforts to engage their spouses in interaction because they are preoccupied with family life and want their husband's partnership in that endeavor. Husbands may withdraw because engagement intensifies their work–family conflicts (Friedman, 1991) and because they are preoccupied with the workplace. Gender-specific concerns with work and family life may thereby serve to instigate and aggravate the demand–withdraw pattern of marital interaction.

Generativity

The Concern in Context

Adults in midlife may become preoccupied with generativity, described by Erikson (1963) as making a difference in the lives of those who come after them (Lemmer, 1987; Peterson & Stewart, 1993; Whitbourne, 1986). Snarey (1993) distinguished among three kinds of generativity: (1) biological generativity, which involves conceiving, giving birth to, and nursing/nurturing an infant; (2) parental generativity, which involves "carrying out childrearing activities that promote children's ability to develop their full potential" (p. 21), and (3) societal generativity, which involves expanding generativity concerns beyond one's own children to the "actual sustained responsibility for the growth, well-being, and leadership of other adults" (p. 22).

Concerns with parental generativity roughly divide the middle adult years into two subphases. In the earlier phase parents are concerned with raising children. This concern continues while children are in the home. During the latter part of middle adulthood, parents are concerned with launching children. Although parenting continues after children leave home, it becomes less time-consuming and demanding.

Generativity and Intimate Relationships

Having and raising children probably stimulates adult concerns with generativity. This stimulating effect may operate as much with societal as parental generativity. In support of this notion, Snarey, Kuehne, Son, Hauser, and Vaillant (1987) found that men who were involved in caring for children were more likely to mentor outside their families. In contrast, launching children may cause parents to place less of a priority on generativity concerns (Deutscher, 1968).

If adults are more willing to forgo intimate contact with peers during the middle years, perhaps it is because they are concerned with generativity (e.g., Lopata, 1971). A willingness to put children's needs first when they compete with parents' needs for intimate contact with spouses or friends may reflect the normative position of this concern during middle adulthood (Erikson, 1963; Peterson & Stewart, 1993). Once children are launched, generativity concerns may carry less weight, allowing adults to more vigorously pursue other intimate relationships.

Changed Time Perspective and Intimate Relationships

For both women and men, middle age brings a growing realization that one's future is not infinite (Tamir, 1982). There is a new awareness of their mortality as people realize sometime during the middle years that they have passed the midpoint of their lives. Neugarten (1976) described this changing awareness of time as a shift from "time-since-birth" to "time-left-to-live."

This changing time perspective may accompany a period of soul-searching during which adults take stock of their lives. Adults may ask themselves whether what they have been doing for the first half of their adult years, their raison d'etre, is a meaningful way to spend the second half (Levinson, Darrow, Klein, Levinson, & McKee, 1978; Rosenberg & Farrell, 1977–1978; Sheehy, 1976). This midlife self-examination can be uneventful, or, rarely, it can become a crisis (Levinson et al., 1978). Because it is frequently not a crisis, the term *midlife transition* is more descriptive of this inner focus than *midlife crisis* (Rosenberg & Farrell, 1977–1978). Although not in crisis, men in their 40s are more likely to report symptoms of anxiety and depression than younger and older men and to perceive the bleakest future (Tamir, 1982).

The midlife transition may stimulate adults to incorporate traits and activities that have traditionally been attributed to the other sex (Douglas & Arenberg, 1978; Gutmann, 1980; Sinnot, 1984). To the extent that women and men pursue traditional roles in young adulthood, they may neglect pursuits that do not fit in with those traditional roles. As a result, they may find themselves at midlife with needs unfulfilled: Men may have unfulfilled needs for community and generativity while women may have unfulfilled needs for mastery and agency (Cooper & Gutmann,

1987; McAdams & Bryant, 1987). The changed time perspective of midlife may instigate people's desires to fulfill neglected needs and to develop different aspects of themselves. The result of this process may be increased androgyny in both women and men.

The higher levels of marital satisfaction of late adulthood may stem from this increased androgyny. Increased androgyny could result in women's and men's concerns being more similar at midlife and beyond (Pleck, 1981). This increased similarity may ultimately encourage intimacy.

LATE ADULTHOOD (65+ YEARS): LIFE-STAGE-RELATED DEVELOPMENTS IN INTIMATE RELATIONSHIPS

Relationships with Romantic Partners

Late adulthood appears to be a time of renewed marital satisfaction. Research that identified a decline in marital satisfaction through the young and middle adult years (e.g., Condie, 1989; Hicks & Platt, 1970; Spanier, Lewis, & Cole, 1975) found marital satisfaction increases after adolescent children are launched. Levenson, Carstensen, and Gottman (1994) found that older couples' interactions with one another are more affectively positive than those of middle-aged couples, suggesting that the improvement continues into late adulthood. Studies of marriages lasting over 20 years are few, however, and have yielded mixed results (Condie, 1989). Some studies support the aforementioned curvilinear relationship between life stage and marital satisfaction. These have found long-enduring marriages disproportionately satisfying compared with marriages of shorter duration (e.g., Fields, 1983). Other research has found many unhappy long-term marriages (Argyle & Furnham, 1983; Weishaus, 1983). An in-depth study of 17 couples who had been married 50 years or more (Weishaus & Field, 1988) found only 7 who described a curvilinear relationship between time and satisfaction. The other 10 described their relationships as having been stable (although not necessarily satisfying) throughout. Condie's (1989) study of 54 couples who had been married 50 years found that conflict had decreased over the years while equitable sharing of domestic responsibilities had increased. The more satisfied couples shared more leisure time and interests.

Sexual intimacy continues through late adulthood, despite stereotypical notions to the contrary (H. Kaplan, 1990). Common misconceptions are that sexual activity must decline sharply or cease altogether as people reach the later years of life. In direct contradiction, H. Kaplan's (1990) review notes that a great majority of Americans, female and male, remain sexually active until the end of life. Kinsey and coworkers (Kinsey, Pomeroy, & Martin, 1948; Kinsey, Pomeroy, Martin, & Gebhard, 1953) found that 70% of 70-year-olds have sex once every week or so.

Relationships with Grown Children

There is evidence that relationships with children become, for many older adults, their most intimate relationships (Connidis & Davies, 1990; Lopata, 1979; see review by Peterson, 1989). Both men and women have reported that their grown children are their best confidantes. Living long distances apart seems to exert little effect on expressions of affection or on frequency of contact between grown children and their parents (E. Peterson, 1989).

Evidence nevertheless exists that older adults who rely less on grown children for intimate contact have higher levels of well-being (E. Peterson, 1989). Those who look primarily to grown children as companions and confidants have poorer morale (Blau, 1973), feel less socially integrated (Messer, 1968), and have more dissatisfaction with life (D. Adams, 1971) than those who depend more on friends (E. Peterson, 1989). Further, childless older adults do not show poorer adjustment than those who are parents. For example, older gay men who maintain close connections with a gay community enjoy a rich network of intimate relationships (Dressel & Avant, 1983). Similar results have been found for lesbians, particularly if they are open about their sexual orientation (Raphael & Robinson, 1980).

Relationships with Friends

There are two predominant views of aging and friendship currently in the literature (Adams, 1987). By emphasizing the impact of older adults' decreasing number of choices and shrinking life space on their friendships, one view predicts a contracting friendship network in late adulthood. Supporting this view is a study by B. Brown (1981) that showed that the friendship network of older adults declines, leaving behind a very small core of "good, old friends." In contrast is the view that as long as one is healthy and has reasonable financial resources, old age can provide new friendship opportunities (e.g., Rawlins, 1992). For example, Atchley (1985) mentioned a commonly observed "honeymoon phase" following retirement. During this phase people try out many activities they had no time for before, including reinvesting in friendship. Unfortunately, the studies supporting each viewpoint were cross-sectional and may therefore represent cohort differences rather than effects of aging (Adams, 1987).

Work by R. Adams (1987) suggests that the expansion or contraction of the friendship network in old age may be best interpreted within the context of social class. Adams found that among "high society" women, friendships did become fewer, just as B. Brown (1981) had found. Those that remained, however, were the close ones (in other words, only casual friends seemed to have dropped from the network). Many of the women ascribed this change to increased time for meaningful friendships and the absence of competing occupational commitments. The latter included the maintenance of collegial relationships that were not classified as true friendships. For some of the women in Adams's study widowhood provided further opportunities to build more intimate (and more rewarding) friendships than they had when their husbands were alive.

In contrast, the group Adams called the "marginal women" (i.e., those who were less socioeconomically advantaged) lived in smaller, denser, but quite intimate networks during midlife. They found that old age (and involvement with publicly funded programs for older adults) had expanded their networks. These women made *more* casual friends than before, with the result that the average level of intimacy in their friendships decreased. That is, this decrease did not seem to stem from loss of close friendships but from the addition of more casual friendships.

Adams noted that her results did not differ particularly from earlier studies. Rather, her inclusion of an important contextual factor (social class) and her more detailed analysis of the network (intimate *and* casual friends) yielded a more realistic picture of friendship in late adulthood. From the perspective of Adams's framework, change is inextricably linked to the woman's experience in middle age and to the social context in which she builds her life.

Continuing a lifelong pattern, women's friendships in old age are more intimate than men's (Gold, 1989; Rawlins, 1992). Intimate self-disclosure in friendships continues to be very important to many older women, both Euro- and African-American (Lewittes, 1989). Older men also value intimate communication but seem less likely than women to turn to friendships as a source of intimate contact (Connidis & Davies, 1990). When older men describe their most intimate friendships, however, they describe them in much the same way women do (Albert & Moss, 1990; Peretti & Lowrey, 1984–1986). Women may place more value on the intimacy of the friendship, while men place more value on companionship (Albert & Moss, 1990; Jerrome, 1992).

People's preferences for old long-term friendships may become more pronounced during late adulthood (Dickens & Perlman, 1981; Lowenthal et al., 1977; Rawlins, 1992). Long-term friends share memories and experiences that new ones do not, and older adults can, for a variety of reasons, be more wrapped up in reminiscing than their younger counterparts. Maintaining a circle of longtime friends is not easy for some older adults, however. Many find themselves having to continue making new friends because of a need to relocate (Shea, Thompson, & Blieszner, 1988). Shea et al. found that relocation did not disrupt old friendships too much. Whether near or far, they were important and continuing sources of love and affection. While old friends could be distinguished from new ones because they shared more self-disclosure and reminiscing, many older adults were nevertheless hopeful that their new friendships could also become very close. They had, in fact, for many of the people Shea et al. talked with.

NEEDS, CONCERNS, PREOCCUPATIONS, AND INTIMACY IN LATE ADULTHOOD

Intimate contact in old age has traditionally been seen in the context of the normative losses of late life (Lewittes, 1989; Lowenthal & Haven, 1968). Much of this literature seeks to understand factors in older adults' lives that buffer them from the stresses and strains of old age (R. R. Bell, 1981).

Research has supported the notion that older adults who have intimate relationships (or confidantes) and people they can call on for assistance (social support) are happier, less lonely, and better able to handle stress (e.g., Lopata, 1979; Lowenthal & Haven, 1968; Rawlins, 1992). The presence of a spouse or intimate friends predicts better physical and mental health in old age (Dean, Kolody, Wood, & Ensel, 1989; Lowenthal & Haven, 1968; Peretti & Lowrey, 1984–1986).

Despite the prevalence of these extrinsic benefits, there is no reason to think that intimate contact has fewer intrinsic rewards in late adulthood than in earlier phases of the life cycle. Therefore, whenever possible, this section discusses adults' intimate interactions and relationships outside as well as within their buffering role. Further, it explores the impact of intimate relating on older adults' normative gains and losses. The life-stage-related concerns and stresses addressed in the following sections are: (1) the dropping of roles and retirement, (2) widowhood, (3) religious participation, (4) health and physical change, and (5) concerns with integrity. Each of these life-stage-related concerns appears to affect and be affected by the intimate interactions and relationships of late adulthood.

The Dropping of Roles and Retirement

The Concern in Context

Later adult life involves a decrease in role-related behavior. Most notably, the roles of parent and worker change dramatically when children become independent adults themselves and when adults retire from the work force. As a result, older adults, especially the oldest adults (age 75+) describe their daily life as significantly less stressful than their younger counterparts do (Pellman, 1992).

Like many transitions in life, retirement is both a loss and an opportunity. Retirement involves dropping what is for some people their most engaging and engrossing roles (Morgan, Parnes, & Less, 1985). Many people mourn the loss of their work roles and have difficulty finding meaningful activity once they are no longer in those roles (Lewittes, 1989). More often, the postretirement years are described as satisfying once the transition has been made (McCallum, 1986). The surge of activity that often follows retirement is indicative of the opportunities this transition introduces. Newly retired people are often eager to explore interests and activities they lacked time for during their younger years (Lewittes, 1989). Perhaps most adults experience some combination of loss and relief, both missing their former roles and looking forward to new ones.

Relationships with Romantic Partners

Little is known about the impact of retirement on marital relationships because for many years retirement has been conceptualized primarily as an individual life transition (Szinovacz, 1989). Retirement is a couple event, however, as evidenced by the many couples who time their retirements to coincide. Further, since employment of both spouses has become the norm among middle-aged couples in the United States (Gilbert, 1993), in the future most couples will be planning how to enjoy their joint retirement.

The upswing in marital satisfaction often observed in late adulthood may be explained in part by the potentially positive impact of retirement on marital relationships. If the demands of work and parenting interfered with a couple's ability to enjoy intimate interaction, retirement can herald the end of such conflicts. Couples can enjoy previously neglected interests and friendships together when they retire.

Like any transition, however, retirement has the potential to create difficulty in the marital relationship. Traditional expectations about marital roles, combined with an inability to adjust those roles, can compromise individual partners' adaptations to retirement (Hood, 1986). Lip-man (1961) noted that husbands who see their provider role as their pri-mary or sole contribution to their marriage are more likely to be de-pressed following retirement than husbands who see their marital role as more "expressive." The ability of spouses to support one another (Lip-man, 1960, 1961; Keating & Cole, 1980) and to engage in open negotia-tion regarding expectations and hopes for retirement may be a necessary contributor to a satisfying adjustment to retirement for married couples.

Relationships with Friends

Impending retirement may stimulate friendship formation. Weiss and Lowenthal (1975) found that both men and women made new friends before and following the retirement transition, with women's friendships becoming more complex and multidimensional than they were during the middle adult years. A person's tendency to make new friends may de-pend on how much the workplace was a source of friends before retire-ment (Rawlins, 1992). Friendships based primarily on common instru-mental goals or interests may drop out of the network, leaving room for friendships based more on socioemotional connections between people (like intimacy). The need for emotional support from friends seems to be minimal, because retirement, on average, is a pleasant transition (McCal-lum, 1986).

Widowhood

The Concern in Context

Adjusting to the death of a spouse may be the most difficult normative adjustment many adults make during their lives (Holmes & Rahe, 1967). Because women routinely outlive their husbands, 11 out of every 12 peo-ple widowed are women (McCallum, 1986). Owing to this overwhelming preponderance of women among the widowed, much of the research in this area has sampled only women.

The death of a spouse creates major upheaval for those who experi-ence it (Lopata, 1979; McCallum, 1986). Widows go through a period of bereavement that can last for a year or more. They must master tasks that were previously the spouse's responsibility. For widows who have been homemakers, the death of a spouse may mean the end of a lifelong occu-pation (Pitcher & Larson, 1989). Finally, widows must rebuild their so-cial lives as single people.

Relationships with Family and Friends

The presence of other satisfying and intimate relationships appears to be an important buffer between the widow and the physical or emotional illnesses that can follow the loss of a spouse. The presence of intimate relationships in the network predicts shorter, less severe depressions following the spouse's death (Dimond, Lund, & Caserta, 1987). After the first year, widows are generally as integrated into their communities as comparable nonwidowed women, and are equal to them in the degree to which they seek emotional support and experience stress (Pellman, 1992).

Close relationships can also be a source of stress when friends and kin respond to the widow's grief insensitively. Common complaints among widows are that friends and acquaintances attempt to run their lives and tell them what to do, even to the point of telling them how to grieve (Pitcher & Larson, 1989). The strain of the loss may cause tempers to flare among family members who are making the arrangements that follow the death of a loved one.

Despite the conflicts, widows tend to list their children as their most important "emotional supporters" (Lopata, 1979). Grown children provide the widow the most respect, make her feel important, and contribute most to her feelings of enjoyment. Possibly, grown children are best able to fulfill widows' needs for what R. S. Weiss (1986) called a "reliable alliance," or a relationship we can count on during difficult times to provide instrumental and emotional aid. This may be our most crucial interpersonal need during a crisis. The perception by widows that their children are their most intimate partners following bereavement may be accounted for in part by the crucial need for a reliable alliance that children fulfill.

Intimate friends may become a more important resource after the early bereavement period. Friends, especially other widows, are important sources of intimate conversation and companionship, perhaps because they have a positive impact on widows' morale (Arling, 1976) and serve as an important buffer against loneliness (Lewittes, 1989). The quality of interactions between friends determines whether they are perceived as supportive. In McCallum's (1986) study of 327 Australian widows, interactions that encouraged the expression of feelings were considered most helpful.

Widowhood can create changes in the friendship network. A spouse's death may result in the discontinuation of relationships with his or her friends and work associates and with couples with whom the couple socialized (Lopata, 1979). The loneliness widows face, even within a stable network, may arise from lapses in friendships that depended on the couple-to-couple relationship for their continuance (McCallum, 1986).

Romantic Relationships

A significant majority of widowed women do not plan or wish to remarry (Lopata, 1979), as compared to widowed men, who are more likely to seek and find romantic partners (McCallum, 1986). There are many factors that contribute to this: Women say they enjoy their independence and doubt they could find a man as good as their late husband (Lopata, 1979). Moreover, they fear that another man may become ill, just as their late husband did, and they do not want to love and lose again. Unlike male widows, who often live longer if they remarry (McCallum, 1986), female widows who marry do not seem to have any health advantages (Lopata, 1979). Further, female widows may be sensitive to gender-specific community and family pressures that restrict the range of options they have for meeting and getting to know potential mates. Finally, female widows may not remarry simply because there are so few single men in their cohort. Men die 7 to 8 years earlier than women, and men's second marriages may be to women who are younger than they are (Lopata, 1979; Sontag, 1972).

When female widows do form romantic relationships, they tend to be with men they have met since their husband's death and to involve at least weekly contact (Lopata, 1979). Unless women are living with these men, however, they do not mention them as important members of their support systems. New husbands, on the other hand, are important intimate partners and companions (Lopata, 1979).

Religious Participation

The Concern in Context

Adults may become more concerned with spirituality as they get older. An analysis of archival data from 3,648 American adults of all ages was conducted by Cornwall (1989) and revealed age-related trends in religious observance: Church/synagogue attendance increases steadily throughout the life span for men whereas it levels off for women during their early 60s. Frequency of personal prayer and feeling close to God increases steadily for both men and women. In all cases and at all ages women tend to be more religious than men.

Religious Participation and Intimate Relationships

When religious participation is accompanied by social activity at the individual's place of worship, it has the potential of facilitating the formation of intimate relationships (Cornwall, 1989; Lopata, 1979; McCallum,

1986). Jerrome (1992) studied the role of Christian-church-affiliated fellowship groups on the friendships of older women and men in Britain. She found that within the women's groups small circles of tight-knit friends could enjoy group activities together. The women formed strong attachments to their fellowship groups and to the leaders, as well as to their own circle of friends.

Church fellowships may be better places for women to enjoy old friends than to make new ones (Jerrome, 1992). While newcomers joined the groups for their spiritual benefits (prayer and Bible study) and perhaps for card games, many complained that groups were cliquish. Once a group of old friends identified themselves as a unit, they used a variety of exclusionary techniques to ensure that new group members did not intrude. While setting boundaries on subgroup membership seemed to foster and maintain the intimacy among members within the group, it excluded others.

Jerrome (1992) also observed fellowships of men and found less emphasis in these groups on exclusivity. Exchanges within the larger group were characterized by self-disclosure, mutual support, and companionship. Intimacy in the men's group came in the form of reminiscences. Sometimes stories involved shared experiences, which seemed to reinforce the strength of the bonds among group members.

Health and Physical Change

The Concern in Context

People become preoccupied with physical changes and declining health as they get older. It is safe to say that the physical changes associated with aging are rarely welcomed and are likely to be a concern or preoccupation at some point for each person during late adulthood.

Changes in strength, stamina, and physical appearance actually become noticeable earlier in adulthood, in the years between 40 and 65 (Bee, 1992). Most adults notice that their bodies have become less predictable and tire more easily. In late adulthood additional changes in height, weight, and body shape occur (Bee, 1992). Some older adults develop chronic illnesses that, while not fatal by any means, can cause discomfort and limit activity (e.g., arthritis, osteoporosis). More serious illnesses, of course, will further restrict activity.

Relationships with Friends

Adults' preoccupations with health will undoubtedly affect their interactions with friends. Friends may find themselves talking about their own health and gossiping about others' bouts of illness or infirmity. Older adults who are healthy may spend their time providing assistance to sick friends and offering reassurance, comfort, and material aid.

Whether they are preoccupations or not, however, health and stamina mediate any relationship that exists between older adults' psychological needs and their ability to seek out friends to fulfill those needs. The most obvious impact is that of good health: The longer adults survive, the more likely they are to outlive their friends (Matthews, 1986). Conversely, poor health affects older adults' ability to maintain friendships by limiting their mobility, energy level, and mood. The effects of declining health may therefore be felt most keenly when older adults seek to share companionable activities. Intimacy can be affected, too, however, when "friends start slipping mentally" (Matthews, 1986, p. 117). As one 90-year-old respondent in Matthews's study of old-age friendship noted, sometimes just remembering a lunch date is a challenge for her friend.

Relationships with Romantic Partners

The impact of changes in an adult's physical stamina seems to be felt first in the sexual relationship (H. Kaplan, 1974). Changes in the frequency of sexual activity and in the intensity of sexual feeling are normal results of the aging process. These changes are different for women and men. For men, the intensity of genital sexual feeling begins declining in young adulthood and is followed later by decreases in frequency of orgasm and increases in length of the refractory period. By age 66, most men need more prolonged and direct genital stimulation than previously to sustain an erection (Kaplan, 1974). For women, maximum intensity of sexual feeling and frequency of orgasm seem to occur much later, between ages 30 and 40, and decline quite slowly thereafter.

If men's concerns are more likely to interfere with a couple's sexual relationship than women's, it may be because men's sexual changes are more obvious. A husband may feel inadequate when he compares his own changing sexual stamina with his wife's, which may not be declining noticeably (Kaplan, 1974). It is feelings of inadequacy, more than the physical changes of aging, that may inhibit a husband's enjoyment of sexual intimacy.

Whether changing sexual functioning will have a detrimental, neutral, or even positive effect on a couple's sexual intimacy is dependent on the quality of their relationship. Couples need intimate communication to keep one another informed of their changing sexual preferences and needs. Kaplan (1990) has observed that couples who remain sexually active do so because they can adapt to the normal changes of aging by varying their sexual activity. The data of the 1953 study by Kinsey et al. show that many couples can accommodate successfully.

Integrity

The Concern in Context

The imminence of death may create in the very old a preoccupation with remembering, reviewing, and reintegrating their "one and only lifetime" (Butler, 1974; Erikson, 1963). Optimally, people feel that they have left a positive imprint on the world while passing through it and are not preoccupied with regrets and remorse about what they could have or should have done (Erikson, 1963).

Integrity and Intimate Relationships

Empirical work on integrity in old age is difficult to find, and the role intimate partners play in helping the older adult construct a sense of integrity is not well documented. Intimate partners, particularly friends and romantic partners, may assist one another in what Butler (1974) called the "life review." The life review allows older adults to achieve a sense of integrity, meaning, and perspective (Lipman, 1986). Friends and romantic partners may aid and encourage each other to construct and reconstruct the memories of a lifetime. During a life review, older adults may bring up memories and reminiscences that have caused regret. A fresh perspective can encourage acceptance.

Old friends who have a shared past may especially cherish opportunities to reminisce. Older adults prefer spending time with long-standing friends over new friends (e.g., Bell, 1981), perhaps because shared reminiscing is an important function of old-age friendship. Together, through trading or embellishing one another's stories, old friends can verbalize the many links between the person of yesterday and today. Perhaps together friends can gain a sense of continuity and of legacy.

SUMMARY AND CONCLUSIONS

This chapter addresses the bulk of the life span, beginning before midlife and continuing into late adulthood. In contrast to changes that occur earlier in life, life-stage-related changes during middle and late adulthood are often gradual and only roughly correspond to chronological age. Comparisons between one epoch of the life span and another, however, reveal some patterns. Unfortunately, the research data are quite limited in many areas. How pervasive certain concerns are at different life stages still needs to be documented. Research results indicating life-stage-related changes in intimate relationships need to be replicated in many cases.

Intimate contact does not seem to increase in the romantic relationships of middle adulthood. In fact, the high levels of intimacy in early marriage rarely persist. Marital satisfaction and relational intimacy typically decline after the first year or two (Lowenthal et al., 1977). Declines in satisfaction may be especially pronounced for women when they unexpectedly confront sex-typed roles following the birth of a child (Ruble et al., 1988) and when their needs for intimacy are not met (Hite, 1987).

Opportunities for intimacy between romantic partners and between friends also decline following the transition to parenthood (Belsky et al., 1985). By middle adulthood, people report having less time for friends than at any other time in their lives (Cohen, 1992). While women's friendships remain more intimate than men's, on average, both sexes report less time for friends than they would like (Dickens & Perlman, 1981). In contrast, young adults' relationships with their parents may benefit from the transition to parenthood (Frank et al., 1988).

Adults report that relationships with their children are both a joy and a burden (Bretherton et al., 1989). Parents usually think more about their children's welfare than their own within those relationships (Whitbourne, 1986). When asked, however, they acknowledge that children meet many of their interpersonal needs (Ambert, 1992; Carbery, 1993).

Late adulthood, compared with the middle adult years, is a time of resurgence in intimate relationships. Satisfaction and intimacy in marital relationships seem to increase, especially after children are launched. For older adults with romantic partners, sexual activity continues, although perhaps less frequently (H. Kaplan, 1990). Relationships with grown children become older adults' most intimate relationships (Connidis & Davies, 1990). Relationships with friends, especially for women, are rewarding (R. Adams, 1987) and coincide with higher levels of well-being and life satisfaction.

Among the research areas reviewed in this chapter, the stress-buffering effects of older adults' intimate relationships have received the most attention. For example, a growing body of evidence demonstrates the importance of intimate relationships to widows. Intimate interactions with grown children and friends clearly help widows cope constructively with bereavement, lifestyle changes, and reintegration into their communities as single people (Dimond, Lund, & Caserta, 1987).

Clearly, there is much still to be learned about the changes in intimate relationships that accompany different adult life stages and about the concerns and stresses that may elicit (or be elicited by) these changes. A few areas stand out as deserving more attention.

Currently, the interplay between adults' intimate relationships and working conditions is deservedly getting extensive attention in the literature (e.g., Barnett & Marshall, 1991; Barnett, Marshall, Raudenbush, & Brennan, 1993; Stoltz-Loike, 1992). It seems that Americans are working longer hours and having increasing difficulty integrating their work and family lives. Long hours and time conflicts create their own stress-related symptoms—and, perhaps, illnesses (Geller & Hobfoll, 1994). What has received less attention, however, is the impact of work–family conflicts on intimate interaction itself. Given the important benefits that people gain from intimate interaction, we should not ignore the implications of less time for it on people's well-being. Research should also attempt to identify working conditions that promote good relationships, not only between workers and their families but between coworkers. There is evidence that the presence of person-qua-person relationships in the workplace is associated with higher levels of job satisfaction (Fox & Hesse-Biber, 1983). Perhaps there are beneficial effects on intimate relationships outside of work as well.

We know little about relationships between adults and their parents. While there is evidence that older adults enjoy intimate relationships with their grown children (E. Peterson, 1989), there is little information about those relationships from the younger adults' perspective. Anecdotal data suggest that strife and conflict in relationships with parents create considerable unhappiness and stress for adults (e.g., H. Lerner, 1989). More information about factors that contribute to healthy functioning and intimacy in these relationships could therefore be useful.

Finally, more work should be devoted to understanding the parent–child relationship from the parents' point of view. As others have pointed out (Bretherton, 1991; Hartup, 1986), parents are themselves experiencing changes in their most prominent concerns, needs and preoccupations. These seem likely to affect the parent-child relationship. Although parenting practices and styles are frequently examined in light of their impact on children's development (e.g., Duck, 1993a), researchers are just beginning to consider how parents' concerns and preoccupations affect these parenting practices. Research examining the impact of parents' marital relationships (e.g., Cummings & Davies, 1994) and mood states (e.g., Downey & Coyne, 1990) on parenting practices and parent–child relationships is beginning to show promise (Vondra & Belsky, 1993). Attachment theorists have begun work exploring parents' preoccupations with their own upbringing as it affects their interactions with their children. Haft and Slade (1989), for example, suggested that

parents who retain strong unpleasant emotions about their own upbringing may misattune to their children's affect in order to preserve their own
emotional equanimity. They found that the need to maintain emotional
equanimity emerges because, by parents' own reports, witnessing children's affect can flood parents with childhood memories and the negative
emotions associated with them. This work has also revealed, however,
that parents can "rework" their memories and the associated emotions
and thereby avoid insensitive interactions with their own children
(Bretherton, 1990). When researchers understand better what parents'
needs and concerns are and how parents typically go about addressing
those need and concerns, the determinants of effective parenting should
become more apparent.

What clearly emerges from the reviews in this chapter and the last is
that adulthood is characterized by as many, if not more, life-stage-related
changes in intimate relationships as is childhood. Changes in life-stage-
specific demands, and therefore concerns, of adults may determine which
relationships are most intimate, which are most important, which demand the most time and energy, and which are most rewarding for any
given adult. These changes may then influence which relationships most
affect and reflect adults' adjustment to the normative concerns of each
life stage. The impact of intimate relationships on adults' well-being
would therefore seem to depend on life-stage-related developments in
adults' lives.

PART THREE

INTIMACY PROCESSES

Intimate Interactions

Two soft, unmistakably feminine arms were clasped about
his neck; a warm cheek was pressed against his, and
simultaneously there was the sound of a kiss . . . [and] all of
him, from head to foot, was full of a strange new feeling
which grew stronger and stronger. . . . He wanted to dance,
to talk, to run into the garden, to laugh aloud. . . . He
quite forgot that he was round-shouldered and
uninteresting, that he had lynx-like whiskers and an
"undistinguished appearance."

—ANTON CHEKHOV, *The Kiss*

In this chapter I look more closely at intimate interactions themselves
and the processes by which intimate behaviors elicit intimate experiences
in those who participate in them. It is important to understand how intimate behavior elicits intimate experience, because intimacy's beneficial
effects on individual health and well-being likely stem from effects of intimate experiences that are repeated over time. In other words, perhaps
intimate interactions have enduring positive outcomes for individual
adaptation and relationship functioning because of the positive feelings
and perceptions of understanding they involve.

Theory and research support the notion that both aspects of intimate experience—positive affect and perceptions of understanding—can
enhance individual well-being. The healing effects of positive affect have
been well documented (Carson & Butcher, 1992). Some positive outcomes from intimate experiences would be expected, then, because by definition they include positive affect. It is unlikely, however, that the beneficial effects of intimate experiences would come from positive affect
alone. After all, the literature reviewed in the introduction to this book
indicates specific health benefits from relationships that are *intimate* as

opposed to only enjoyable or otherwise positive (e.g., Brown, Bhrolchain, & Harris, 1975).

A number of theorists have converged on the notion that perceptions of being understood are important to well-being. Cooley's (1902) notion of the "looking glass self" refers to the important impact of others' feedback on a positive, clearly defined self-concept. Sullivan (1953) said that "validation" (i.e., being understood and accepted) is critical to the development of a healthy personality. Kohut (1980) believed that a need for "empathic mirroring," similar to Sullivan's concept of validation, is innate and present from birth. Rogers (1974) said, "The individual human being has a profound need to be fully known and fully accepted . . . [there is a stress now] on the development-inducing and growth-promoting character of the basic human encounter" (p. 11). Both the positive affect and the perceptions of understanding that intimate interactions provide are therefore likely to enhance well-being.

Because intimate interactions, and intimate experiences in particular, exert beneficial effects on individual well-being, it is important to understand when, how, and under what circumstances people are likely to have intimate experiences. Researchers have recognized the importance of identifying links between interaction behavior and experience for over a decade. Reis (1984a) wrote, "There is an important distinction to be drawn between social support and social interaction. . . . How does the occurrence of the [latter] lead to the perception of the [former]? At some level, feeling supported must be based on the conduct of actual interaction" (p. 29). The same question can be raised about the association between experiencing intimacy and intimate behavior. The following example illustrates the links between intimate behavior and experience:

> Katie has been listening to an uninspiring lecture for nearly an hour and has found her eyelids dropping more than once. Suddenly, the speaker catches her attention by making a substantial factual error. Amused and now awake, Katie, without reflection, looks in the direction of her close friend and colleague, Grant, who is sitting several rows away, to see if he caught the error. To her delight, he has simultaneously turned in her direction. When their eyes meet, both mime raised eyebrows and wide-open eyes in feigned horror. Both smile and turn back to the speaker. Katie's feelings of warmth and amusement persist for several minutes.

Katie and Grant have experienced a moment of intimacy. Their interaction was intimate because what they shared was totally private. Katie's experience of intimacy consisted of positive feelings (warmth toward Grant) and a perception that she and Grant understood each other's meaning (see Duck, 1994a). Their intimate behaviors were all non-verbal. Each used eye contact to seek out the other and then used a facial expression to express and thereby share amusement.[1]

In this chapter I draw from the literature on intimate interactions to identify nonverbal and verbal behaviors that may affect experiences of intimacy. Because the literature rarely addresses experiences of intimacy per se, studies of attraction and liking, for example, have been used to provide clues about behaviors that elicit intimate experiences.

In the bottom half of Figure 8.1 is a simple account of the direct effects of intimate behavior on intimate experience. I have depicted A's behavior as evoking an experience of intimacy in B. B's experience of intimacy, in turn, prompts B to behave intimately with A. B's intimate behavior then evokes an intimate experience in A, who is inspired to continue behaving intimately. This simple account of mutual influence draws from theories of communication such as the one described by Raush et al. (1974). In their model, each behavior by Partner A is associated with a finite set of possible responses from Partner B. Each response in the set has its own probability of occurrence, given Partner A's initial behavior. Because each partner's behavior constrains the other's, their interaction constitutes a mutual influence system. Raush et al. also emphasize the role played by the partners' thoughts and feelings. Partners' interpretations and emotional reactions to one another affect how they behave, further constraining the range of interactions they can have. These internal events are therefore critical mediators of the association between Partner A's and Partner B's behavior.

This chapter does more than address simple interrelationships between intimate behavior and intimate experience, however. It also considers the impact of *contextual factors* on these interrelationships. Contextual factors determine whether behavior influences experience and how much and in what direction it does so.

The top half of Figure 8.1 depicts the contextual factors that influence intimate interactions. This discussion includes contextual factors because simple, direct links between interactions and experiences are rare. Associations between behavior and experience almost always depend on something: the physical surroundings, the personalities involved, the cultural backgrounds of the partners, and so forth. Nevertheless, studies of intimate interaction have often treated contextual factors as background, that is, as elements that are acknowledged but barely discussed (Duck, 1993b; Duck & Miell, 1986; Parks & Eggert, 1991). These factors are so important, however, that relationships between behavior and experiences of intimacy can rarely be discussed without reference to them.

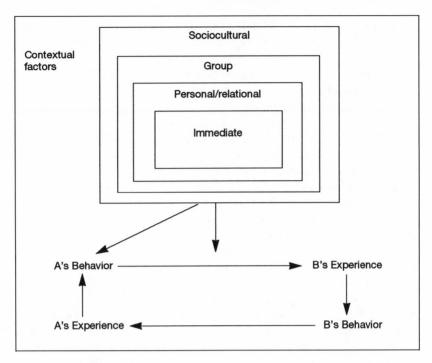

FIGURE 8.1. Intimate behavior and intimate experience in context.

Figure 8.1 depicts two ways that contextual variables may exert an impact on intimate interactions. First, these factors may affect the behavior of interaction partners directly; this effect is indicated by the diagonal arrow. Second, context *modifies* the relationship between behavior and experience; the vertical arrow depicts this effect.

This chapter therefore proposes a second notion, namely, that the benefits of intimacy can only be understood in context. In other words, no behavior or adaptation is effective in all contexts. To shed light on this proposal, in this chapter I address a range of contextual factors that could contribute to behavior and experience in intimate interactions. With that objective in mind, I have developed a typology of contextual factors. This typology borrows heavily from a scheme proposed by R. Adams and Blieszner (1992, 1994). In this scheme contextual factors can be placed on a continuum of immediacy or distance relative to the space-and-time frame of the interaction (R. Adams, 1993). On this continuum more immediate contextual factors are embedded within more distal ones. The purpose of the typology is to ensure that a range of contextual factors receives attention.

My discussion of contextual factors has two other objectives for which Adams and Blieszner's (1994) framework is relevant. First, I propose that both psychological and social structural factors impinge on intimate interactions. Adams and Blieszner constructed their model to serve as a framework for the integration of psychological and sociological variables. In their framework psychological variables are "personality, motives, and personal preferences . . . that is, *psychological dispositions*" (p. 168, emphasis in original). Social structural factors are "differing levels of power, prestige and wealth and thus different opportunities for and constraints on behaviors . . . cultural expectations about how people should act; role demands; and the availability, accessibility or appropriateness of spending time in various types of contexts" (Adams & Blieszner, 1994, p. 168). The mutually embedded contextual factors depicted in Figure 8.1 include both psychological and social structural variables.

Second, like Adams and Blieszner, I hope to encourage researchers to look beyond "proxy variables" to directly assess concepts of interest. According to Adams and Blieszner, proxy variables are easily obtainable measures that stand in for factors that are more relevant to a particular framework but are difficult to measure. An individual's sex, for example, is a typical "proxy variable" for constructs such as different levels of power, prestige, and wealth, as well as for different personality characteristics.

I have used Adams and Blieszner's framework as a springboard for the development of a typology of contextual factors. I created the four-category framework in Figure 8.1 with several objectives in mind: (1) to organize the literature on intimate interactions and to expose the gaps in our knowledge; (2) to maximize opportunities to consider psychological and social structural variables within the same framework; and (3) to show by means of its hierarchical structure how such immediately accessible variables as sex and race serve as windows onto higher-level contextual variables such as group and sociocultural norms. The four levels of context to be considered here are as follows: the immediate level, the personal/relational level, the group level, and the sociocultural systems level.

At the *immediate level* are the contextual factors closest in space and time to the interaction itself. The nature of the occasion and the physical surroundings exemplify immediate contextual factors. Other examples are the purpose of the setting, the number and characteristics of people present, time of day, proximity allowed by the physical layout, degree of privacy, and so forth. In the example of the intimate interaction between

Katie and Grant, the immediate context of a crowded lecture hall may have served to intensify their experience of intimacy. The nature of the occasion and the physical layout of the environment presented many obstacles to contact (e.g., the necessity for quiet, the physical distance between them, the large number of other people present, and the potential difficulty of getting each other's attention). Their pleasure at sharing understanding may therefore have been intensified by surprise they felt in experiencing the interaction.

At the *personal/relational level* are contextual factors specific to these particular individuals in this particular relationship. The personal/relational level includes the individual histories and characteristics of each participant (e.g., expectations, assumptions, and vulnerabilities), the history and definition of their relationship (e.g., marital partners, friends, new acquaintances), and the outcomes of those histories (e.g., relationship satisfaction). Because of their individual histories and inherited proclivities, people may develop certain characteristic ways of thinking and behaving (motives and traits) that affect their intimate interactions across partners (Cook, 1994). For example, an individual with a fear of intimacy may hesitate to self-disclose even with a trustworthy partner (Descutner & Thelen, 1991). An individual with a secure attachment style should be willing to seek comfort from a friend or romantic partner when feeling anxious (Simpson et al., 1992).

The type of relationship and the partners' history together are also likely to affect their intimate interactions. Some of these effects may be direct. For example, a husband's disclosure of sad feelings may not be met with sympathy from his wife if he is chronically depressed and she has grown weary of listening (Coyne, 1976). In Katie and Grant's case, a long-standing collegial relationship increased the likelihood that each would be interested in the other's reaction and would therefore look in the other's direction.

Some effects may be indirect. Relationship history may affect relationship norms, which in turn affect interaction. For example, let us say that Katie and Grant had established a norm of not engaging in intimate interaction when one of them is facing a deadline, a norm that grew out of negative experiences they had when trying to maintain contact while one was pressed for time. That norm would now determine when Katie and Grant are likely to have intimate contact.

The *group level* refers to the social groups and networks in which the individual and the dyad are embedded. Some of these groups may be embedded within one another, and dyads may be embedded within many groups. Groups seem most likely to affect intimate interaction via group norms. For example, a brother and sister exist within the context of the same family; family rules that discourage intimate interaction could set limits on the depth of their self-disclosures to one another (Cook, 1994). The norms of a professional organization to which Katie and Grant belong would create conditions that could either facilitate or impede intimate interactions between them. For example, the organization's annual meetings might provide opportunities for its members to socialize, and Katie and Grant might take advantage of these opportunities.

Larger social groups also have norms that are likely to affect intimate interaction. For example, individuals in the United States with a Hispanic background describe themselves as less self-disclosing than individuals with a Western European background (LeVine & Franco, 1981). Findings like these suggest that broad cultural groups may have different interaction norms that affect dyadic interactions.

Finally, the broadest contextual level is what I call the *sociocultural systems level*. Sociocultural factors frequently manifest themselves as norms and are the most abstract. They are best expressed in broad statements about appropriate and expected behavior within a culture. Sociocultural norms are difficult to assess because they are often unarticulated and are therefore outside awareness. Exposure to alternatives is often the only means by which sociocultural norms become evident to people. When these norms do become explicit, people can be highly resistant to violating them, and they react negatively to others who do (P. Andersen, 1993). Sociocultural norms are accepted as human nature, "the way things are," or "the facts of life" (P. Andersen, 1993). People may view them as moral imperatives.

The third purpose of this chapter is to discuss mechanisms by which associations between intimate behavior, intimate experience, and context come to exist. Raush et al. (1974) have argued that one partner's behavior in an interaction shapes the other's experience by activating a certain set of schemas within the other. A schema (or a working model or template) is an organized cognitive structure that gives meaning to experience (P. Andersen, 1993; Baldwin, 1992; Cross & Markus, 1993; Geis, 1993). It arises from previous experience and serves to integrate new experiences and old. These organized structures consist of affective and cognitive components and serve as links between the partner's behavior and internal experience (P. Andersen, 1993; Reis & Shaver, 1988). In my example, Katie interpreted the fact that Grant sought her out (visually) as an indication that he wanted to share his experience with her. Further, her interpretation of his facial expression was, "We are on the same wavelength!" Both interpretations were imbued with positive affect. Katie's interpretations, then, were the conduit by which Grant's behavior had a positive effect on Katie.

Just as behavior's impact on affect is determined by the schema that is activated in the interaction, so is the impact of context on affect influenced by contextual schemas. Different contextual factors elicit sets of schemas that, through observation and direct experience, contain expectations, assumptions, and feelings about those contexts (e.g., Fiske & Taylor, 1991; Markus & Zajonc, 1985). Gender is an especially potent example of such a contextual factor (e.g., Lott & Maluso, 1993). It is one of the first categories that children learn (e.g., Kohlberg, 1966) and one of the first components of the self-concept to be established (Slabey & Frey, 1975). It is also a central category for thinking about others (Cross & Markus, 1993). Gender-related schemas shape people's perceptions and actions without their awareness and exert profound effects on interactions (S. Fiske, 1993; Geis, 1993). Schemas affect interaction in part because they filter what we see and hear and what escapes our notice (Beall, 1993). These filtered perceptions then affect our behavior.

Schemas, then, may serve as "interpretive filters" (Reis & Shaver, 1988) that select certain aspects of interactions and people for our attention, imbue behavior and situations with meaning, and shape the final product of the person–situation interaction (Beall, 1993). The final product is, at the individual level, the ongoing stream of each participant's thoughts and feelings (intimate experience). At the dyadic level it is interaction behavior (intimate behavior). The more thoroughly we understand how individuals attribute meaning within their interactions, the better our understanding of how behaviors, persons, and contexts affect intimate experience (Duck, 1994a).

There are three specific objectives for this chapter. First is to review the literature on intimate behavior and experience and generate hypotheses about associations between these two aspects of intimate interactions. Second is to review the literature on contextual factors with the purpose of generating hypotheses about how they directly affect intimate behavior or how they modify its relationship with intimate experience. Third is to present inferences, based on existing research, about the processes by which one person's behavior and the context in which it occurs might elicit another person's schemas, which then filter attention and guide behavior. The first part of this chapter addresses nonverbal behavior, the latter half verbal behavior.

NONVERBAL BEHAVIOR

Nonverbal behavior likely plays "an underestimated role . . . in the quality of [intimate] communication" (Keeley & Hart, 1994, p. 135). Keeley and Hart defined nonverbal communication as "signs and symbols . . . that qualify as potential messages by virtue of their regular and consistent use and interpretation" (p. 136). Nonverbal behavior may contribute as much to people's intimate experiences as verbal behavior, perhaps even more.

Research suggests that several types of nonverbal behavior can have direct effects on intimate experience (e.g., Keeley & Hart, 1994; M. Patterson, 1988). The bulk of the evidence, however, shows that the nature of these effects depends heavily on the interaction context. Thus far, the immediate context has received the most attention in the literature on nonverbal behavior (e.g., Kleinke, 1986).

Three categories of nonverbal behavior can be labeled as intimate. First, nonverbal "involvement behaviors" include physical proximity, gaze, touch, body lean, facial expressiveness, postural openness, gesturing, head nods, and vocal cues such as intonation, speech rate, and pauses (M. Patterson, 1984). These are called involvement behaviors because they display attentiveness, interest, and participation in interaction. Second, touch can be an intimate behavior; touch seems to intensify and is also prompted by intimate experiences (Thayer, 1988). Finally, the extensive and prolonged bodily contact involved in sexual activity is a third type of intimate nonverbal behavior.

Nonverbal Involvement and the Experience of Intimacy

The impact of nonverbal involvement behavior is illustrated in the following description of two distinctly different interactions:

> An-Mei and Kathy sit across from one another at a small table in a sidewalk café. They each lean forward across the table as they converse, barely taking their eyes away from one another's faces. Both are smiling as they talk. Two tables away sit Rebecca and Charles. Rebecca is leaning forward and gazing at Charles, but she is not smiling. Charles sits back in his chair, does not smile, and gazes not at Rebecca but around the room or over her head.

All we know about the interactions of our four protagonists is based on the nonverbal involvement behaviors each is displaying. Despite this limitation, most of us could make reasonable inferences about the interactions based only on those behaviors. Perhaps we would guess that An-Mei and Kathy are enjoying one another's company, that each is interested in what the other has to say, and that they like one another. Similarly, using the same kind of information, we might surmise that Rebecca and Charles are not enjoying each other and that Charles is withdrawing from Rebecca; few of us would assume that their current interaction is intimate. That such different inferences can be made about these two conversations is a testament to the potent informative value of nonverbal involvement behaviors.

Interest in nonverbal behavior arose when theorists and researchers observed its previously unacknowledged but powerful impact on communication (Argyle & Dean, 1965). According to Mehrabian (1971), this interest originated when research on meaning expanded beyond its verbal aspects (e.g., Osgood, Suci, & Tannenbaum, 1957). Researchers soon discovered how seemingly small gestures (looking away, moving away) conveyed potent messages that could override the meaning of such verbal content as "I'm not mad at you" (Bateson, Jackson, Haley, & Weakland, 1956). Research on nonverbal interaction behavior has continued efforts to identify systematic linkages between behavior, context, and people's reactions to one another. The work has been surprisingly divorced, however, from theory and research on intimate relationships.

Each nonverbal involvement behavior has a demonstrated impact on the experience of intimacy. High levels of mutual gaze have been associated with phenomena such as liking (Argyle, Ingham, Alkema, & McCallin, 1973), love (Z. Rubin, 1970), sexual involvement (Thayer & Schiff, 1975), friendship (Couits & Schneider, 1976), and positive evaluations of interactions (Burgoon, Buller, Hale, & deTurck, 1984). Closer seating distance conveys friendship and liking (Gifford, 1991). Forward body lean conveys attentiveness and emotional involvement while backward lean communicates indifference and detachment (Mehrabian, 1969). Smiling is a universally recognized indicator of liking, although, as M. Patterson (1982) pointed out, it is not completely reliable.[2] In the main, however, nonverbal involvement behaviors are associated with intimate experience, that is, with liking, attraction, and enjoyment in interactions.

Intimate nonverbal behaviors are best understood as a subset of involving behaviors, because nonverbal involvement behaviors do not *exclusively* communicate personalness. These behaviors can communicate other messages, such as dominance submission (Kleinke, 1986) and general positivity and rapport (Tickle-Degnen & Rosenthal, 1990). People can also summon them at will for impression management purposes (M. Patterson, 1987). In other words, not all involving interactions are intimate, but all intimate interactions are involving (assuming they are face-to-face).

Touch and the Experience of Intimacy

Touch seems to greatly affect intimate experience, perhaps because it eliminates the space between people. More than any other nonverbal interaction behavior, touch may intensify experiences of intimacy (Thayer, 1986). Certain kinds of touch have been identified that may be sufficient in and of themselves to create an intimate experience (assuming they are wanted or invited). Based on daily recordings of university students' experiences with touch, Jones and Yarbrough (1985) identified three types of touch that nearly always foster intimate experience. All convey positive affect and carry a nonverbal relational message. "Inclusion touches" (e.g., shoulders or knees touching) are sustained touches that convey or draw attention to the act of being together; they are tactile statements of togetherness, usually involving lower body parts (legs, knees, hips, side-by-side hugs), and nearly always occur between lovers, spouses, or close friends rather than between family members. Sexual touches (e.g., long strokes of the hand up and down the body) express physical attraction or sexual intent; involving holding, caressing, or both, these are prolonged, involve multiple body parts, and move from one part of the body to another. A third type of touch, "affection touches" (e.g., hand on a shoulder, squeezing an arm), always communicates affection, in part because these touches are positive and in part because they do not express any other specific meaning. These affection touches express general positive regard for the other and include a wide range of behaviors.

The extent to which touch elicits intimate experience may depend on which parts of the body are touched. College students viewed face touching, for example, as more personal than handshakes, arm touches, or arms around the shoulder or waist (Burgoon, 1991). Jones and Yarbrough (1985) distinguished between "nonvulnerable" body parts (in the United States this includes hands, arms, elbows, shoulders, and upper-middle back) and "vulnerable" body parts (all others). The former are body parts that, by convention, can be touched by those with whom one does not have an intimate relationship.

Experiences of intimacy may be intensified when touch is sustained or prolonged. In some cultures, such as the United States and New Zealand, certain kinds of sustained affectionate touch (e.g., watching television while in one another's arms) occur rarely, except between lovers and spouses, even though these touches are not sexual.

Certain kinds of touch, then, may foster experiences of intimacy, particularly when they are sustained and involve vulnerable parts of the body. It is likely true as well that positive feelings and the perception of being understood, which constitute intimate experience, prompt people to touch one another.

Sexual Interaction and the Experience of Intimacy

People commonly define sexual interactions as intimate interactions. Sprecher and McKinney (1993) note that when researchers ask people what intimacy means to them, they are likely to include sexual contact among their answers (Helgeson et al., 1987; Waring et al., 1980). Researchers commonly include sexual intimacy in typologies of intimacy (Holt, 1977; Schaefer & Olson, 1981; Tolstedt & Stokes, 1983).

There are several ways in which dyadic sexual behavior can provide intimate experiences for participants. First, intimate behavior involves sharing that which is private. Sexuality is private behavior in most of the known societies on earth. Therefore, people experience the sharing of sexuality as intimate. Sprecher and McKinney (1993) noted that "all of the actions that typically occur in the sex act—being nude in front of one's partner, expressing to the partner what feels good, actually having sex, experiencing an orgasm—are considered to be very intimate self-disclosures" (p. 100). By participating in sexual activity with a particular partner, one is sharing personal, private aspects of the self that are not known to other kinds of intimate partners, such as family members and close friends. In many cultures the relative exclusiveness of sexual sharing contributes to its value as an intimate experience.

Conclusions

The foregoing review indicates that the relationship between nonverbal intimate behavior and intimate experience is robust. The investigations conducted thus far are limited, however, to a few intimate experiences (liking, attraction). There has also been little attempt to explore schemas that might link nonverbal behavior and intimate experience. As the next section suggests, these schemas may be elicited as much by the context of the behavior as by the behavior itself.

NONVERBAL INVOLVEMENT AND INTIMACY IN CONTEXT

The current research literature suggests that context influences whether certain nonverbal behaviors will occur and whether these behaviors will evoke experiences of intimacy. Most of the contextual variables scholars have explored thus far are at the immediate contextual level (i.e., in Figure 8.1, those in the central rectangle of the diagram). The following dimensions of immediate context appear to exert independent effects on partners' behavior within interactions and/or to modify the relationship between behavior and experience.

Nature of the Occasion

Occasions vary in their level of structure. Some occasions have clearly defined purposes and roles for the individuals involved while others do not. Structured occasions, with specific instrumental purposes, prescribe certain kinds of nonverbal behavior.

Highly structured occasions may elicit situational schemas (i.e., sets of expectations about the situation itself and the interpretations of behavior that follow from those expectations). Situational schemas may block or prevent intimate experiences, even when nonverbal behavior potentially elicits such experience. For example, touch serves a clearly structured purpose on occasions such as a visit to the physician or hairdresser, participating in a sport, or helping an infirm relative across the street. Situational schemas associated with haircuts, physical exams, and so forth would likely preclude interaction participants experiencing intimacy in association with touch. In support of this view, Tickle-Degnen and Rosenthal (1990) reported that nonverbal involvement behaviors are more facilitative of rapport in nonhelping than in helping interactions (i.e., conversations with therapists, nurses, or counselors). Perhaps schemas involving professional helpers invoke interpretations such as "She has to pay attention because of her role" instead of "She pays attention because she is interested in what I am saying and cares about me." As a result, the impact of nonverbal involvement behaviors on intimate experiences in professional "helping occasions" may be diluted.

By definition, unstructured occasions should have no particular situational schemas associated with them. Interaction partners should therefore not be constrained from interpreting nonverbal behavior as intimate. Perhaps this is why many touches that convey no other specific meaning convey affection (Jones & Yarbrough, 1985).

Most research on nonverbal intimate behavior takes place in the laboratory, with researchers imposing varying amounts of structure on participants. A common research procedure involves experimenters asking college students to talk about a prearranged topic for a specific time and purpose. This highly structured task probably maximizes participants' awareness that they are participating in a psychology experiment (as op-

posed to believing that they are just conversing freely), and would thereby elicit in them a "psychology experiment schema." This schema, in
turn, would affect how participants interpreted each other's behavior.
Even if both are sitting close together and self-disclosing personal information, this schema seems likely to block or minimize any intimate experience the partners might have. This is because they are more likely to attribute their interaction partners' behavior to the demand characteristics
of the situation than to any genuine liking the partner might feel. Yet,
with a few exceptions, the effects of structuring have not been systematically addressed. In order to observe people in an unstructured situation,
Ickes (1982) has surreptitiously videotaped pairs of friends as they were
supposedly waiting for an experimental procedure to begin. No method
has been devised yet for using Ickes' procedure to observe intimate interaction.

Function/Structure of the Physical Setting

Bedrooms, living rooms, automobiles, bars, classrooms, and church sanc-
tuaries—these settings have different functions and offer correspondingly
different opportunities for intimate interaction. The function of the setting likely exerts an independent influence on the kind of intimate behavior that will occur within it. A certain amount of sexual touching, for
example, is normal in a bar but not in a church (except, perhaps, during a
wedding ceremony).

There is evidence that the physical arrangements within the setting
directly affect nonverbal involvement behavior. For example, when two
strangers converse, a moderately close seating distance elicits the fewest
adjustments to nonverbal involvement behavior (Keeley & Hart, 1994).
When seating distance is manipulated in the laboratory (i.e., when unacquainted people are required to sit closer together or farther apart than
would be customary), people often adjust their nonverbal involvement
behaviors, such as gaze and body lean, in an apparent effort to compensate (Argyle & Dean, 1965; Gifford & O'Conner, 1986; Kleinke, 1986;
Wada, 1990). When their fellow participant sits too close, people avert
their gaze; when the other participant sits too far away, people will lean
farther forward or adjust their own seating to be closer. The physical
arrangements in a room may therefore directly affect nonverbal intimate
behavior.

The function of the physical setting may also modify the relationship between behavior and intimate experience. Consider this example:
Juan is attracted to coworker Mariela and imagines that it would be nice

to be closer to her. If she were to sit near him and lean toward him at a party, he would likely experience this positively and interpret it as a sign of budding involvement. In contrast, Mariela may sit only an inch or two away from him in a meeting room at work, but because of that room's function Juan does not experience intimacy in response to the behavior.

Mood

Participants' moods may directly affect involvement behavior in interactions. For example, depressed persons tend to gaze and smile less during interaction than nondepressed persons (Hops et al., 1987; Kleinke, 1986). Mood may also affect the relationship between behavior and experience. Depressed persons interpret critical reactions from others more negatively than do persons with normal mood and are more likely to remember negative exchanges (e.g., Hoehn-Hyde, Schlottmann, & Rush, 1982; Kowalik & Gotlib, 1987). Depression may modify the relationship between intimate behavior and experience, therefore, by increasing the likelihood that behavior will elicit negative schemas, thereby reducing the likelihood that behavior will elicit positive affect. Firm conclusions await further investigation.

Interaction Partner Attractiveness or Likability

Research evidence currently shows that the attractiveness of interaction partners exerts independent effects on nonverbal involvement behaviors such as proximity, smiling (Burgoon et al., 1984), and gaze in both U.S. (Kaplan, Firestone, Klein, & Sodikoff, 1983; Kleinke, Meeker, & La Fong, 1974) and Japanese samples (Wada, 1990). Moreover, same-sex pairs of previously unacquainted college students will move closer to one another if they come to like one another more as they interact (M. Patterson, 1982).

Limited evidence indicates that attraction and/or liking may be salient moderators of the relationship between behavior and experience. Violations of conventional norms for interactions between strangers, such as avoiding gaze, are less likely to interfere with experiences of intimacy when one's interaction partner is attractive or liked (Kleinke, 1986). In addition, Burgoon (1991) found that certain kinds of touch elicit more pronounced experiences of intimacy when they come from attractive, rather than unattractive, people. An arm around the shoulders in a same-sex dyad is viewed as significantly more affectionate when the toucher is attractive than when he or she is not.

Gender

Few contextual variables have been studied more than gender, and few have been found more likely to affect intimate behavior. At the immediate contextual level gender refers to sex (i.e., whether the persons interacting are female or male). At this level gender appears to (1) exert direct effects on nonverbal behavior, (2) modify the association between behavior and intimate experience, and (3) interact with other contextual variables in its effect on behavior–experience relationships.

Independent effects of gender on nonverbal behavior show that women engage more frequently in involvement behaviors than do men. Women engage in higher levels of gaze and persist in a face-to-face orientation more than men do (Abele, 1986; Gifford, 1991; Kleinke, 1986; Wada, 1990). After reviewing the literature, M. Patterson (1982) concluded that women also maintain closer interaction distances and engage in more frequent touching than do men. When male subjects were forced (by the experimental situation) to sit at predetermined relatively close distances, they appeared to compensate by reducing their level of gaze, particularly in same-sex dyads (Rosenfeld, Breck, Smith, & Kehoe, 1984). Female subjects maintained involvement behaviors at closer sitting distances than did male subjects.

The relationship between nonverbal behavior and the experience of intimacy is also significantly modified by participant sex. As evidenced by their self-disclosure levels, female subjects experienced more intimacy with a stranger who gazed at them than with one who did not gaze as much, while male subjects' responses were just the opposite (Ellsworth & Ross, 1975). In one study women tended to prefer a stranger who gazed more and tended to gaze more themselves when feeling more positively (Kleinke, Bustos, Meeker, & Standeski, 1973); this pattern was not observable in men.

The effects of gender are themselves modified by other contextual factors. Research on gaze (Rosenfeld et al., 1984) and on touch (Andersen & Leibowitz, 1978) indicates that the sex composition of the dyad, rather than the sex of either individual, affects gender-related patterns in nonverbal involvement. These studies found that men gaze and touch less than women do when interacting with a man but behave similarly to women when interacting with a woman.

Gender also modifies the impact of relationship type on nonverbal intimate behavior. Most studies of the direct effects of gender on nonverbal involvement involve interactions between strangers (e.g., Kleinke et al., 1973; Rosenfeld et al., 1984; Wada, 1990). Within established rela-

tionships gender effects appear to be reduced. In one study the level of acquaintance and type of relationship between the interaction partners
modified the effect of gender on touching (Guerrero & Andersen, 1991).
In established romantic relationships, women and men touch one another with comparable frequency whereas in new and developing relationships women, compared with men, refrained from initiating touch.

There is evidence, then, that gender affects how much and what
type of nonverbal intimate behavior will occur between interaction partners. At the immediate level, however, gender offers little in the way of
explanatory value. As I will show in subsequent sections, gender effects
serve intimacy researchers better as indicators of the effects of higher-level contextual factors than as explanations unto themselves.

Personal/Relational, Group, and Sociocultural Contexts

The contextual factors discussed thus far have all been immediate-level
variables. Research exploring the influence of higher-level contexts on
nonverbal intimate behavior is presently sparse enough to combine into a
single section. There are, nevertheless, a few studies suggesting that these
higher-level contextual levels affect nonverbal intimate behavior and
modify its relationship to intimate experience.

At the personal level a trait called "communication apprehension"
has predicted nonverbal involvement behavior. Communication apprehension refers to the tendency to get nervous and apprehensive in social
interaction. Communication-apprehensive people are more likely to
avert eye contact and to lean backward and are less likely to touch each
other during interaction than are individuals with little communication
apprehension (P. Andersen, 1993; Burgoon & Koper, 1984).

General attitudes toward touch may also affect nonverbal intimate
behavior. People who describe themselves as "touch avoidant" are, not
surprisingly, less likely to touch others (Andersen & Leibowitz, 1978).
Touch avoiders maintain greater physical distance during interactions as
well (Andersen & Sull, 1985) and have more negative attitudes toward
others who touch them than do "touch approachers" (P. Andersen,
1993).

Relationship type and history may also affect the presence and impact of nonverbal intimate behavior. Couples in love gaze at one another
more than do pairs of strangers (Z. Rubin, 1970) and engage in more affectionate touching (Jones & Yarbrough, 1985). In contrast, couples who
are experiencing high levels of conflict in their relationship gaze at one

another less, touch one another less, and sit farther apart than nondistressed couples (Beier & Sternberg, 1977).

Aspects of nonverbal behavior may also change as a function of relationship length. Complaints about mates who are no longer attentive are commonplace (Huston & Vangelisti, 1991). Sexual contact seems to decrease in frequency over time as well (Blumstein & Schwartz, 1983).

Contextual factors at the group and sociocultural level may affect intimate interactions through their association with powerful situational norms. Members of groups and cultures internalize social norms in the form of cognitive/affective situational schemas, which serve as blueprints for interpretations, emotions, and behavior within a particular class of situations (P. Andersen, 1993; Geis, 1993). Individuals differ, of course, in their willingness and ability to comply with group and sociocultural norms (Brown & Gilligan, 1992). The impact of these norms, then, is likely dependent on individual conformity to them.

People are aware of some group norms and of their own efforts to conform to or resist conforming to them. For example, Chapter 4 discusses gender-specific peer group norms that may encourage or even dictate certain kinds of nonverbal involvement behaviors (Tannen, 1990b). Brown and Gilligan (1992) found that adolescent girls are explicitly aware of peer group interaction norms and are actively engaged in shaping (or not shaping) their own behavior to match those norms. They are also aware of classmates' behavior toward norm violators, which is often rejecting, excluding, and defaming. As one writer aptly put it, when a man behaves in defiance of gender-specific interaction norms, it is "an act of courage . . . [because of the] judging, jeering band of other men in his mind . . . [that he is] playing to" (A. Gottlieb, 1993, p. 57). The violation of group norms, then, can carry heavy interpersonal costs for the individual who attempts to break the mold. After all, the "judging, jeering band of other men" is not only in one's mind (Thorne & Luria, 1986).

Sociocultural norms may also exist outside awareness yet still exert considerable influence on how people behave and interpret others' behavior. As P. Andersen (1993) noted, schemas containing sociocultural norms are often disguised as views about the way things are or should be. When exposure to alternatives brings unexamined norms into focus, people may express resistance to violating those norms and may react negatively when others do so (P. Andersen, 1993; Cross & Markus, 1993; Markus & Kitayama, 1991). As P. Andersen (1993) described it, "Americans believe that Arabs stand too close. Swedes think the French use too much eye contact. . . . The Japanese think Westerners talk too much" (p. 17).

Nonverbal Intimate Behavior and Intimate Experience: Concluding Thoughts

The preceding review suggests that nonverbal involvement behaviors evoke intimate experiences. As the review indicates, what little we know about nonverbal intimate behavior must often be gleaned from studies whose original intent was not to study intimacy. Consequently, information about its impact on intimate experience is uneven. For example, empirical research supports a link between nonverbal intimate behavior and affective intimate experience, such as liking, attraction, and enjoyment of the interaction. Scholars currently know little, however, about the impact of nonverbal behavior on perceptions of being understood. Similarly, research indicates that several factors in the immediate context, such as partner attractiveness and the structure and function of the physical setting, modify the influence of nonverbal intimate behavior on intimate experience. Furthermore, research indicates that the impact of the immediate context on intimate behavior can be further modified by other contextual variables, particularly gender. Research on other levels of context, however, is in its infancy.

I have proposed that nonverbal involvement behaviors contribute to experiences of intimacy because they are associated with positive schemas. Perhaps people apply these positive schemas to their interaction partners when their partner displays intimate nonverbal behaviors. There is reason to believe, for example, that in the United States such nonverbal involvement behaviors as maintaining gaze and turning toward the speaker signal attentiveness. Perhaps attentiveness schemas elicit interpretations like "She is really trying to understand me" or "She respects and values me." To the extent that they do, attentiveness is likely to be powerfully rewarding (Ivey, 1971) or, in Reis and Shaver's (1988) terms, "validating" (i.e., likely to encourage the speaker to think positively about himself or herself).

The impact of nonverbal behavior on the experience of intimacy may to some extent lie in its involuntary quality. M. Patterson (1988) noted that nonverbal behaviors can serve as signs of a person's internal experience (feelings, emotions, and motives). Our nonverbal interaction behavior is to some extent a direct manifestation of our internal state, bypassing our conscious control in its expression of that state (Duck, 1994a; Robbins & Haase, 1985). Although, as M. Patterson points out, people can manipulate these nonverbal signs to some extent in the interest of impression management, our control over these behaviors is less than the control we have over our verbal behavior. Perhaps because it emerges without (or despite) our conscious efforts at control, we are often unaware of our own nonverbal behavior. This lack of conscious control and our conversation partner's awareness of the uncontrolled quality of non-verbal behavior may contribute considerably to its impact on experience in interactions.[3]

VERBAL BEHAVIOR

Self-disclosure has overwhelmingly served as a focal point for research on verbally intimate behavior. Much of this research has been devoted to identifying its relevant dimensions (e.g., Chelune, Skiffington, & Williams, 1981), describing the impact of individual differences on self-disclosing behavior (e.g., Shaffer & Tomarelli, 1989), and predicting the conditions under which self-disclosure is likely to occur (e.g., Prager, 1986). Therefore, a large proportion of the following sections discuss self-disclosure.

The first part of this section reviews literature on direct effects of verbal intimacy on intimate experience. Three dimensions of self-disclosure are explored: content, depth, and immediacy; this is followed by a discussion of verbal responsiveness. This section proceeds with an eye toward identifying gaps in our knowledge that merit further study.

Self-Disclosure and the Experience of Intimacy

Self-disclosure, the revelation of personal and private information about the self, seems to be a central component of verbal intimacy (e.g., Waring, 1981; Waring et al., 1980). Married couples describe "sharing private thoughts, dreams, attitudes, beliefs, and fantasies" (Waring et al., 1980, p. 473) as central to intimacy in their relationships. College students rate self-disclosure as one of the most important components of intimacy (Helgeson et al., 1987; Monsour, 1992; Roscoe, Kennedy, & Pope, 1987). Unlike nonverbal indicators of involvement, which often occur below the level of conscious awareness, self-disclosure appears to be deliberate. People disclose, in part, to establish rapport with another and to provide a basis for a continuing relationship (Archer, 1987; Derlega & Grzelak, 1979; Prager et al., 1989).

Research evidence suggests that self-disclosure facilitates positive feelings between interaction partners (Altman & Taylor, 1973; Guerrero, Eloy, & Wabnik, 1993; S. Hendrick, 1981; see review by Dindia, 1994). Jourard (1959) initially proposed that reciprocal exchanges of self-disclosure would facilitate liking and attraction between strangers. Research supporting this premise shows that, at a moderate level of personalness, self-disclosure reciprocity increases liking and the expectation that a relationship will develop (Falk & Wagner, 1985; Jourard, 1959; Sunnafrank, 1988). Self-disclosure has been found to increase in breadth and depth, although not necessarily in simple linear fashion, as relationships develop (Altman & Taylor, 1973; Derlega, Metts, Petronio, & Margulis, 1993; Spencer, 1994).

Self-disclosure and liking are also associated within established relationships. Friends who regularly disclose personal, private information to one another like one another more than do those who are undisclosing (e.g., L. Miller, 1990). Verbal intimacy is also highly valued in romantic relationships by both men and women (Merves-Okin, Amidon, & Bernt, 1991; Rubin, Hill, Peplau, & Dunkel-Schetter, 1980). Self-disclosure is predictive of partners' satisfaction with their relationship (Burke, Weir, & Harrison, 1976; Cole & Goettsch, 1981; Hendrick, 1981; Levinger & Senn, 1967; Sprecher, 1987; Tolstedt & Stokes, 1984).

A few studies have indicated that self-disclosure enhances perceptions of understanding. Ickes, Stinson, Bissonnette, and Garcia (1990) found that self-disclosure enhanced mutual knowledge and understanding in previously unacquainted pairs of college students. Diaz and Berndt (1982) found that adolescent friends who had disclosed more to one another knew each other better. Shapiro and Swenson (1969) reported similar results with a sample of married couples. These studies often gauge understanding by asking partners to predict each other's responses to certain questions. Since perceptions of understanding do not always correlate perfectly with actual understanding (Acitelli, Douvan, & Veroff, 1993), future research exploring the link between self-disclosure and understanding should assess partners' *perceptions* in addition to their ability to predict.

The depth (or personalness) of self-disclosure varies along several dimensions, each of which seems to have direct effects on partners' intimate experiences. Scholars have paid particular attention to three such dimensions: (1) topic or content of disclosure, (2) emotional expressiveness of disclosure, and (3) immediacy of disclosure.

Topic or Content of Disclosure

People seem to agree about how personal or private certain kinds of disclosures are (Solano, 1986; Strassberg & Anchor, 1975; Taylor & Altman, 1966). Researchers have assumed that disclosures revealing one's vulnerabilities (e.g., "The most serious personal problem I have had during the last year was . . . "; Falk & Wagner, 1985, p. 561) should be perceived as most personal (L'Abate & Sloan, 1984). Disclosures that "lend little if any insight into . . . feelings or character" (Shaffer, Pegalis, & Cornell, 1991, p. 8), such as disclosures about tastes ("My favorite food is double chocolate fudge cake"), interests ("I enjoy fishing"), and preferences ("I'd rather see an opera than a rock-and-roll concert"), are perceived as less personal. Possibly, the more dependent one is on the discloser's report to gain the information, the more private it is. Disclosures about how one generally behaves, for example, are not as personal as disclosures about one's beliefs, motives, feelings, or fantasies (Lazowski & Andersen, 1990). Negative disclosures may be more personal than positive ones, but may also lead to less liking (Gilbert & Horenstein, 1975).

Emotional Content of Disclosure

There is evidence that people can make almost any topic of conversation more personal by embellishing their talk with expressions of feeling and emotion (e.g., Lazowski & Andersen, 1990; Morton, 1978). The most personal disclosures seem to combine the revelation of personal facts and the expression of feelings and emotions about the information (Howell & Conway, 1990; Morton, 1978). Revealing emotional reactions may be one way disclosers share the meaning personal information holds for them and the importance they attach to it (Morton, 1978). As Duck (1994a) has argued, this sense of shared meaning, rather than the shared personal information per se, may contribute most to experiences of intimacy for both partners.

We may understand better why disclosure of emotions augments intimate experience by making a distinction between *emotional expression* and *emotional communication*. Emotional expression (called "spontaneous expression" by Buck, 1989), based on innate tendencies to display certain kinds of motivational or emotional information, is largely involuntary. For example, raising one's voice, changing one's facial expression, shedding tears, and clenching one's jaw can all be involuntary responses to emotions. Emotional communication, in contrast, is learned and voluntary. It is socially based and composed of symbols. Verbalizations like "I'm uncomfortable with this" or "I'm overjoyed" or "I was so upset" are examples of emotional communication. Both emotional expression and emotional communication can inform us of an interaction partner's emotional state concerning the matter at hand.

There are nevertheless a couple of reasons why emotional communication, but not necessarily emotional expression, should invoke an intimate experience. First, listeners should make different attributions about emotional communication than about emotional expressions. Theoretically, partners should only interpret as emotional communications information that is deliberately shared or behavior that allows the partner to witness emotions. Without deliberateness, the signs of emotion are only signs and are therefore unlikely to be interpreted as acts of sharing. As Derlega et al. (1993) have argued, "The attributions we use to explain why someone is telling us something . . . revealing are an important part of what the self-disclosure will mean to the relationship" (p. 27).

Second, only emotional communication, and not emotional expression, should invite the listener to participate in an interaction either about the emotion itself or about a conversation topic associated with the emotion. Because it is deliberate, emotional communication invites the listener to participate in whatever way seems responsive at that moment: talking about the communication, probing, giving advice, commiserating, hugging, laughing, or just making eye contact. In contrast, emotional expression does not invite the listener's involvement. The listener may even feel compelled *not* to react to or comment on such "leakage." Visible emotional reactions without emotional communication about their meaning may even be a source of distance (i.e., may generate negative affect and misunderstanding.[4]

Sharing positive feelings about one's interaction partner is a particularly valued intimate behavior (Helgeson et al., 1987). The communication of positive information and feelings is more conducive to liking and attraction among college students than negative disclosure (Lazowski & Anderson, 1990). Communicating positive feelings toward the partner has the potential of conferring instant validation, particularly if the recipient of that communication believes the discloser truly understands her or him (Reis & Shaver, 1988). Communicating positive feelings toward one's partner may also contribute to intimate experience because of the immediacy of the message, which will be discussed next.

Immediacy of Self-Disclosure

Mehrabian (1971) described immediacy in communication as a silent message within a message that indirectly conveys how much distance speakers place between themselves and what they are saying. According to Mehrabian, immediacy in communication brings something into the present, while nonimmediacy puts it into the past. Speakers can convey immediacy with pronoun use (*this* and *these* vs. *that* and *those*), adverb use (*here* vs. *there*) and verb tense (present vs. past).

Self-disclosing communication may vary in immediacy. The language of disclosure can increase immediacy with personal references (i.e., using *I* instead of *you* or *it*) and the use of the present tense. The attribution of responsibility to self ("I want to see you again") rather than to some external agent ("If my boss gives me some time off, I'll call") increases immediacy by decreasing distance between the self and the message. Using the active versus passive voice decreases the distance between the speaker and the event or point of interest (Altman & Taylor, 1973; Mehrabian, 1971; Montgomery, 1984b). Indirectness, as in "There must be a problem here" versus "I have a problem I need to talk to you about," can decrease immediacy.

If immediacy in self-disclosure affects intimate experience, this is likely due to the relationship between immediacy and liking. Mehrabian's (1969, 1970) early work on nonverbal immediacy indicated that people who like one another approach one another in a variety of ways, such as moving closer or leaning toward, touching, or reaching out to touch each other. Montgomery (1984a) found that immediacy in verbal communication contributes significantly to people's perceptions of another's openness, beyond the personalness of self-disclosure content. Less information is available, however, about the impact of verbal immediacy.

Because of their high impact potential, high-immediacy conversations, by definition, have to engender positive feelings to promote intimate experience. This is because any negative feelings they engender would likely have a strong impact and would therefore preclude any experience of intimacy. Perhaps for this reason, high-immediacy self-disclosure may be rare or even taboo in some close relationships. One example is intentional metacommunication, in which partners talk about their own interaction and their moment-to-moment feelings. This is apparently rare, even in very close relationships (Baxter & Wilmot, 1985). High-immediate conversations may not have to occur frequently to have an impact on intimate experience, however. Derlega et al. (1993) noted that at times a single highly immediate disclosure, such as "I love you," can transform the definition of a relationship. People in close relationships may deliberately recall and replay high-immediacy conversations to reexperience the intimacy these conversations originally generated (e.g., "Remember when you first asked me to marry you?").

Despite a long history of research on self-disclosure and its impact, little is known about the importance of immediacy in intimate interactions. Nevertheless, writers continue to mention immediacy as an ingredient that fosters intimate experience (e.g., Beach et al., 1990; Sternberg, 1988). Whether immediacy fosters intimate experience may depend on characteristics of the relationship partners. For example, because it focuses conversation on the present moment and the people at hand, high-immediacy self-disclosure seems likely to be associated with stronger emotions and therefore more passion than less immediate self-disclosure. As a result, partners' preferences for a more passionate versus a more companionate relationship may predict the impact of verbal immediacy (Sternberg, 1988). Further, the ability to use immediacy as a positive force may depend on partners' skills and comfort with handling strong emotions (and each other). Fitzpatrick (1988) found that those who value openness and tolerate both high levels of relational intimacy and high levels of conflict may benefit more than their traditional counterparts from verbal immediacy. There is some evidence that married couples vary in their use of high-immediate conversation (Acitelli, 1993) and in their desire to incorporate it into their relationship (Jacobson, 1989). A better understanding of the way immediacy in communication fosters (or inhibits) intimate experience could help marital therapists make decisions about when to encourage such communication in distressed couples.

VERBAL RESPONSIVENESS AND THE EXPERIENCE OF INTIMACY

Like nonverbal involvement, verbal responsiveness may enhance experiences of intimacy by conveying to interaction partners that they are paying attention to and valuing one another (Reis & Shaver, 1988). Called conversational responsiveness (Berg, 1987) or attentiveness (e.g., Carkhuff, 1972, 1973; Egan, 1975; Ivey, 1971), verbal responsiveness purportedly communicates that the listener is "interested in and understanding of that communication" (Miller & Berg, 1984, p. 193). A listener's verbal responsiveness may determine whether the listener gets enough information to understand the speaker's meaning. People may disclose more fully and completely to responsive listeners (Egan, 1975). If verbal responsiveness does increase listener understanding, it could be a necessary ingredient for promoting intimate experience.

Perhaps more than any other aspect of intimate behavior, emphasis has been placed on verbal responsiveness as a skill that can be learned but is not automatically present in a caring, interested listener (e.g., Egan, 1975). While nonverbal involvement can be communicated by a finite set of behaviors (e.g., maintenance of gaze, forward lean, head nodding), verbal responsiveness is more complex. It comes in several different forms and may be most effective when tailor-made for its recipient.

Berg (1987) suggested three facets of interaction behavior that may contribute to perceptions of recipient responsiveness: content, style, and timing. According to Berg, responsive content is that which addresses the communicator's interests and previous communication. Responsive style is enthusiastic and willing while unresponsive style conveys indifference or reluctance. Verbal phrasing and voice intonation, pitch, and modula-

tion, should all contribute to responsive style. Timing refers to the occurrence of the response relative to the other's communication.

Research has supported Berg's notions about responsive content and
intimate experience. For example, findings indicate that college students
like new acquaintances better when they reciprocate self-disclosures and
respond to disclosures with sympathy and a willingness to talk more about
the topic (Berg & Archer, 1980; Dindia, 1994). Listeners whose responses reflect the discloser's perceptions and feelings are more attractive as
potential friends and are perceived by disclosers as more understanding
and sympathetic than listeners whose responses reflect their own perceptions.

Tannen (1990b) suggested that the context of the communication
may determine what kind of timing is responsive. In some contexts, rapid
switches and interruptions are seen as signs of involvement (Tannen,
1990b), while in other contexts the discloser perceives the recipient as
more responsive when the latter permits him or her to finish before
speaking.

Literature in therapeutic psychology has long recognized the importance of verbal responsiveness. Rogers (1959) saw it as a key ingredient in
psychotherapeutic effectiveness. Research has, to some extent, supported
Rogers's notion that therapist responsiveness is necessary, if not sufficient, for therapeutic progress (e.g., Barkham & Shapiro, 1986; Wexler &
Rice, 1974). Its role in facilitating intimate experience has not, however,
received the research attention that self-disclosure has.

Verbal responsiveness may have received less attention than self-disclosure because of the focus of earlier research on intimate interaction.
Jourard's (1959) theory of self-disclosure and liking and Altman and Taylor's (1973) theory of social penetration generated much of the self-disclosure research in the '60s and '70s. Both of these theories are principally concerned with the individual behavior of self-disclosure rather than
with the intimate interactions of which intimate behavior is a part. Now
that scholarly interest has expanded to include dyadic intimate interactions within personal relationships (e.g., Duck, 1994a), research should
widen its focus to investigate the role of verbal responsiveness.

Given the definition of intimate experience in Chapter 1 (which includes both positive affect and perceptions of being understood by and
understanding of another), a discloser is unlikely to experience intimacy
in the absence of verbal responsiveness from his or her interaction partner (e.g., Sprecher, 1987). It seems instead that both kinds of intimate
behavior—self-disclosure and verbal responsiveness—must be present in
a verbally intimate interaction; neither seems likely to foster intimate experience without the other.

Verbal Intimacy in Context

The purpose of this section is to explain how a contextual perspective can shed new light on verbal intimacy research. Duck (1993b) recently argued forcefully for the need to expand personal relationships research beyond the dyad to include the social, economic, and political forces that constrain the "options people recognize and the choices they make" (p. 2). This section considers those contextual factors that affect intimate interaction (behavior and experience) itself. Since much of the literature on verbal intimacy deals with self-disclosure, most of this section focuses on new ways of understanding the reasons and circumstances under which one person will self-disclose to another. As much as possible, I address contextual factors (at all levels) that directly affect verbally intimate behavior and those that modify its impact on intimate experience in interactions. Self-disclosure research up to this point has, however, focused largely on contextual factors at the personal/relational level. This chapter's discussions of the immediate, group, and sociocultural levels are therefore more speculative.

The Immediate Context

Information on how verbal intimacy is influenced by the immediate context is currently quite limited. The immediate context refers to variables that are close in space and time to the interaction itself. Participant mood is one such variable; one study suggested that partners who are in a happy mood at the time of their conversation self-disclose more than those who are in an unhappy mood (Cunningham, 1988). Attraction is another; partners who feel more attraction to each other self-disclose more (Dindia & Allen, 1992). Rubin and Shenker (1978) studied another immediate contextual variable—physical proximity—and its effect on self-disclosure among college students. They found that roommates disclose more frequently to one another than hall mates, regardless of the sex composition of the dyad or the level of friendship. Proximity, however, exerted most of its effect on impersonal levels of disclosure and had little or no effect on personal topics. While these studies indicate that verbal intimacy is affected by the immediate context, the substantial body of work on nonverbal behavior and immediate context has no counterpart in the research on verbal intimacy.

One immediate contextual variable that has received extensive attention in the literature is participant gender. Available evidence suggests that participant gender exerts a direct effect on self-disclosure (Dindia & Allen, 1992). After a review of the literature, Dindia and Allen concluded that it is interactions between two women that are likely to be highest in self-disclosure depth, followed by interactions between a woman and a man; interactions between two men seem likely to elicit the least personal self-disclosures. A closer look at studies reviewed by Dindia and Allen reveals that men and women are less likely to differ in the breadth of information they disclose than in the depth (e.g., Rubin & Shenker, 1978). Men disclose as broadly as women but restrict their disclosure to less personal topics like matters of personal taste or topics of common interest, such as sports (Aries & Johnson, 1983; Chelune, 1976; Grigsby & Weatherley, 1983; Pederson & Breglio, 1968).

The effects of gender are considerably more complex than this summary of direct effects implies, however. Gender also interacts with other contextual variables, modifying their impact on verbal behavior and on the relationship between verbal behavior and intimate experience. Moreover, the effects of *most* higher-level contextual factors addressed here are modified by gender. Therefore, each of the following sections—on the personal/relational, group, and sociocultural contextual variables that affect verbal intimacy—includes a separate exploration of gender as it interacts with the other contextual factors in that category.

The Personal/Relational Context

Important contextual determinants of verbal intimacy reside within the individuals who participate in intimate interaction: personality, attitudes and beliefs, and goals. Personality refers to the "distinctive patterns of behavior (including thoughts and emotions) that characterize each individual's adaptation to the situations of his or her life" (Mischel, 1981, p. 2). Definitions of personality usually include motives and goals. Motives are affectively charged preferences for certain kinds of experiences; they function individually and in relation to one another as stable dispositions within individuals. A goal is "a mental image or other end point representation associated with affect toward which action may be directed" (Pervin, 1989, p. 474). The relationship between personality and intimate behavior has received considerable attention in the research literature.

In order to highlight the pervasive effects of gender on relationships between intimate behavior and personal/relational contextual factors, I have divided my discussion of these factors into gender-independent and gender-related effects. First, I address the personal side of the personal/relational context, and discuss gender-independent effects of specific personality traits, motives, and goals on self-disclosure, verbal responsiveness, and related intimate behaviors. Next, I discuss how the effects of each of these factors are modified by gender. My discussion of the relational side of the personal/relational context primarily addresses relationship type and its impact on self-disclosure. The final section presents interactive effects of gender and relational variables.

Personality. A few personality traits seem to have a consistent relationship with self-disclosing behavior. In an earlier review of the relationship between personality and self-disclosure, Archer (1979) noted that scores on introversion (Jourard, 1971), neuroticism (Jourard, 1971), conventionality (Burhenne & Mirels, 1970; Kent, 1975), and locus of control (Ryckman, Sherman & Burgess, 1973) were negatively correlated with the extensiveness of disclosure to several partners (assessed via the Jourard Self-Disclosure Questionnaire [JSDQ]). Studies conducted since Archer's review indicate that the following personality traits are also associated with self-disclosure: sensation-seeking (Franken, Gibson, & Mohan, 1990; Hendrick & Hendrick, 1987), self-esteem (Cramer, 1990a, 1990b), attachment style (Mikulincer & Nachshon, 1991), trait anxiety (Post, Wittmaier, & Radin, 1978; Prager, 1986), locus of control (Prager, 1986), empathy (Todd & Shapira, 1974), and gender-role orientation (e.g., Winstead, Derlega, & Wong, 1984). Relationships between general adjustment and self-disclosure are positive (Altman & Taylor, 1973; Brown & Harris, 1978; Carpenter & Freese, 1979). Scholars have found relationships between self-reports of self-disclosure and personality characteristics but not between personality and observed self-disclosing behavior (Cozby, 1973). Private self-consciousness and self-monitoring tendencies are interesting exceptions, which I discuss next.

People's tendencies to monitor themselves seem to predict how they will self-disclose to certain partners. There is evidence for two different, somewhat independent, self-monitoring tendencies. *Private self-consciousness* refers to the tendency to attend to and monitor "the more private and covert aspects of oneself" (Davis & Franzoi, 1987, p. 60). Davis and Franzoi argued that private self-consciousness encourages verbally intimate behavior for two reasons. First, the introspections engaged in by privately self-conscious people should increase their self-knowledge and make their inner selves more accessible to sharing. Second, privately self-conscious individuals, like most people, talk to others about what is interesting to them, and what is interesting to them is their own inner life. Privately self-conscious people, then, should be more inclined to self-disclose than their less self-conscious counterparts. Davis and Franzoi reported that adolescents and young adults high in private self-consciousness do disclose more, mainly in interactions with close friends and romantic partners.

People also demonstrate individual differences in their tendency to monitor themselves during interpersonal interactions, a tendency M. Snyder and Simpson (1984) called *self-monitoring*. This public self-monitoring appears to ensure that one behaves appropriately, given the norms for a particular situation (M. Snyder, 1979). Because reciprocation of self-disclosure with a new acquaintance is a well-established interaction norm in many cultures (e.g., Chaikin et al., 1975), individuals who closely monitor their normative behavior should be more likely to reciprocate self-disclosure in this context. Research supports this notion; individuals who are high in public self-monitoring reciprocate disclosure more than their low-self-monitoring counterparts when conversing with new acquaintances (Shaffer, Smith, & Tomarelli, 1982; Shaffer & Tomarelli, 1989). Perhaps as a result, they have more frequent and intense intimate experiences in the early stages of their dating relationships than do low-self-monitoring individuals (Snyder & Simpson, 1984).

Despite these findings, it is rare to find direct relationships between personality and self-disclosing behavior. Researchers examining asssociations between individual personality and verbal intimacy have recently discovered person–situation interactions that explain behavior better than personality alone (e.g., Snell, Miller, Belk, Garcia-Falconi, & Hernandez-Sanchez, 1989). For example, Machiavellianism correlated with more personal self-disclosure content among college-age males only when the social context (defined by the experimenters) called for them to influence their interaction partners. It did not affect disclosure when they were asked to get to know their partner better (Dingler-Duhon & Brown, 1987).

The results of several studies suggest that personality traits affect self-disclosure through their impact on a person's awareness of and adherence to norms for appropriate self-disclosure in a given context. College students high in neuroticism, for example, may be less able than nonneurotic students to disclose appropriately in interactions with strangers. In a study by Chaikin, Derlega, Bayma, and Shaw (1975) neurotic college students did not follow norms for reciprocating self-disclosure with a stranger the way that nonneurotic college students did. In another study, neurotic college students were less likely than nonneurotic students to disclose to a stranger at a moderately personal, and therefore normatively appropriate, level (Chelune & Figueroa, 1981). Intimacy capacity may also predict awareness of and adherence to self-disclosure norms. Prager (1986) found that individuals high in intimacy capacity regulated their self-disclosures to provide more personal information to a close friend than to a new acquaintance; individuals low in intimacy capacity did not discriminate.

Those personality traits that predict a person's ability to self-disclose selectively may be traits associated with adjustment (e.g., neuroticism, intimacy capacity, self-monitoring). If this is the case, it appears that there is a connection between self-disclosure and mental health that is different from the direct relationship originally proposed by Jourard (1971). Present research suggests that an ability to discriminate how much to disclose, to whom, and under what circumstances may be associated with good adjustment. This ability may serve as both an antecedent to and an outcome of mental health.

The final part of this section concerns individual motives and goals that are likely to affect a person's intimate behavior. A body of work by McAdams and his colleagues (e.g., McAdams, 1984, 1988a; McAdams & Constantian, 1983; McAdams & Powers, 1981) supports the notion that individual differences exist in people's desires for intimate contact and that these individual differences are predictive of behavior.

Intimacy motivation is defined by McAdams (1984, 1988a) as a persistent desire for experiences of self merging with others. By definition, people who are high in intimacy motivation (1) view relationships as sources of positive affect and (2) value talk for its own sake, particularly reciprocal and noninstrumental talk (McAdams, 1984). Viewed another way, intimacy motivation refers to the strength of a person's need for intimacy. Intimacy motivation is assessed from the thematic content of stories written in response to Thematic Apperception Test (TAT) cues (McAdams, 1982b; see Chapter 2).

Research supports McAdams's (1984) premise that intimacy motivation is reflected in the frequency and likelihood of intimate behavior. College students high in intimacy motivation are more likely than their low-scoring counterparts to engage in intimate interactions (McAdams & Constantian, 1983). McAdams and Constantian's study indicates that both men and women who score high on intimacy motivation are more likely to be engaged in intimate interaction when contacted during the day via a pager. McAdams and his colleagues also found that intimacy motivation predicts specific behavior in interactions, both in groups (McAdams & Powers, 1981) and in dyads (McAdams, Jackson, & Kirshnit, 1984). In groups, individuals high in intimacy motivation encourage the expression of positive affect, reciprocal dialogue, spontaneous interaction, and laughter more than do their less intimacy-motivated counterparts. Intimacy motivation also predicts certain nonverbal behaviors, such as smiling, tender touching, and laughing. Individuals high in intimacy motivation seem to prefer dyadic, as opposed to large group, interaction and engage in more self-disclosure and responsive listening than do those with lower intimacy motivation. The topics they discuss are more personal and private, and they invite the same from their interaction partners (Craig, Koestner, & Zuroff, 1994; McAdams, Healy, & Krause, 1984).

Perhaps research on intimacy motivation can shed some light on the mechanisms that link interaction behavior and experience. One possibility is that intimacy motivation reflects positive schemas about intimate contact. At least two possible manifestations of such schemas come to mind. First, highly motivated individuals should be more inclined to interpret behavior in interactions according to their wishes and expectations for intimate contact. One way to determine how prevalent such interpretations are would be to ask people to keep diaries. In their diaries people could record their interpretations of their own and others' behavior in interactions over a period of time (using, for example, the measure developed by Duck et al., 1991, or the one by Wheeler and Nezlek, 1977). Another way would be to ask people to recall their interpretations of events occurring during a particular interaction, using a stop-and-start videotaping technique like the one described by Ickes (1988). Second, because of these interpretations, highly motivated individuals should organize their behavior to maximize the likelihood that their intimacy needs will be met. The strength of intimacy needs is reflected in the frequency and intensity with which people experience gratification and pleasure in the presence of intimate contact, and the loneliness or other deficit states (e.g., depression) they experience in its absence (e.g., Buhrmester, in press). Researchers could use either a diary method or an interaction recall method to discover what people actually say and do in response to their interpretations.

Intimacy motivation may also serve to lower the intimacy-potential threshold required for a particular interaction to elicit intimacy-related schemas. According to McAdams (1984), "intimacy motives appear to inform thought, feeling, and behavior by conferring upon relationships a particular thematic meaning" (p. 41). Intimacy motivation, then, may correspond to a set of schemas that increases a person's readiness to evaluate social interactions according to their potential for fulfilling intimacy needs. To illustrate this process, consider the example of Aletha, who is a highly intimacy-motivated person. When Aletha talks with Marion, she interprets her steady gaze, easy laugh, and unaffected manner as indications that she might be available for intimate interaction of some kind. Yolanda, who is not particularly intimacy motivated, may interpret the same characteristics as indications that Marion will be easy to work with. Intimacy-motivated people should also evaluate interactions that fulfill intimacy needs more positively than do people who are less intimacy motivated. Further study of intimacy motivation, then, may enhance understanding of the psychological mechanisms that link intimate behavior with intimate experience.

There are other individual goals and purposes that can affect the likelihood of intimate behavior. It is usually not true that partners engage in interaction solely because they are seeking to fulfill a need for intimacy (Buhrmester & Furman, 1986; Derlega & Grzelak, 1979; Prager, Fuller, & Gonzalez, 1989). Perhaps more frequently, people enter intimate interactions to achieve multiple goals and purposes (Duck & Sants, 1983; Miell & Duck, 1986; L. Miller, 1990). Some of these goals may be more salient at the time than needs for intimacy. People may seek intimate interactions because they are likely to make progress toward several goals through these interactions (see Part II of this book).

When people seek intimate interactions for other purposes, their intimacy needs may nevertheless be met. It is likely that only some needs that intimate interactions fulfill are the result of purposeful pursuit of need fulfillment. The rest are likely fulfilled serendipitously along the way (Derlega & Grzelak, 1979). Some needs (like intimacy needs) may sometimes exist outside awareness (Tracy, 1991), decreasing the likelihood still further that their fulfillment is the result of deliberate goal-directed activity. People do not have to actively seek intimacy, then, for their intimacy needs to be fulfilled (e.g., see Derlega & Grzelak, 1979; Buhrmester & Prager, 1995).

Whether their purposes are conscious or not, people's intimate behavior seems to vary in accordance with their goals for the interaction. Specifically, people's reasons for seeking interaction are associated with the depth of their self-disclosure content. Prager et al. (1989) found that when college students' interactions fulfilled needs for self-expression (catharsis of strong feelings) and social validation (reassurance of worth and value), their self-disclosures were more personal than in interactions that served other purposes (e.g., developing and nurturing a relationship, eliciting reciprocal disclosure from another). People's goals and purposes, then, may exert an independent effect on personalness of self-disclosure.

Events occurring within the interaction may, conversely, affect people's goals. Partners may shift their goals several times over the course of an interaction on the basis of what they can realistically hope to gain from it (Sanders, 1991).

The final personality characteristic to be discussed in this section has been associated less with disclosers than with those who listen to another person's disclosures. Empathy refers to a set of characteristics and competencies traditionally associated with verbal responsiveness, or a person's ability to express caring and interest to a disclosing partner. Scholars and clinicians alike have long suspected that a person's experience with self-disclosure is dependent upon the listener's ability to express empathy (Rogers, 1951). Several decades of research have investigated the impact of empathy in psychotherapeutic interactions (Hill & Corbett, 1993). Despite research efforts, the extent to which the listener's (or therapist's) empathy is necessary or sufficient to benefit a discloser seeking support is still an open question (Hill & Corbett, 1993). The plethora of mixed results is due in part to a multiplicity of outcome measures and to confusion regarding the definition of empathy.

Recent work on empathy suggests that empathy encompasses cognitive, affective, and behavioral components (Davis & Kraus, 1991; Eisenberg et al., 1994; Gladstein, 1983; Harman, 1986). Perspective taking, the cognitive component, is the ability to comprehend or predict another person's thoughts, intentions, and emotional states. Empathic concern, the affective component, is a tendency to experience feelings of warmth, compassion, and concern for a distressed other. Empathy also implies an ability to avoid uneasiness and self-oriented concern in the presence of a distressed other (Davis & Kraus, 1991). Behaviorally, empathy includes the ability to describe with accuracy another's immediate affective experience, that is, to express one's understanding of another effectively enough for the other to feel understood (Rogers, 1980). It also includes the ability to use the other's responses to modify any inaccuracies in one's own understanding of the other (Harman, 1986). Empathy, then, is a set of cognitive and behavioral skills used in the presence of genuine caring and compassion for another.

Perhaps because empathy is difficult to define, the importance of empathy in intimate interaction outside the therapeutic context has received surprisingly little attention until recently (Jordon, Kaplan, Miller, Striver, & Surrey, 1981; Paul & White, 1990). One of the difficulties with the concept of empathy is that, like intimacy, it includes both intrapersonal and interpersonal components. Social and developmental psychologists have studied the affective and cognitive aspects of empathy as aspects of personality (e.g., Eisenberg et al., 1994; Strayer & Schroeder, 1989). Clinical psychologists have studied empathy's behavioral aspects in therapeutic interaction (e.g., Carkhuff, 1972, 1973; Egan, 1975). Of significance for the study of intimacy is Barkham and Shapiro (1986)'s finding that when psychotherapeutic outcome is operationalized as client's (or recipient's) perceptions of being understood, counselors' empathic communication is correlated positively with outcome. Advice giving, for example, is not. Scholars have yet to examine the ways that cognitive and affective aspects of empathy are translated into interaction behavior, nor have we examined the effects of that behavior on intimate experience.

Gender and Personality. The inspiration for much of the research on gender, personality, and intimate behavior has been a desire to understand why, in many parts of the Western world, girls and women disclose more than boys and men. One of the most favored explanations has been that sex differences in self-disclosure actually stem from personality traits that differ systematically between women and men. Gender, at the personal/relational level, has been described as a set of sex-typed personality traits, called *psychological masculinity* and *psychological femininity* (Spence & Helmreich, 1978). Masculine and feminine personality traits earned their names through their association, in the minds of American undergraduates, with typical or ideal behavior of either men or women but not both (Rosenkrantz, Vogel, Bee, Broverman, & Broverman, 1986). Research conducted primarily with American college undergraduates has entertained two principal hypotheses: One says that women disclose more because they have internalized more feminine sex-typed traits through socialization. Feminine sex-typed traits (e.g., compassion, gratitude, nurturance, and kindness) emphasize the maintenance of harmony and connection in interpersonal relationships. By the same logic, this hypothesis says that men disclose less because they have internalized masculine sex-typed traits (e.g., strength, competitiveness, assertiveness, and ambition) and are therefore reluctant to appear vulnerable.

The hypothesis that feminine and masculine sex-typed personality characteristics predict self-disclosing behavior has only weak support. Relationships between feminine sex-typed traits and self-disclosure tend to be positive, particularly in interactions between strangers (Jourard, 1959, 1961; Jourard & Lasakow, 1958). Just as often, however, no association is found between femininity and self-disclosure (Bem, 1977; Grigsby & Weatherley, 1983; Winstead et al., 1984) or results are inconsistent (Naurus & Fischer, 1982).

Masculine sex-typed traits are more reliably associated with self-disclosure than are feminine sex-typed traits, but there is no clear pattern of results. Some studies provide evidence for a negative relationship between masculinity and self-disclosure: Negative relationships have been found in interactions between previously unacquainted male college students (Grigsby & Weatherley, 1983; Winstead et al., 1984), between adolescent boys and their friends (Jones & Dembo, 1989), and between young men and their fathers (Snell et al., 1989). However, other studies show a positive relationship between masculinity and self-disclosure (Bem, 1977; Naurus & Fischer, 1982) or no association at all in certain relationships (Hill & Stull, 1987; Snell et al., 1989).

Some scholars have explored a second hypothesis, namely, that sex typing (rather than masculinity or femininity per se) predicts lower levels of self-disclosure (Hill & Stull, 1987). Sex-typing is the extent to which the individual describes him/herself with same sex-typed traits while rejecting opposite sex-typed traits. Androgyny refers to the simultaneous endorsement of same and opposite sex-typed traits. Studies comparing sex-typed and androgynous individuals on their self-disclosing behavior have also yielded mixed results. In the laboratory with strangers, androgynous male and female college students disclose more personal information than do sex-typed students (Dingler-Duhon & Brown, 1987). Androgynous students also report disclosing more in their personal relationships (Stokes, Fuerer, & Childs, 1980). Grigsby and Weatherley (1983), however, found no relationship between androgyny and self-disclosure. Others found that androgyny predicts for one sex (not always the same one!) but not the other (Hill & Stull, 1987).

It would be surprising if masculine or feminine sex-typed personality traits alone predicted self-disclosure in all relational contexts. Androgyny theoretically fosters flexibility and appropriateness in responding to a variety of situations (Kaplan & Sedney, 1980). In this regard, androgyny may be analogous to some other personality traits in that it is associated with sensitivity to self-disclosure appropriateness rather than absolute levels of self-disclosure. An investigation of this hypothesis might shed light on why studies investigating relationships between androgyny and self-disclosure have yielded such disparate results.

People's responsiveness to situational pressures that call for gendered behavior may also explain why gender differences in self-disclosure occur. Bem (1983) has argued that "gender schematic" individuals interpret their world in light of gender-related stereotypes. That is, they have "a generalized readiness . . . to organize information—including information about the self—according to the culture's definitions of males and females" (p. 232). Gender-schematic individuals may distinguish more readily than others between situations that call for gendered behavior and those that do not.

Certain patterns of self-disclosure should be evident if gender schematicity does contribute to sex differences in self-disclosure. Specifically, individuals who are more gender schematic should avoid self-disclosure most in situations in which it is gender inconsistent (e.g., a man does not disclose about his marital troubles to a same-sex friend). They should avoid it less in more gender-neutral situations (e.g., a male professor shares his experiences from graduate school with a dissertation student) or gender-consistent situations (e.g., a man discloses to a woman his feelings of sexual attraction for her). In contrast, patterns of self-disclosure in less gender-schematic individuals should be less constrained by gender-related pressures in situations. More research is needed to learn if these hypotheses have merit.

The motives and goals that individuals bring to self-disclosing interactions may vary by gender, and may thereby contribute to gender differences in self-disclosure. Female–male differences in intimacy motivation may contribute to differences in self-disclosure. One study, conducted with high school and college students, found that females score higher on TAT-assessed intimacy motivation than do their male age-mates (McAdams, Lester, Brand, McNamara, & Lensky, 1988). Other studies, however, have shown no gender differences in intimacy motivation (McAdams, 1988b). In addition, no gender differences have been found on fear of intimacy (Mark & Alper, 1980). Whether links exist between sex differences in intimacy motivation and sex differences in self-disclosure has yet to be determined empirically.

To the extent that women and men seek intimate interactions for different purposes, they may reveal information that is more or less personal. Prager et al. (1989) found that the reasons for disclosing that were more typical of women than of men—self-expression and social validation—were also reasons associated with more personal and private disclosures. Moreover, in this study gender differences in reasons for disclosing accounted for a significant proportion of the total gender-related variance in disclosure personalness. This suggests that women's disclosures are more personal than men's because women pursue different goals in their intimate interactions with others.

The study by Prager et al. (1989) suggests that men and women may be prompted to disclose for different reasons. There is evidence that male college students disclose more personal information, particularly with women, when their goal is not intimacy but a more instrumental aim. Shaffer and Ogden (1986) found that men disclose more in interactions when they believe they will have to work with their interaction partner on a project in the future. Perhaps they believe that the higher levels of disclosure will aid their working together. When experimental instructions dictate that they get to know their partner better, men disclose more with female partners than with males. Interestingly, when their purpose is to get to know a female partner better, males disclose more than females do with partners of either sex (J. Davis, 1978; Derlega, Winstead, Wong & Hunter, 1985). Gender-related self-disclosure patterns may be reversed, then, as a function of the reasons for disclosing.

Partners' Relationship. Perhaps the most potent influence on ver-bally intimate behavior is the type of relationship interaction partners have. There is evidence that type and length of relationship directly af-fect the content and affective tone of self-disclosure (e.g., Falk & Wag-ner, 1985; L. Miller, 1990; Morton, 1978; Prager, 1986). Type and length of relationship also exert a powerful influence on people's judgments about the appropriateness of self-disclosure within a particular interac-tion (e.g., Catalbiano & Smithson, 1983).

Starting in adolescence, the breadth and depth of self-disclosure content increase as relationships progress from those involving casual ac-quaintances and friends to those involving close friends and romantic partners (Altman & Taylor, 1973; Falk & Wagner, 1985; Hale, Lundy, & Mongeau, 1989; Hornstein & Truesdell, 1988; L. Miller, 1990; Prager, 1986; Rawlins & Holl, 1987; Vanlear, 1987). It is also true that people are more expressive of their emotions with close friends than with casual friends or acquaintances (Dosser, Balswick, & Halverson, 1983; Highlen & Gillis, 1978). In fact, it is the presence of confiding interactions that most distinguishes close relationships from more casual ones (Hays, 1988).

There are other indications that partners' interactions in close rela-tionships are more intimate than those between casual acquaintances. Compared with casual friends, close friends display more nonverbal in-volvement when conversing (Stinson & Ickes, 1992), are more deliberate in arranging to have conversations with one another, and seek more ex-clusivity and privacy when they do converse (Hays, 1989). Interactions between close friends are viewed as more beneficial and enjoyable than other interactions, at least among college students (Hays, 1989). They are more likely than interactions with casual acquaintances to be de-scribed as emotionally supportive (Cramer, 1990; Hays, 1989) and mean-ingful (Reis, Senchak, & Solomon, 1985).

Partners respond to one another's self-disclosures differently depend-ing on what kind of relationship they have. The well-documented reci-procity effect, whereby interaction partners reciprocate self-disclosures of the same depth, appears to be unique to interactions between individuals just getting acquainted (Derlega, Wilson, & Chaikin, 1976; Morton, 1978). Intimate interactions between close friends or romantic partners tend to be less structured and more complementary.

The structured self-disclosure reciprocity observed in interactions between new acquaintances likely reflects the important role played by sociocultural interaction norms in organizing exchanges between unacquainted individuals. Adherence to sociocultural norms, including reciprocity of self-disclosure, may serve several purposes in initial interactions between strangers. Reciprocity may allow partners who do not know one another to show that they are fair-minded (i.e., willing to divide the rewards of the interaction equitably). As others have pointed out (Derlega & Grzelak, 1979; Reis & Shaver, 1988), there are rewards associated both with providing and receiving personal information in an interaction. Reciprocity may allow those rewards to be distributed equitably. Reciprocity may also allow partners to show that they are trustworthy (i.e., will not make fun of or openly disapprove of their partner's disclosures). Finally, exchanging personal information may allow partners to establish commonalities about which they can converse further. Following the norm of reciprocity, then, may lay a positive foundation for future interaction.

A study by Ickes, Stinson, Bissonnette, and Garcia (1990) suggests that reciprocity of disclosure may be the most efficient means strangers have to get to know one another. Ickes et al. found that in mixed-sex dialogues between strangers one partner's expressiveness and disclosures are predictive of the other's ability to accurately assess what the first partner is thinking about and feeling during the interaction. In a later study with pairs of male college students, Stinson and Ickes (1992) replicated this finding with stranger pairs but found that it did not apply to dyads of close friends. Even inexpressive friends assessed one another's thoughts and feelings accurately. The strangers, compared with the friends, were completely dependent on the current interaction to gauge their partner's responses to the exchange. Strangers who reciprocated self-disclosure knew each other better at the end of the dialogue than strangers who did not.

If, as I have implied above, formal norms serve as conversation guides solely in the absence of trust and mutual knowledge, friends, romantic partners, and family members can probably dispense with strict reciprocity. The longevity of more intimate relationships may also allow for a different kind of reciprocity. As relationships persist over time, equity of listening and sharing should occur in the long run, eliminating the need for equity within a single interaction (Clark & Reis, 1988). Evidence exists that friends do indeed reciprocate self-disclosure over time rather than within the same conversation (Miller & Kenny, 1986).

Gender and Relationship Type. As important an influence as relationship type is on verbal intimacy, research suggests that we cannot understand its impact without also considering the influence of gender (Dindia & Allen, 1992). Gender appears to determine how much relationship type will influence verbal intimacy, although relationship type exerts the same type of effect on both women's and men's behavior. As was mentioned earlier, women tend to disclose more extensively and personally than men in a variety of relationship contexts (Dindia & Allen, 1992). Conversely, the extent of that gender difference and the consistency with which it occurs depend on the relationship context.

It is within the context of same-sex friendships that sex differences in verbal intimacy are most reliably observed. The gender composition of close friendships appears to directly affect intimate behavior and magnifies differences between the interactions of friends and more casual acquaintances (Stokes et al., 1980). Within same-sex friendships, young women consistently report sharing more personal, private disclosures than men and doing so more frequently (Aries & Johnson, 1983; Davidson & Duberman, 1982; Reis et al., 1985; Tschann, 1988). Women are also more likely than men to express their feelings to friends (Highlen & Gillis, 1978). Women are more likely than men to report that they understand their same-sex friend's meanings through gestures and facial expressions alone (Davidson & Duberman, 1982).

In contrast, the context of a heterosexual romantic relationship appears to diminish women's tendency to disclose more than men. Although some studies show women disclosing more than their male partners (Hendrick, 1981; Sprecher, 1987), these differences are moderate compared to those observed between same-sex friends (e.g., Rubin et al., 1980). In addition, several studies have shown men and women disclosing comparably to romantic partners, and about similar topics (Antill & Cotton, 1987; Chelune, Rosenfeld, & Waring, 1985; Komarovsky, 1967; Prager, 1989). Moreover, husbands' and wives' tendencies to disclose to one another are positively correlated (Antill & Cotton, 1987; Hendrick, 1981; Levinger & Senn, 1967).

Sexual orientation also seems to attenuate gender-related patterns in verbally intimate behavior. Nardi and Sherrod (1994) found no differences in amount or depth of self-disclosure between gay and lesbian nonsexual same-sex friendships. This was in contrast to findings from the same study that suggested similarities between gays and lesbians and their same-sex heterosexual counterparts in the areas of conflict management and sexuality.

The Group and Sociocultural Contexts

Group and sociocultural norms may strongly constrain the kinds of behaviors that are acceptable and desirable within certain situations (Allan, 1993). Existing research on group and sociocultural norms and verbal intimacy has mainly addressed gender-related effects; this section is devoted to a discussion of those effects. Two sociocultural norms are worth considering here. First is the norm that people should reserve very personal disclosures for sharing with highly selected people (Derlega & Grzelak, 1979; Worthy et al., 1969). Second is the related norm that designates a moderately personal level of self-disclosure as optimum in conversations in which people are getting acquainted. In the latter case, these moderately personal revelations should be neither so personal that the discloser seems indiscriminate for disclosing them nor so impersonal that the listener is unable to know the discloser better. Together, these two sociocultural norms should ensure that interactions involving very personal disclosures are labeled intimate. These norms should also affect people's judgments about whether a particular self-revealing message is appropriate within its context.

A diverse group of studies has documented agreement among college students regarding what is appropriate self-disclosure in interactions between strangers (e.g., Cunningham, Strassberg, & Haan, 1986). What these studies have in common is that they ask college students to make judgments about and react to self-disclosing messages of other students. In many of them, disclosures spoken or written by confederates are manipulated to be more negative or personal than would ordinarily be expected between unacquainted people. In my view, because participants in these studies do not know each other, students' judgments should reflect their understanding of sociocultural norms rather than their reactions to specific individuals.

What emerges most clearly from these studies is that students' judgments of self-disclosure appropriateness are dependent on participant gender (e.g., Caltalbiano & Smithson, 1983). Norms for appropriate self-disclosure, at least among American and British college students, may be different for male–male, female–female, and female–male dyads (e.g., Banikiotes, Kubinski, & Pursell, 1981; Chelune et al., 1981).

I review the results of this research here with the purpose of making explicit some gender-specific sociocultural norms governing self-disclosure in Western culture. While conclusions drawn from this body of work must be tentative, owing to the varied methods and purposes of the studies reviewed here, there are some trends worth noting. First, norms regarding the optimum level of depth of information exchanged in stranger interactions seem to be different for male–male, female–female, and male–female dyads. Males who disclose very personal information to other men are viewed as less well adjusted (Derlega & Chaikin, 1977), are less well liked (Lazowski & Anderson, 1990), and are less likely to be chosen for a potential friendship (Caltalbiano & Smithson, 1983) than men who disclose less personal information. In contrast, more personal disclosures enhanced both men's and women's enjoyment of interactions with a female partner (Banikiotes, Kubinski, & Pursell, 1981; Caltalbiano & Smithson, 1983; J. Davis, 1978). Moreover, research participants view females who disclose personal problems as better adjusted than males who do (Derlega & Chaikin, 1977). Perhaps because male students are not expected to disclose as much as their female counterparts, their behavior is judged as more intimate even when it is no different from women's (Chelune et al., 1981).

Second, there is evidence that college students' appropriateness judgments are affected by whether the content of self-disclosure is consistent with or in opposition to sociocultural definitions of femininity and masculinity. In a study by Cunningham et al. (1986) men's views of other men's disclosures were especially likely to be negative when the content deviated from traditional masculinity norms. In this study men liked both male and female disclosers less when they described themselves using cross-sex-typed adjectives from the Bem Sex Role Inventory (Bem, 1974). Women's judgments, in contrast, appeared to be less affected by the sex typing of disclosure content.

Both women and men are responsive to gender-role norms when choosing what to disclose to whom. Snell and his colleagues (Snell et al., 1986; Snell, Belk, Flowers, & Warren, 1988) found that men were considerably more reluctant to disclose information about their feminine side to another man than to a woman. When men's and women's willingness to disclose to a male interaction partner were compared, however, men were more willing than women to discuss their masculine side. A similar pattern of findings was reported by Blier and Blier-Wilson (1989) regarding the emotions that men and women are willing to express to male and female recipients; that is, both women and men edit their disclosures to men more than they do to women. Perhaps this suggests that people are responsive both to the sociocultural norms themselves regarding what is appropriate to disclose and to the fact that men's judgments are more affected than women's by those norms.

An interesting study by Snell (1989) illustrates the ways in which variables at one contextual level can modify the impact of variables at another level. Snell's research indicates that social anxiety (a personal-level factor) mediates the relationship between sociocultural gender role norms and self-disclosure. In his study socially anxious undergraduates of both sexes were less willing than nonanxious students to disclose cross-sex-typed personal information, particularly with opposite-sex friends. Socially anxious males, more than nonanxious males, were especially unwilling to disclose personal information about their expressive (or feminine) side to same-sex friends. Snell's results indicate that gender role norms (a sociocultural factor) affect students' willingness to disclose certain kinds of information about themselves to certain partners. However, those with social anxiety (a personal/relational factor), which reflects excessive concern about social disapproval, are the ones most likely to adhere to those norms. Students' personal characteristics, then, can modify the impact of sociocultural norms on their behavior. Given the evidence that adhering to gender-related norms reduces the risk of disapproval from peers, especially male peers (Cunningham et al., 1986), the conforming behavior of socially anxious students can be viewed as a response to social risk.

Analyses at the group contextual level may shed light on how sociocultural norms come to carry weight in individual decisions about what to disclose to whom. Groups enforce social norms in two ways: (1) by providing (or failing to provide) support and positive reinforcement for conforming behavior and (2) by actively punishing nonconforming behavior through belittlement, exclusion, and even banishment.

It is likely that children's same-sex peer groups play a powerful role in enforcing sociocultural gender norms (Bardwick & Douvan, 1971; Buhrmester & Prager, 1995; Maccoby, 1990a). Girls' peer groups appear to support behavior that facilitates closeness and harmony, including self-disclosure, but to punish behavior that calls attention to or attempts to distinguish the self (Brown & Gilligan, 1992; Maccoby, 1990a). Boys' groups, in contrast, denigrate vulnerability, and therefore self-disclosure, but support and encourage behavior that conveys toughness, competitiveness, and self-aggrandizement. Boys' peer groups, then, do not offer the same opportunities for intimate interaction that girls' groups do (Buhrmester & Prager, 1995). Further, the punishment boys mete out to one another when vulnerabilities are exposed may lead many boys to avoid self-disclosure with other boys altogether (Jones & Dembo, 1989).

SUMMARY AND CONCLUSIONS

This chapter's purpose is to further our understanding of the conditions under which people are most likely to have intimate experiences. The importance of this issue resides in the (as yet untested) presumption that intimate experiences have health-enhancing effects, which explains in part the association between intimacy and well-being.

The chapter pursues three objectives. First, it reviews and organizes theory and research establishing linkages between the behavioral and the experiential components of intimate interactions. Second, it identifies contextual factors that may directly affect intimate behavior or modify its relationship to intimate experience. Third, it suggests that people's expectations about situations and their interpretations of behavior (i.e., their schemas) may explain why certain contextual factors modify associations between intimate behavior and intimate experience.

This chapter reviews studies indicating that both nonverbal and verbal interaction behaviors seem to affect intimate experience. Involvement behaviors, like gaze and physical proximity, affect experiences such as liking, attraction, and emotional engagement (e.g., Kleinke, 1986). Touch further intensifies affective aspects of intimate experience (Burgoon, 1991). Verbally intimate behavior, such as self-disclosure, serves to establish rapport (Falk & Wagner, 1985), increase relationship depth and involvement (Derlega et al., 1993), and maintain (or reflect) satisfaction in ongoing relationships (S. Hendrick, 1981). Some research suggests, then, that intimate behavior exerts a direct and simple effect on partners' experiences of intimacy.

Direct and simple effects, however, are the exception rather than the rule. Most research indicates that links between intimate behavior and intimate experience depend on contextual factors. Some of these contextual factors directly affect the likelihood of intimate behavior. Immediate contextual variables such as the nature of the occasion (Tickle-Degnen & Rosenthal, 1990), the structure of the physical setting (Wada, 1990), partners' moods (Kowalik & Gotlib, 1987), and dyad gender composition (Gifford, 1991) seem to affect nonverbal involvement behaviors in interactions. Research on verbal behavior has concentrated more on personal/relational factors. It indicates that variables such as private self-consciousness (Davis & Franzoi, 1987), public self-monitoring (Shaffer & Tomarelli, 1989; M. Snyder, 1979), intimacy motivation (McAdams, 1988a), and the nature of the partners' relationship (Ickes et al., 1990) increase the likelihood and depth of self-disclosure.

Scholars have arguably paid more attention to gender-related factors and gender differences than to any other contextual factor. Fortunately, this body of work has shed some light on gender-related patterns in intimate behavior. At the immediate level is a fairly well established pattern in which women display more intimate behavior, both nonverbally

(Abele, 1986) and verbally (Duck & Wright, 1993). Once other contextual factors are considered, however, this gender-related pattern often attenuates or disappears altogether. At the personal/relational level, sex-typed personality traits seem to explain some gender-related variance in self-disclosure patterns (Stokes et al., 1980), although not systematically. Differences between women's and men's interaction goals may also explain why women's disclosures tend to be more personal (Prager et al., 1989). When men's and women's goals are similar, their behavior is more similar.

Other contextual variables attenuate gender effects as well. There are indications that gender interacts with relationship length, for example, so that gender differences in touching are observable in short-lived but not in more established relationships (Guerrero & Anderson, 1991). Gender also interacts with sexual orientation in the context of same-sex friendship, so that lesbian friends do not self-disclose more than gay friends (Nardi & Sherrod, 1994).

As this review indicates, we have much to learn about intimate interactions. A few gaps in our knowledge stand out. Sexual contact, while clearly exerting a profound impact on intimate experience, is the form of nonverbal intimate behavior scholars know least about (Sprecher & McKinney, 1993). While knowledge about human sexual anatomy, physiology, and behavior has accumulated, human sexuality research has not substantially encompassed the study of human sexual experience. Sexual experiences potentially evoke not only physical pleasure and gratification but also strong emotions about the partner, about oneself and one's body, and about one's relationship with one's partner. There is reason to believe that they play an important role in establishing attachment relationships between adults (L. Rubin, 1983; Sprecher & McKinney, 1993). Sexual experiences may even maintain relationships in the face of other difficulties. In short, there is currently a dearth of knowledge about the psychological and relational aspects of sexual interaction, which may represent a serious gap in our understanding of intimate interactions.

A neglected area in the research on verbal intimacy is verbal responsiveness. Although scholars and clinicians alike have recognized its importance to intimate experience (Berg, 1987; Egan, 1975), few conclusions can be drawn about its impact on experience at present. Initial efforts might concentrate on simply describing it in interactions. For example, videotaped interactions could be rated in two ways: (1) descriptively, using coding schemes that classify behaviors in which the listener reflects content, expresses concern, reflects emotion, suggests new perspectives, and so forth, and (2) subjectively, according to how much raters would enjoy talking to the person on tape. Correlations between the two sets of ratings might help identify key responsive behaviors.

There are contextual factors that deserve more research attention. For example, empathy represents a set of individual characteristics: perspective taking, empathic concern, and responsive behavior. Each of these characteristics of empathy could be important to intimate interactions. Perhaps because it is difficult to define and operationalize empathy, there is little information available about its role. Future research would do well to identify the components of empathy and the situations in which each component is important to intimate interaction. If empathy is as vital for promoting intimate experience as theorists like Rogers (1959) have suggested, then it is an important set of competencies for people to obtain.

Researchers also need to consider sociocultural contextual factors. Gender differences have proved to offer an invaluable window onto the kinds of effects sociocultural norms can have on intimate interactions. A speaker's gender significantly affects people's judgments about a self-disclosing person (Catalbiano & Smithson, 1983). People's willingness to disclose reflects the same gender-related norms (Snell, 1989). Research on children's reactions to gender role deviance suggests that at one time or another defying gender role norms has had negative social consequences (Thorne & Luria, 1986). As researchers more clearly articulate norms and the consequences of breaking them, they can better illuminate the nature of their effects on people's intimate behavior (P. Andersen, 1993).

Finally, this chapter proposes that cognitive/affective structures such as schemas be explored as mechanisms linking intimate behavior with intimate experiences. Ideas about situations and people are likely to be mentally organized as schemas. Again, the study of gender differences may prove to be a valuable approach, in this case to understanding schemas that people develop about situations. Schemas based on previous experiences with defying gender role norms may affect expectations in subsequent situations (e.g., Bem, 1983). Expectations of negative consequences could intensify people's efforts to confine themselves to "sex appropriate" behaviors. The current review suggests that gender-related schemas may be carried into intimate interactions and may restrict people's behavior and experiences in situations that, by some definitions, should encourage free self-expression and authenticity (e.g., Dahms, 1972; Jourard, 1971). Explorations of these cognitive/affective links between behavior, situations, and experiences may ultimately advance our understanding of the ways intimate interactions exert their beneficial effects on our health and well-being.

CHAPTER   NINE

Intimacy in Relationships

There is so much abundance in the people I have: . . .
Marie , Dawn, Arlene, Father Dunne, and all in their
short lives give to me repeatedly, in the way the sea places
its many fingers on the shore, again and again, they know
me, they help me unravel, they listen with ears made of
conch shells, they speak back with the wine of the best
region.

—ANNE SEXTON, *The Big Heart*

Intimate relationships may benefit as much as the individual partners
from the presence of intimate interactions, or relational intimacy. Relational intimacy should exert a direct, positive impact on relationship
functioning because of its own reward value (Reis & Shaver, 1988;
Thibaut & Kelley, 1959). Relational intimacy has reward value because
people feel accepted and appreciated when their most personal selves are
received with warmth and sensitivity.. The more frequently relationship
partners have such rewarding interactions, the more likely they are to
perceive the relationship as rewarding. Further, partners develop positive
expectations of one another as a result of these rewarding interactions
(Chelune, Robison, & Krommor, 1984). These expectations may be a
source of positive affect about the relationship even when partners are
not actively engaged in interaction.

Relational intimacy should also affect relationship functioning indirectly through its positive associations with other relationship-enhancing
factors such as affection, trust, and cohesiveness. Specifically, positive affect from an intimate interaction should generate affection for the partner. In addition, experiences with sensitive responding and authenticity
from a relationship partner should elicit trust. Finally, cohesive experiences should provide opportunities for intimate interactions. This chap-

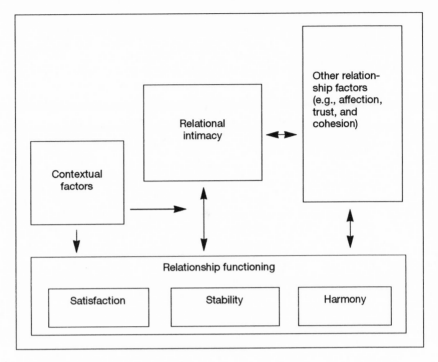

FIGURE 9.1. Model of relational intimacy within intimate relationships.

ter's first goal is to describe several processes by which relational intimacy contributes to intimate relationship functioning.

The extent to which intimate relationships function well likely depends on the contexts within which they are embedded. Neither intimate interactions (see Chapter 8) nor intimate relationships (e.g., Allan, 1993; Duck, 1993b) can be understood in isolation from their contexts. Further, contextual factors likely modify the impact of relational intimacy on intimate relationships. For example, the importance of relational intimacy to marital functioning may depend on the partners' personality characteristics (e.g., intimacy motivation) and their cultural background (e.g., cultural models and norms about the benefits of marriage). The second section of this chapter considers the impact of several contextual factors on intimate relationship functioning.

Figure 9.1 portrays the proposed association between relational intimacy and intimate relationship functioning. Relational intimacy, in the center of the figure, likely affects relationship functioning directly (the vertical line) and indirectly (the horizontal line) via its effects on other relationship factors. Contextual factors affect relationships directly and modify the impact of relational intimacy on relationship functioning.

INTIMATE RELATIONSHIP FUNCTIONING

Before moving on to my discussion of relational intimacy and intimate relationship functioning, I would like to specify a working definition of relationship functioning. The three major indicators of intimate relationship functioning in the literature at this time are as follows: (1) persistence/stability (functional relationships tend to resist dissolution); (2) reward value (the partners in the relationship are satisfied and evaluate it positively); and (3) harmony or freedom from discord (partners in functional relationships do not engage in destructive or dysfunctional conflict).[1]

Stability, satisfaction, and harmony should be positively intercorrelated, although they do not necessarily co-occur. Levinger (1965), for example, noted that satisfaction and stability may be orthogonal in some marital relationships. In "half-shell marriages," partners may be happy with one another but find it difficult to live together. In "empty-shell marriages," they stay together though they are not particularly satisfied with the relationship. Studies by Gottman and Levenson (1992) and by Lavee and Olson (1993) found only weak correlations between marital satisfaction and stability.

I have included these three indicators in my definition of relationship functioning because research on close relationships has used each extensively. For example, marital research has used partners' ratings of satisfaction with the relationship as an outcome variable for several decades (Hicks & Platt, 1970). Dissolution and divorce are also used at times as indicators of dating or marital relationship failure (e.g., Bentler & Newcomb, 1978; Gottman, 1993; Rusbult, Johnson , & Morrow, 1986) and as indicators of the failure of friendships (Hays, 1988; Rawlins, 1992). Finally, the presence of excessive or dysfunctional conflict is evidence of poor relationship functioning in studies of dating relationships (Rusbult et al., 1986), cohabiting couples (Kurdek & Schmitt, 1986a), married couples (O'Leary, 1987), and parent–adolescent relationships (J. Sroufe, 1991). For purposes of this chapter, then, relationship functioning refers to one or more of these three specific indicators.

I hope to avoid the implication that an intimate relationship is necessarily a perfect relationship. Intimate relationships, as Hatfield (1988) put it, "are a mixed bag of rewards and frustrations" (p. 207). Nor are intimate relationships necessarily more than minimally functional (nonintimate relationships, on the other hand, can be quite functional).

Relational Intimacy and Intimate Relationships

A positive association between relational intimacy and relationship functioning has been well established (Clark & Reis, 1988). Relational intimacy is associated with relationship growth (Dosser et al., 1983; Falk & Wagner, 1985; Nardi & Sherrod, 1994). It distinguishes more rewarding from less rewarding relationships (e.g., Burke et al., 1976; Chelune, Sultan, Vosk, & Ogden, 1984; Derlega et al., 1976; Merves-Okin et al., 1991) and contributes to relationship satisfaction (Acitelli & Antonucci, 1994; Fitzpatrick, 1988; Waring & Russell, 1980). A more detailed discussion of the processes by which intimate interactions create positive experiences for those who participate in them can be found in Chapter 8.

Scholars have debated whether greater amounts of relational intimacy inevitably lead to (and/or result from) higher levels of relationship functioning. On the one hand, there is evidence that partners in more functional relationships have more intimate contact (i.e., more frequent, extensive, and/or personal interactions; e.g., Miller, Lefcourt, & Ware, 1983; Sprecher, 1987). Satisfaction with friendship (Hays, 1989) or marriage (Jourard & Lasakow, 1958; Levinger & Senn, 1967; Tolstedt & Stokes, 1983) tends to be positively correlated with amount of verbal intimacy. On the other hand, there is evidence that the association between verbal intimacy and relationship functioning plateaus at higher levels of intimacy (Gilbert, 1976).

Too much intimacy in the form of self-disclosure may interfere with the fulfillment of other important needs in a relationship and may thereby damage it (e.g., A. Weiss, 1987). Gilbert (1976) and others (e.g., Cozby, 1973) argued that self-disclosure should have a curvilinear relationship with satisfaction, so that when self-disclosure exceeds some optimum amount, satisfaction should decrease. Gilbert's reasoning was that needs for security and stability in the relationship cannot be met if certain types of personal information, particularly information that is threatening to the relationship, are shared. Such disclosures, (e.g., disclosing about one's attraction to others to one's romantic partner) might threaten the future of the relationship (LaFollette & Graham, 1986). They could also open up areas of conflict the partners are not interpersonally skilled enough to cope with.

Along similar lines, Derlega and Chaikin (1975) argued that withholding self-disclosure should benefit an intimate relationship if the content of the disclosure is punitive. They contended that some disclosures may be put-downs or may be delivered in an untimely fashion. Far from fulfilling intimacy needs, these disclosures could interfere with the fulfillment of partner's needs for positive regard in the relationship and could therefore be destructive. Assuming that these arguments have merit, how can we account for the bulk of the research, which shows a linear, positive relationship between relationship satisfaction and self-disclosure? This persistently positive relationship may in part be due to the way researchers usually measure self-disclosure. Rarely do we ask partners if they have disclosed, for example, their views about one another's bad or disgusting habits or character flaws or their opinions about other volatile and unpleasant topics. If these kinds of negative disclosures were assessed, the positive correlation between self-disclosure and relationship satisfaction would likely be attenuated. However, partners' ability to resolve the conflicts evoked by negative disclosure might be a better predictor of satisfaction than their ability to withhold negative disclosures.

These arguments remind us that relational intimacy should not be equated with self-disclosure (see Chapter 1 for further discussion on this point). While self-disclosure can be positive or negative, sensitive or insensitive, intimacy is associated with positive experiences by laypersons and scholars alike (Helgeson et al., 1987; Reis & Shaver, 1988). Research on negative interactions, while important in its own right, is unlikely to resolve the conflict between the curvilinear hypothesis and the consistently observed positive correlation between relational intimacy and satisfaction.

In sum, more relational intimacy seems to be associated with better functioning in intimate relationships. While it is theoretically possible for partners to engage in more intimate relating than would be beneficial for their relationship, most evidence points to a linear, positive correlation between relational intimacy and relationship satisfaction.

The influence that relational intimacy and relationship satisfaction exert on each other is likely simple and direct, at least in part. Intimate interactions are rewarding, and frequent, rewarding interactions of any kind are likely to enhance relationship satisfaction.

It is also likely, however, that relational intimacy exerts effects on relationship satisfaction because of its impact on other aspects of intimate relationships. Affection (love), trust, and cohesiveness are three likely concomitants of relational intimacy that in turn enhance relationship functioning and increase the likelihood of continued intimacy.

Affection, Love, and Intimate Relationships

The research evidence to date certainly indicates that partners in intimate relationships have affection and/or love for one another, particularly in romantic relationships and friendships. A positive association between love and intimacy has been well documented among adolescents, college students, and adults (e.g., Davis & Latty-Mann, 1987). What remains to be determined is how relational intimacy and love are linked.

My multitiered conceptual structure for intimacy (intimate interactions, intimate relationships, see Figure 1.2) can be used to create a coherent model of the linkages between relational intimacy and love (or affection). Drawing from that conceptual structure, I can identify four types of links between intimacy and love: (1) links between intimate experiences and loving emotions, (2) links between intimate behavior and loving emotions, (3) links between intimate interactions and love relationships, and (4) links between intimate relationships and loving emotions. By allowing for distinctions between intimate interactions and relationships, the model encourages exploration into the circumstances under which different associations between intimacy and love might apply. I shall illustrate this momentarily.

In order to talk meaningfully about relational intimacy and love, we must also have an organized concept of love. Like intimacy, love likely serves best as a superordinate category. Recall from Chapter 1 that the purpose of superordinate categories is to group together basic categories whose members have a few highly significant attributes in common. The basic categories then serve to most effectively discriminate between similar (but not identical) phenomena while allowing trivial differences to remain. A review of the literature on love suggests that the basic categories of love are (1) love as emotion (e.g., Shaver, Schwartz, Kirson, & O'Connor, 1987; Solomon, 1981) and (2) love as a type of relationship (e.g., Aron & Aron, 1993; Sternberg & Barnes, 1988).[2]

First when we talk about love as an emotion and when we talk about intimacy as the affective aspect of people's experiences in intimate interactions, intimacy and love can be synonymous. The literature suggests that the emotion of love is likely a common form of intimate experience. Intimacy can refer to intimate experiences, an important component of which is positive feelings and emotions about one's relationship partner (e.g, affection).

Support for these notions lies in conceptualizations of love and intimacy that seem to equate the two. For example, Dion and Dion (1988) viewed deeper involvement in a romantic love relationship as synonymous with heightened relationship intimacy. Dion and Dion's model seems to equate relationship intimacy with the loving emotions people feel toward their romantic partner. Likewise, Sternberg and his colleagues (Sternberg, 1988; Sternberg & Grajek, 1984) equate the emotional aspects of love with intimacy. In Sternberg's triangular model of love, intimacy is the "liking" component and includes affective concepts like happiness, warmth, affection, tenderness, closeness, and attachment. Loving emotions, called different names by different theorists (Berscheid & Walster, 1978; Davis & Todd, 1982; Sternberg & Grajek, 1984) are often equated with intimacy (Olson, 1990; Sternberg, 1988; Waring, 1981).

Second, loving emotions may prompt intimate behavior. Supporting this view are definitions of love as a primary emotion (Arnold, 1960) and as a powerful motivational force in human existence—that is, "[The lovers'] overwhelming impulse is to push themselves closer together" (Solomon, 1988, p. 193). Marston, Hecht, and Robers (1987) believed that love was primarily a subjective experience, a combination of feelings and motivations. On the basis of interviews with college students, they identified five "love experience" clusters, each of which included a particular type of intimacy. The authors extrapolated from the interviews the idea that, for each cluster, love serves to motivate the partners to engage in certain intimate behavior. The intimate behavior in turn creates and enhances the feelings of love. For example, "collaborative love," the first cluster, is characterized by feelings of increased energy and intensified emotional responses and motivates partners to engage in supportive communication. Feelings of security and comfort characterize "secure love," the third cluster, which motivates partners to talk about personal topics.

Third, relational intimacy is, most likely, a common characteristic of love relationships. I suggest that when theorists talk about intimacy as a dimension of love, they are acknowledging the importance of intimate interactions to love relationships. For example, in a factor analytic study whose purpose was to identify the dimensions of love, Critelli, Myers, and Loos (1986) found that "communicative intimacy" emerged as a distinct component.

According to the framework discussed in Chapter 1, love relationships that are characterized by relational intimacy are also intimate relationships. Not all love relationships are intimate relationships, however. Based on a factor analytic study of several measures of love and intimacy, Hendrick and Hendrick (1989) reported that some types of love are highly correlated with measures of intimacy (i.e., Eros, erotic love, and Mania, obsessive love) while others (i.e., Storge, low-key, companionable love, and Pragma, pragmatic love) are not. Their research suggests that some, but not all, love relationships involve relational intimacy.

The literature suggests that relational intimacy is not only a frequent characteristic of love relationships but that it likely enhances the functioning of those relationships. Hatfield (1988), for example, argued that it is important to acquire the skills and competencies required to successfully participate in intimate interactions because intimate interactions are the "ultimate rewards" in intimate relationships (p. 207). When partners develop competency in the skills necessary for intimate encounters, the affection and love in their relationship should be enhanced (e.g., L'Abate & Sloan, 1984).

The final link—between intimate relationships and loving emotions—may partially explain the mechanism by which increasingly frequent and expected intimate interactions become conceptualized as intimate relationships. In this process, described in Chapter 8, intimate behavior generates intimate experience. Intimate experience, as noted earlier, can come in the form of loving feelings and emotions. As the sequence of intimate behavior and loving emotions is repeated over time, the person may develop an intimate relationship schema. This schema includes a set of positively valued memories and expectations of intimate contact with a particular partner. At some point, the activation of that schema is likely to arouse feelings of love even in the absence of intimate interaction. For example, a particular kind of smile from a partner may activate the schema because of its association with memories of previous interactions. A statement from one partner to another, such as "Let's go out to dinner this weekend," may activate the schema because the partner expects intimate interaction over dinner. In the context of an intimate relationship these schema activations may be sufficient to arouse feelings of affection or love.

Trust and Relational Intimacy

It has long been believed that the extensive and personal information people self-disclose as they become more involved in relationships contributes to, and grows out of, trust between the partners (Altman & Taylor, 1973; Derlega & Grzelak, 1979; Rogers, 1951). Both scholarly and lay definitions of intimacy include trust (Roscoe et al., 1987). Adolescents claim that a major distinction between a friend they can confide in and one they cannot is the trustworthiness of the former (Rawlins & Holl, 1987). There is, nevertheless, little information available about the role trust plays in enhancing and maintaining relational intimacy.

Self-disclosing communication is an arena in which trustworthiness can be tested and either demonstrated or proven inadequate. As a result of self-disclosing interactions, one person can discover whether another will respond sensitively to the personal material revealed, and display acceptance and understanding (Reis & Shaver, 1988). The repeated demonstration of this sensitivity is what theoretically allows trust to develop.

Once people have formed an intimate relationship, there is reason to believe they expand their expectations of trustworthiness. People expect a relationship partner to keep a confidence, particularly when the information could be damaging to their reputation if shared with others (Buhrmester & Prager, 1995; Rawlins & Holl, 1987). Further, a relationship partner is expected to refrain from using personal, private information to hurt or punish (Kelvin, 1977). It is not enough to respond sensitively during an interaction if the responder later hurls the discloser's vulnerabilities at him or her during an argument. Finally, as intimate relationships progress, partners come to know more about each other's personal, private thoughts and feelings (Hatfield, 1988). They can use this information to try to persuade, cajole, or otherwise solicit the other's cooperation. They can also use it to coerce, intimidate, and threaten. As an intimate relationship becomes more central to the partners' lives (i.e., as interdependence increases), partners have increased opportunities to prove to one another the extent, and the limitations, of their trustworthiness.

Cohesion in Intimate Relationships

The literature on cohesion and intimacy (sparse as it is) has focused on exploring linkages between the two in specific types of intimate relationships, for example, friendship and marriage. (The literature on love and intimacy, in contrast, has leaned toward devising theoretical principles that apply to all relationships.) This section on cohesion and intimacy, summarizes the findings on several different kinds of relationships and infers a theoretical account from the specific findings.

Like love and intimacy, the concept of cohesion has a history of varied definitions (Pittman, Price-Bonham, & McKenry, 1983; Spanier et al., 1975). Originally used to describe processes in small group interaction (Festinger, Schachter, & Back, 1950), *cohesion* has been defined as "commitment, help, and support family members provide for one another" (Moos & Moos, 1983, p. 254) and "the emotional bonding that family members have toward one another" (Olson & Portner, 1983, p. 299). The following discussion will rely on Spanier's (1976) definition, which is the amount of pleasant partner togetherness in the intimate relationship (see also Beach & Tesser, 1988; Kerr & Bowen, 1988).

Despite the significant contributions that both relational cohesiveness and relational intimacy make to the functioning of intimate relationships, surprisingly little is known about how these two phenomena are interrelated. Cohesion, for example, has a demonstrated positive association with relationship functioning in both friendship (Buhrmester & Furman, 1987; Hays, 1989; Oliker, 1989; Swain, 1989) and marriage

(Baxter & Dindia, 1990; Reissman, Aron, & Bergen, 1993). There are likely multiple ways that cohesion and relational intimacy facilitate one another.

Beach and his colleagues (Beach et al., 1990; Beach & Tesser, 1988) distinguished between cohesion and intimacy that suggests ways the two may be related. According to Beach et al. (1990), intimacy and cohesiveness can be distinguished on the dimension of depth.[3] In their view cohesive activity is pleasant for relationship partners to share, whether it involves conversation or parallel work activity. The conversation or activity is not necessarily personal or private. As a result, the concept of cohesiveness encompasses a broader range of activity than that of intimacy. Intimate interaction could be one type of cohesive activity.

The distinction made by Beach et al. suggests that intimate and cohesive interactions do not necessarily occur on separate occasions. Cohesive partners enjoy one another's company and seek out togetherness. Cohesiveness and intimate interaction should be linked, then, because some time spent together should lead to intimacy.

Although the potential exists for relational intimacy to promote cohesiveness just as cohesiveness promotes relational intimacy, I propose that these two processes are not equally dependent on one another. The continued presence of relational intimacy is quite dependent upon partners' willingness to spend pleasant time together. In contrast, partners can enjoy ample cohesiveness without engaging in intimate interaction. Research thus far, which has largely been correlational, has not yet substantiated this claim.

The processes by which cohesive experiences support periodic or extended intimate exchanges may be best discovered in studies of day-to-day interactions within relationships (Duck et al., 1991). In the realm of everyday interaction, relationship partners who are enjoying pleasant time together may have periodic intimate exchanges mixed in with other kinds of talk, all within a single encounter. The extent to which cohesive experiences and intimate experiences flow easily into one another and back again may turn out to be a marker of highly functional relationships.

In sum, an important route to understanding what contributes to the quality of intimate relationships is the study of their critical components. I have suggested that relational intimacy has an especially potent effect on, and is affected by, the affection, trust, and cohesion in the relationship.

Intimate Relationships in Context

Like the interactions that compose them, intimate relationships exist within the embedded contextual structures described in Chapter 8 (also see Adams & Blieszner, 1994; Duck, 1993b). Except for the immediate context (which addresses only a single point in time), each contextual level identified in Chapter 8—the personal/relational level, the group level, and the sociocultural level—likely plays a role in determining how an intimate relationship will function.

I propose here two ways contextual factors may affect the functioning of intimate relationships (i.e., the partners' satisfaction with the relationship, the stability of the relationship, and/or the degree of harmony or destructive conflict within the relationship). First, contextual factors may exert direct effects on the functioning of the intimate relationship. For example, the functioning of a mother–child relationship appears to be directly affected by the quality of the mother's marital relationship (Belsky, 1979), the financial circumstances of the mother, and the availability of child care arrangements (Ambert, 1992).

Secondly, contextual factors may modify the strength of the association between relational intimacy and relationship functioning. In other words, context may affect where an intimate relationship lies on a continuum of intimacy importance. At one end of this continuum are intimate relationships whose functioning is only minimally dependent on relational intimacy. For example, a married couple may frequently engage in intimate interactions but their marital satisfaction and the stability of their relationship may depend more upon how they share child care than on the quality of their intimate interactions (Risman & Schwartz, 1989). At the other end of this continuum are intimate relationships in which the quality of relational intimacy heavily influences partners' satisfaction. Close friends who cannot see each other frequently may find that the maintenance of their relationship is heavily dependent on the quality of their intimate interactions when they are together.

Possibly, contextual factors could alter a relationship's position on this intimacy-importance continuum. For example, grandparents who live in the same town might, by their willingness to be involved in the care of their grandchildren, relieve the parents of some child care responsibility. The grandparents' presence in the couple's local network, then, may result in the couple's marital satisfaction being more heavily affected by the quality of their intimate interactions than by their participation in child care.

What follows is a review of personal, group, and sociocultural contextual factors that appear to affect intimate relationships. These contextual factors may either exert direct effects on the functioning of intimate relationships or modify the importance of relational intimacy to relationship functioning. Because of the pervasiveness of gender-related effects on relationships and the number of contextual factors that influence gender-related effects, that literature is discussed separately.

The Personal/Relational Context

Personality. The possibility that personality exerts direct effects on the functioning of intimate relationships has received more attention in recent years. Personality traits and social competencies reflect a person's adaptations to the people, circumstances, and stresses of his or her life (Mischel, 1981).

The impact of some personality characteristics seems most pronounced in the context of forming new relationships. Specifically, personality traits may interfere with relationship formation. Examples of this include shyness and social anxiety (Bruch, Kaflowitz, & Pearl, 1988; Davis & Oathout, 1992), poor social skills (Canary & Cupach, 1988; K. Miller, 1990), and reciprocation wariness and mistrust (Cotterell, Eisenberger, & Speicher, 1992). Others exert more effect on the deepening of relationships. People that Miller et al. (1983) called "openers" seem to have a knack for encouraging disclosure and therefore fairly intimate conversation with others. College students who are high self-monitors are more likely to change dating partners early in a relationship and, perhaps consequently, are less likely to be involved in enduring intimate relationships (Snyder & Simpson, 1984). Finally, some characteristics have impact primarily on the quality of existing relationships. For example, people who are high in private self-consciousness are more likely to self-disclose to their personal relationship partners, and self-disclosure is positively associated with relationship satisfaction (Davis & Franzoi, 1987). An internal locus of control, with respect to one's marriage, increases the likelihood of conflict engagement and persistence until problems are solved, which in turn increases marital satisfaction (Miller, Lefcourt, Holmes, Ware, & Saleh, 1986). An internal locus of control, realistic, age-graded expectations of children, and an active coping style predict warmth, acceptance and approval in parent–child relationships (Belsky, 1984). Perspective-taking capacity (Davis & Oathout, 1992; Long & Andrews, 1990; McGuire & Weisz, 1982; K. Miller, 1990), neuroticism and openness to experience (Shaver & Brennan, 1992), empathy (Davis & Oathout, 1992), intimacy motivation (McAdams, Healy, & Krause, 1984), intimacy capacity (Prager, 1989, 1991), and self-esteem (Hendrick, Hendrick, & Adler, 1988) all affect the quality of an intimate relationship.

The association between individual characteristics and the quality of intimate relationships is most likely the result of a two-way causal effect. On the one hand, people seem to bring certain characteristics with them to their relationships, starting from birth. For example, infants seem to be born with certain temperamental differences that may affect the quality of their relationship with their parents (Dunn, 1993; Thomas &

Chess, 1977). On the other hand, intimate relationships can shape individual characteristics. There is evidence that parent–child relationships,
for example, may alter the impact of infants' growth and development on
their temperamental characteristics, such as negative and positive emotionality (Belsky, Fish, & Isabella, 1991).

Personality should also affect the contribution of relational intimacy
to total relationship functioning. Possibly, the stronger and more important the partners' needs for intimate experience are, the more critical are
intimate interactions to a high-functioning relationship.

There is reason to believe that people's needs for intimate experience vary in strength and importance (Buhrmester & Prager, 1995;
McAdams, 1982b). Theorists have long believed that individual differences in need strengths exist, along with differences in how important
needs are in relation to one another (Murray, 1938). Several writers have
argued that fulfillment of needs can result in experiences of relief, satisfaction, pleasure, and even joy while frustration of needs results in deficit states, such as loneliness (in the case of intimacy deprivation)
(Buhrmester, in press; Maslow, 1968; McAdams, 1988a; Shaver & Hazan,
1985; Sullivan, 1953; R. Weiss, 1973). Individuals may differ in the
amount of intimacy they need to avoid experiencing loneliness; conversely, they may differ in the amount of intimacy they can enjoy before
experiencing saturation. Assuming for the moment that such individual
differences do exist, they can be said to represent variations in need
strength.

It is my hypothesis that the strength of partners' intimacy needs
modifies the association between relational intimacy and the functioning
of their relationship. The more frequent intimate interactions the partners require to avoid loneliness and the deeper their enjoyment before
reaching saturation, the stronger the association should be between the
amount of relational intimacy and the partners' satisfaction with their relationship. Two specific predictions emerge from this argument. One,
partners with stronger needs should expend more effort toward ensuring
intimate contact with their partners. In support of this contention,
McAdams, Healy, and Krause (1984) found that college students higher
in intimacy motivation engaged in more listening and more encouragement of their interaction partner to talk. Two, partners whose needs are
not as strong should be satisfied with relatively infrequent intimate contact in their relationships. For them, the association between intimacy
and relationship satisfaction could be weak.

Attitudes and Beliefs. A growing body of research supports the notion that individual attitudes and beliefs exert direct effects on intimate
relationship functioning (Epstein, 1986; Fletcher, Fincham, Cramer, &

Heron, 1987). Several findings have emerged from this research. First, there is evidence that expectancy violations are associated with relationship dissatisfaction. Romanticized expectations about marriage, which are unrealistic and liable to be violated, seem to be associated with dissatisfaction, especially for women (Belsky & Rovine, 1990; Kurdek, 1991a; Ruble, Fleming, Hackel, & Stangor, 1988). The wider the discrepancy between peoples' expectations and their partners' behavior, the more likely they are to be dissatisfied with their relationship (Hackel & Ruble, 1992; Ruble et al., 1988). The exception, not surprisingly, occurs when positive expectations are exceeded, which tends to result in higher levels of satisfaction (Kelley & Burgoon, 1991). Some research shows that violations of expectations about relational intimacy are especially predictive of relationship dissatisfaction (Davis & Todd, 1985; Kelley & Burgoon, 1991; Rogers-Doll et al., 1992).

Second, certain kinds of dysfunctional beliefs about intimate relationships seem to predict dissatisfaction and disharmony in those relationships. Research in this area has concentrated mainly on dysfunctional beliefs held by marital partners (Baucom & Epstein, 1990). Eidelson and Epstein (1982) found that endorsement of commonly held dysfunctional beliefs about the nature of intimate relationships predicts marital distress. Subsequent research has supported their findings (Eidelson & Epstein, 1982; Emmelkamp, Krol, Sanderman, & Ruphan, 1987; Gaelick, Bodenhausen, & Wyer, 1985; Pretzer, Epstein, & Fleming, 1991). Dysfunctional beliefs were also found to be associated with marital partners' reports of communication problems (Epstein, Pretzer, & Fleming, 1987) and with wives' negative confrontations during conflict (Bradbury & Fincham, 1992). Endorsing an exchange (quid pro quo) as opposed to a communal orientation in one's marital relationship tends to predict dissatisfaction as well (Broderick & O'Leary, 1986). A belief that one's own sexual performance is the most important determinant of one's partner's enjoyment of sex may interfere with sexual intimacy (McCarthy, 1987). Changes in relationship beliefs have been found to accompany changes in marital satisfaction over a 3-year period (Kurdek, 1991a).

Third, people's attributions about relationship events may affect (or reflect) their relationship satisfaction (Fincham, 1989; Pretzer et al., 1991). One of the most consistent findings to emerge from this research is that marital partners who attribute their spouse's negative behavior to global personality characteristics, rather than situation-specific factors, are more likely to be unhappily married (Bradbury & Fincham, 1990; Fincham, 1989). Attributions regarding the spouse's negative intent or blameworthiness concerning a particular undesirable behavior have also been useful in distinguishing between distressed and nondistressed married couples (Bradbury & Fincham, 1987; Fincham, Bradbury, & Scott, 1990).

Since much of this research addresses conflict in marital relationships, more information on attitudes and beliefs and their impact on relational intimacy is desirable. For example, we have yet to learn whether attitudes and beliefs exert direct effects on relational intimacy or whether effects on intimacy are produced indirectly via their impact on marital conflict. Future research might also investigate the impact of dysfunctional beliefs on the functioning of other kinds of relationships, such as friendship or gay romantic relationships. Work investigating the effects of parents' beliefs on parent-child relationship functioning has already begun (Belsky, 1984; Duck, 1993a; MacKinnon-Lewis et al., 1994).

Types of Relationships. The type of marital relationship two people form appears to affect the importance of relational intimacy as a predictor of marital functioning. On the basis of individual partners' self-reported values and behavioral patterns, Fitzpatrick (1988) identified three types of marriages based on their relationship values. "Traditionals" hold conventional values about marriage and place emphasis on companionship and interdependence while deemphasizing privacy and assertiveness. "Independents" hold unconventional views and place simultaneous emphasis on companionship and sharing, and privacy and assertiveness. "Separates" hold conventional values about marriage, while de-emphasizing togetherness, interdependence, and assertiveness. Intimacy is very important to the marital functioning of Traditionals and Independents, and both groups display mutual understanding. Independents have more frequent and more disclosing intimate interactions than do Traditionals or Separates. Separates, in contrast, are satisfied with significantly less intimacy than the other two groups and do not appear to place an especially high value on intimacy. As might be expected, they also show lower levels of mutual understanding.

The importance of intimacy as a predictor of satisfaction and stability in friendship is dependent on whether friends are casual or close (Hays, 1988). As discussed in Chapter 8, the extent to which a friend serves as a confidant and a source of emotional support has been a defining feature of close versus casual friendships (Bigelow & LaGaipa, 1975; Derlega et al., 1976; Hays, 1989). Once a friendship develops to the point where it is considered close, a certain amount of self-disclosure, emotional support, and accessibility appears to be necessary in order to maintain it (Knapp & Harwood, 1977; Rawlins & Holl, 1987), particularly for girls and women (Caldwell & Peplau, 1982; Kon et al., 1978; Reisman, 1990). The presence of relational intimacy in a friendship also seems to offset certain costs (conflict, disagreement) of the relationship (Hays, 1989).

By definition, the importance of erotic or sexual intimacy to relationship functioning is dependent on whether the relationship has been defined as a romantic and sexually active relationship by one or both partners. People in romantic relationships report that sexual intimacy is critical to the total functioning of their relationships (Blumstein & Schwartz, 1983; Patton & Waring, 1985), although not necessarily more important than other kinds of intimate interactions (Tolstedt & Stokes, 1983). Although both wives' and husbands' satisfaction with sexual intimacy is positively correlated with their marital satisfaction, this association may be stronger and more consistent over time for wives (W. Adams, 1988).

The amount of sexual intimacy shared by a couple (assessed as frequency of sexual encounters) is also associated with relationship satisfaction (Birchler & Webb, 1977; Blumstein & Schwartz, 1983; Sprecher & McKinney, 1993), although this association is not as strong for female–female couples (Blumstein & Schwartz, 1983). Within romantic relationships, more frequent and more satisfying sexual intimacy coincides with more affection, more cohesion, and more frequent verbal intimacy (Leigh, 1989; Patton & Waring, 1985; Russell, 1990). Among college students, the association between sexual intimacy and feelings of love and affection was stronger for women than for men (Christopher & Cate, 1984; Hatfield, Sprecher, Pillemer, Greenberger, & Wexler, 1988). This sex difference may disappear by midlife (Sprague & Quadagno, 1989), although some studies show that it persists (Hatfield et al., 1988). Regardless of age, the association between sexual intimacy and love is strong in both women and men.

Data from 1,200 American couples in a study conducted by Blumstein and Schwartz (1983) indicate that frequency of sexual activity varies depending on whether the couple is heterosexual and married, heterosexual and cohabiting, homosexual female, or homosexual male. Both dyad sex composition and relationship stage are associated with frequency of sexual activity. Compared to the other couples in this study, heterosexual cohabitors and gay men had the most frequent sex early in the relationship. Of the couples who had been together 10 years or more, married partners reported having the most frequent sex, and lesbian couples reported having the least frequent sex.

Conclusions about whether relationship dissatisfaction results in less sexual intimacy or vice versa are difficult to come by, because sex frequency is often the only available barometer of sexual intimacy. The use of sex frequency as a measure of sexual activity is not completely unwarranted. As noted earlier, sex frequency is highly correlated with global ratings of relationship satisfaction and with ratings of sexual satisfaction for gay, lesbian, and heterosexual couples. Other aspects of sex may be more important to a person's experience of sexual intimacy, such as length of time spent in sexual episodes, variety of sexual behavior, and verbal expressiveness or tenderness during sex. Other variables, such as sexual gratification and affectional expression, may, once measured, be more highly correlated with relationship satisfaction than is sex frequency (Sprecher & McKinney, 1993). Perhaps sex frequency is an outcome rather than a cause of gratifying sexual practices.

In relationships that are otherwise defined as nonerotic by both partners, the possibility of sexual intimacy can be viewed with fear, or at least ambivalence (Rubin, 1985; Swain, 1992). Scholars have paid some attention to the role of sexual intimacy in friendships between heterosexual women and men (Sprecher & McKinney, 1993). There is evidence that heterosexual opposite-sex friends may have ambivalent feelings about sexual intimacy. They acknowledge that sometimes they like one another "more than just a friend" (Swain, 1992, p. 166). When heterosexual men and women form friendships, they may have to explicitly exclude the possibility of sexual intimacy with one another (L. Rubin, 1985). Even when friends explicitly exclude sexual intimacy, sexual attraction must, as one writer put it, be "continually monitored, contended with, and regulated through negotiation" (O'Meara, 1989, p. 534). Gay men and lesbians seem more willing than heterosexuals to include fleeting, enduring, and previous sexual partners among their friends (Nardi & Sherrod, 1994).

Anxiety about the possible negative impact that sexual intimacy— or talk about sexual intimacy—may have on a friendship is also common (L. Rubin, 1983; Swain, 1992), particularly in friendships between heterosexual males (Swain, 1989). In Swain's (1989) study college-age men reported going to considerable lengths in their communication with each other to avoid implying an interest in sexual intimacy of any kind.

The attention people pay to possible sexual intimacy with friends may stem not from their sexual desires but from what Rawlins (1994) called a "dominant heterosexist ideology" (p. 2). This sociocultural ideology, according to Rawlins, defines "sexual striving . . . as the root metaphor for our being in the world . . . with other persons consequently reduced to sex objects" (p. 2). This ideology, in turn, purportedly influences the "opportunity structure" that either facilitates or discourages friendships (O'Meara, 1994). An opportunity structure that would encourage cross-sex friendship, for example, might include (1) opportunities for proximity, (2) political, economic, and social equality between the sexes, (3) a supportive set of norms defining appropriate means by which such friendships could be initiated, developed, and maintained, and (4) time to develop and maintain the friendship (O'Meara, 1994, p. 5). The lack of an opportunity structure such as the one O'Meara described may result in an absence of sociocultural schemas for cross-sex friendship, leaving women and men with nothing except the inappropriate "dating and mating" set. The lack of an opportunity structure and the resulting lack of culturally derived schemas may explain why sexual intimacy preoccupies friends, or inhibits the formation of friendships altogether.

Relationship Stage. Two questions come to mind when evaluating the impact of relational intimacy on relationship quality over time. The first question is, Does the quality of intimate interactions early in a relationship serve as a reliable predictor/indicator of the relationship's outcome at a later point? The second is, Does the impact of relational intimacy on relationship functioning vary over the course of a relationship? Might intimate contact be more important early in a relationship than later, for example?

Some normative changes in intimate interaction over time in romantic relationships have been documented. As I mentioned in earlier chapters, the amount of relational intimacy, particularly sexual intimacy, appears to be highest early in marital and cohabiting relationships, whether heterosexual, gay, or lesbian (Blumstein & Schwartz, 1986; Kurdek & Schmitt, 1986a). Frequent sexual contact (i.e., three times per week or more) typically drops off after 1 or 2 years, although gay male couples persist with frequent sexual activity more than do other couples. As mentioned previously (Chapter 7), decreases in relational intimacy accompany changes in relationship satisfaction, at least for married couples. Whether variations from these normative patterns bode ill or well for the future of a relationship is unknown.

Our knowledge of the impact that early-stage intimate interaction has on the course and outcome of intimate relationships is extremely limited. There is some evidence that early intimacy predicts the stability of friendship in young adulthood. A pattern of increasing breadth of self-disclosure in college students' friendships predicted which friendships would develop and become close and which would not (Hays, 1985). Similar results were obtained for college students' dating relationships (Sprecher, 1987). Studies have found that close friendships become quite intimate within the first few weeks and remain so (Hays, 1985, 1988) contrary to social penetration theory's prediction of gradual increases in intimacy over time (Altman & Taylor, 1973). Acquaintances who do not begin relating on a more intimate level within a few weeks may decide quickly not to be close friends (Berg, 1984).

Characteristics of early-stage relationships other than relational intimacy can predict the course of a relationship to some extent. For example, in a study of parent–child relationships early attachment patterns were predictive of the quality of parent–child communication 6 years later (Main et al., 1985). In other studies styles of communication and the expression of affect observable at the time of marriage predicted dissatisfaction and instability 1 to 4 years later (Gottman, 1991, 1993; Gottman & Krokoff, 1989; Hays, 1988; Markman, 1981; Smith, Vivian, & O'Leary, 1990).

The impact of intimate communication over time may be modified by other kinds of interactions, such as criticism and complaining. A recent study by Huston and Chorost (1994) suggests that affectional expression by newly wed husbands buffers the effects of their negativity on their wife's marital satisfaction. (Wives' behavior did not exert similar effects on husband's satisfaction.) After two years of marriage, however, affectional expression does not exert the same buffering effects. The extent to which intimate behavior elicits intimate experiences as relationships progress, then, may be modified by the quality of partners' nonintimate interactions.

It is unclear whether the importance of intimacy to relationship functioning increases (or decreases) as relationships progress. Berscheid's (1983) theory of emotion in close relationships suggests that intimacy remains important but that partners' *awareness* of needing intimate contact with one another may decrease over time. Berscheid posited that people in smoothly functioning, emotionally tranquil relationships will underestimate the importance of their relationship and the intimacy it provides. According to Berscheid, the reason why they underestimate is because they are neither overloaded nor deprived of intimate contact; they therefore experience little or no intense emotion in relation to intimacy or its lack. A lack of conflict about intimacy, then, may result in an *apparently* decreasing importance attached to intimacy. However, Berscheid argued that "partner[s] . . . may . . . be seduced by the emotional tranquility of the relationship to discount their emotional investment in it, only to discover, when the relationship is dissolved, how much the relationship meant to them, as evidenced by their severe emotional upheaval" (1983, p. 145).

The Group Context

The Relationship Network. For the last 25 years there has been a growing recognition that dyadic relationships exist within a web of overlapping and interconnecting relationships called a social network (e.g., Bott, 1971; Levinger, 1977; Milardo et al., 1983; Willer & Anderson, 1981). Research shows that the quality and stability of dyadic relationships may depend on and influence the nature of the other relationships in each partner's network (e.g., Cohn et al., 1991; Julien, Markman, Leveille, Chartrand, & Begin, 1994) and the characteristics of the networks themselves (Adams, 1987; Berg & McQuinn, 1986; D. Jones, 1992).

Although relationship networks exert influence on individual dyads in a variety of ways (Duck, 1993b; Julien et al., 1994), the hierarchical structure of relationships within adults' social networks may be especially worth examining in relation to intimacy. Relationships in a network seem to be arranged in a hierarchy of centrality or importance. The place of a relationship in the hierarchy seems to help people decide how to distribute scarce resources like time and attention over several close relationships (Johnson, Huston, Gaines, & Levinger, 1992; D. Morgan, 1990). People therefore may have to make decisions regarding which relationships they will invest these resources in and which they will neglect (Cohen, 1992; Johnson et al., 1992). These decisions likely have an impact on relational intimacy within those relationships.

Other important relationships in an adult's network, particularly with romantic partners, seem to affect the amount of intimacy in friendships (D. Morgan, 1990; Surra, 1985). In North America and Europe, at least, children and romantic partners (or spouses) are frequently given top priority in adults' social networks. This should be visible in at least two ways. First, when the time and energy available for intimate contact is limited, people should devote what they have to those who are highest in the hierarchy (Carbery, 1993; Cohen, 1992; Oliker, 1989; Swain, 1992). When adults face time constraints, then, intimate contact with friends may decrease in frequency or may disappear altogether (L. Rubin, 1985). For example, young adults have reported sharing less intimacy with their friends as a dating relationship progressed to a more intimate relationship (Milardo et al., 1983). Men's friendships are particularly vulnerable to being replaced by a budding romantic relationship (Cohen, 1992; Fischer, 1982; Komarovsky, 1967). Married couples' interactions with friends become more dominated by interactions with other couples (Wellman, 1992), perhaps because this allows them to accomplish two things at once with limited time: maintain the marital relationship and the friendships. Parents not only have difficulty making time for intimate friendships but also struggle to find shared leisure time for one another (Johnson et al., 1992; see Chapter 7).

Second, when a friendship competes with a marriage in other ways, people preserve the marriage at the expense of the friendship. For example, some friendships are seen as threatening to a marriage. Both men and women tend to carefully monitor any adverse effect a cross-sex friendship might have on their marriage (L. Rubin, 1985; Swain, 1992; Tschann, 1988), with some reporting a deliberate withholding of (nonsexual) intimacy that they might otherwise enjoy sharing.

As discussed in previous chapters, existing data suggest that adults do not lose interest in intimate friendships. Interviews with both female and male subjects reveal reports of regret and acceptance by spouses who have less time, and therefore less frequent intimate contact, with their friends (Cohen, 1992; Oliker, 1989; L. Rubin, 1985).

Despite conflicts between intimacy in friendship and intimacy in marriage, couples who maintain high levels of intimacy with friends appear to have more satisfying marriages (Fowers, Tredinnick, Pomerantz, & McIntosh, 1992; Stein et al., 1992). Perhaps friends fulfill intimacy needs when marital relationships do not, allowing spouses to feel satisfied who would otherwise experience loneliness if they had to rely solely on their marriages (Oliker, 1989; Reid & Fine, 1992; L. Rubin, 1985; W. Williams, 1992). Possibly, people can fulfill their needs for intimacy within a variety of relationships. As long as those needs are fulfilled, perhaps people can find satisfaction with their entire network of relationships, regardless of which relationships are most intimate (Levinger, 1977; Milardo & Wellman, 1992; Stein et al., 1992).

The Sociocultural Context

The Value Placed on Intimacy. Cultural values with respect to intimacy likely affect the importance individual dyad members place on intimacy in their own relationships. Broude (1987) provided evidence that values and expectations for intimacy in certain types of relationships vary dramatically from one culture to another. Among Trobriand Islanders, for example, married couples are expected to spend most of their working and leisure hours together enjoying intimacy and companionship. In contrast, the Rajputs of India view marriage as existing primarily for sex and procreation, with intimacy needs met in relationships with family members and same-sex friends. The way that people conduct their relationships should reflect those expectations (Broude, 1987). A fuller understanding of the impact of cultural values on how much people seek out and value relational intimacy awaits further research. This review demonstrates the important impact of contextual factors on intimate relationship functioning. Especially apparent is the interplay between partners' personality characteristics, such as private self-consciousness, need strengths, relationships beliefs, and intimate relationships. Intimacy also affects and is affected by the type and stage of the relationship. The most pervasive effects of context on intimate relationships may be exerted by gender, however. These effects are discussed next.

Gender and Intimate Relationships

The purpose of this section is twofold. First, it organizes and reviews the literature on gender-related patterns in intimate relationships. Gender-related patterns abound in friendships (e.g., Nardi, 1992b; O'Connor, 1992), romantic relationships (e.g., Christensen & Heavy, 1990; Blumstein & Schwartz, 1983), and parent-child relationships (e.g., Blyth & Foster-Clark, 1987). Following J. Wood's (1993) suggestion, this review strives to avoid oversimplifying gender-related patterns through the erroneous equating of conceptually distinct variables. For example, Wood noted that researchers may find gender-related patterns in emotional expressiveness and conclude that men lack feelings of closeness. The current review attempts to draw conclusions about gender-related patterns in intimate relationships without equating concepts that should remain distinct (see Duck & Wright, 1993, for a similar view).

A second purpose of this section is to consider the impact of contextual factors on gender-related patterns in intimate relationships. Research thus far has considered personal/relational contextual variables, such as psychological androgyny (D. Williams, 1985); group-level variables, such as sex-typed communication styles (Maccoby, 1990); and sociocultural variables such as reward structures for communal versus agentic activity (Seidler, 1992). This section addresses each of these contextual levels and considers how it might affect gender-related patterns in intimate relationships.

Gender and Friendship. Gender-related effects on intimate relationships are most apparent in females' and males' same-sex friendships. While males and females seem to have about the same number of best friends (Benenson, 1990), females, from adolescence to late adulthood, characterize their same-sex friendships as more intimate than males do (Blyth & Foster-Clark, 1987; Booth & Hess, 1974; Fischer & Narus, 1981; Hacker, 1981; Lowenthal et al., 1977; Rose, 1985; Winstead, 1986).

A closer look at the research is required to detect what, specifically, girls and women do that leads them (and scholars who study them) to describe their friendships as more intimate. As discussed in Chapter 8, girls' and women's conversations with friends include more personal self-disclosures (e.g., Hacker, 1981; Wright, 1989). Further, girls and women are more likely to share personal feelings with their friends (Caldwell & Peplau, 1982; Duck & Wright, 1993; Sharabany et al., 1981) and to value talk as an end in itself (Raffaelli & Duckett, 1989). Possibly, they express their affectionate feelings to one another more than boys and men do with their friends (Helgeson et al., 1987), both through physical contact and self-disclosure (Monsour, 1992).

The sex differences commonly found in heterosexual samples were not found in Nardi and Sherrod's (1994) study of lesbians' and gay men's friendships. In that study, social support, self-disclosure, shared activities, and the overall importance of friendship were quite similar for women and men. The only gender difference they found was that women were more likely to confront and discuss conflict with their friends than were men. Nardi and Sherrod (1994) did not directly assess whether lesbians' and gay men's friendships are more similar to heterosexual female or male friendships. Evidence from other research, however, indicates that these friendships may resemble heterosexual women's more than men's (Nardi, 1992). Nardi's work showed that gay men and lesbians were as likely to seek support and intimate contact within nonerotic friendships as within romantic relationships, a finding supported in studies of heterosexual women, but not men (e.g., Nardi, 1992a).

Gender-related effects on friendship are attenuated in nonromantic, cross-sex friendships. Men, but not women, tend to describe these friendships as more intimate than their same-sex friendships (Dindia & Allen, 1992; L. Rubin, 1985). Men are more emotionally expressive in their cross-sex friendships than in their same-sex friendships (Monsour, 1992) and disclose more personal information (Dindia & Allen, 1992), particularly about their feminine side (Snell, 1989). They are also more physically affectionate with their female friends (Monsour, 1992). Like women, they are more likely to seek out female than male friends when they need support and, like women, believe their female friends know them better than their male friends do (Buhrke & Fuqua, 1987).

The gender-related patterns in same-sex friendships described above are not universal, either across cultures or within Western culture over time. Similar patterns exist in Western cultures like the former Soviet Union (Kon et al., 1978) and New Zealand (Aukett, Ritchie, & Mill, 1988) whereas men's and women's friendships in India are quite similar

(Berman, Murphy-Berman, & Pachauri, 1988). There is also evidence that American women's and men's expectations for intimate contact with friends has changed since the 19th century (Hansen, 1992).

Gender and Romantic Relationships. Gender-related patterns in romantic relationships are apparent in the ways that women and men approach intimacy (Helgeson et al., 1987; L. Rubin, 1983). First, in both their heterosexual and homosexual romantic relationships, men and women may favor different types of intimate contact: Men favor sexual intimacy a bit more than verbal intimacy while women favor verbal intimacy (Blumstein & Schwartz, 1983; Engel & Saracino, 1986). In a study of predominantly heterosexual American college students, Hatfield et al. (1988) found that men were more likely than women to view physical contact and sex as central features of intimacy. Further, young women, more than men, reported that they were likely to verbally express their warm and affectionate feelings to their romantic partners.

Second, women and men may initiate different kinds of intimate interactions in their marriages. Clinicians' reports indicate that women initiate more verbal intimacy with their husbands than their husbands do with them (Markman & Kraft, 1989). Women encourage their spouses (and children) to seek emotional support from them more frequently than men do. Women also express more empathy in their heterosexual relationships than do men (Goldner, 1987; Gulley, Barbee, & Cummingham, 1992). Men, in contrast, may take more responsibility for initiating sexual intimacy than their wives do (Blumstein & Schwartz, 1983; L. Rubin, 1990).

Third, women are less likely than men to withdraw from conflict in their romantic relationships (Christensen & Heavy, 1990; Gottman, 1994; Komarovsky, 1967; L. Rubin, 1983). Women report using more constructive problem-solving approaches in their dating relationships (Rusbult, Zembrodt, & Gunn, 1982). When wives initiate conflict, husbands may be especially likely to withdraw (Christensen & Heavy, 1990; Heavy, Layne & Christensen, 1993). Women may persist more in their conflict resolution efforts than men do (Rusbult, Ziembnodt, & Gunn, 1982).

Women may, on the average, understand better how important constructive communication about conflict is to relationship functioning. For example, male college students were more likely than females to attribute the breakup of their romantic relationships to the absence of a "mysterious and inexplicable magic in one another's presence" (Baxter, 1986, p. 297). Young women, in contrast, tended to see reasons for breaking up as stemming from specific communication and behavioral problems within the relationship.[4]

Perhaps the most popularized finding in the literature on gender-related patterns in marital relationships is that women are more likely than men to complain that their intimacy needs are not being met adequately (Chodorow, 1979; Hite, 1987; L. Rubin, 1983; Tannen, 1990b). Despite the attention this finding has received, empirical support for it is scanty (but see Veroff, Douvan, & Kulka, 1981). What has been found is that intimate contact is a stronger predictor of women's marital satisfaction than men's (Acitelli & Antonucci, 1994). The possibility that women's intimacy needs are more likely to go unmet than are men's has garnered enough attention to prompt several writers to speculate on the determinants of this pattern, which are discussed in the next section.

In sum, most of the many studies that document gender-related patterns in intimate relationships conclude that women seek and find more relational intimacy within their relationships. In the following sections, I examine factors at three contextual levels (personal/relational, group, and sociocultural) that may modify gender-related patterns in intimate relationships. In doing so I propose some ways that may help us better understand gender differences and similarities in intimate relationships.

Factors Modifying Gender-Related Patterns in Intimate Relationships

Personality. The following individual difference variables have been proposed to explain gender-related friendship patterns: (1) gender differences in pathways to intimacy, (2) gender-related definitions of intimacy, and (3) differences between women and men in the value placed on intimate contact. One argument suggests that if different behaviors, activities, and contexts prompt experiences of intimacy in women and men, then studies that define intimacy solely in terms of self-disclosure may underestimate how intimate men's friendships are (Cancian, 1986; Duck & Wright, 1993; Wood, 1993). There is empirical support for this view. Men may perceive more pathways to intimate experience with friends than women do. Girls and women, for example, distinguish clearly among their friendships on the basis of whether or not they can self-disclose to that friend. Boys and men are less inclined to make this distinction (Blyth & Foster-Clark, 1987; Caldwell & Peplau, 1982; Lowenthal et al., 1977). Boys and men say that sharing activities and interests are just as important pathways to intimate experience as is self-disclosure. Further, they may see sharing activities as creating opportunities for intimacy while girls and women do not (Camarena, Sarigiani, & Petersen, 1990; L. Rubin, 1983; Swain, 1989; Youniss & Smollar, 1985).

Some studies have tested the hypothesis that women and men define intimacy differently, which is then reflected in differing reports about intimacy in friendship. Available evidence suggests, however, that males and females agree on what intimacy is (Helgeson et al., 1987; Reis et al., 1985). Further, they agree that self-disclosure is the primary means for developing intimate relationships (Camarena et al., 1990; Monsour, 1992). Gender-related patterns cannot be attributed, then, to different definitions of intimacy held by males and females.

Women's friendships may be more intimate because women value intimate contact more than men do and therefore pursue it more actively and deliberately with their friends. Specifically, females place higher value on mutual help, support, trust and stability in friendships than males do (Gulley et al., 1992; Oliker, 1989; Rawlins, 1992; Wright, 1982). Women, more than men, distinguish among their friendships based on closeness. Men seem inclined to view friends as close in one respect but not in others; women tend to see friends as either close or not (Wright, 1988). Women differentiate friends from acquaintances on a broader range of characteristics and appear to have clearer ideas than men about the differences between the two kinds of relationships (Wright, 1988). While women and men both value intimacy and its emotional concomitants in friendships, women place more emphasis on it than men do (Duck & Wright, 1993).

Sex differences in how intimate relationships are approached have most frequently been attributed to gender differences in sex-typed personality characteristics. Research shows that psychological masculinity and femininity are more efficient predictors of intimate relationship functioning than is anatomical sex. Mixed results, however, leave open the question of whether femininity or androgyny is the best predictor of relationship satisfaction (Siavelia & Lamke, 1992).

Initially, hypothesized links between sex-typed traits and relationship quality focused on androgyny, a combination of feminine and masculine traits. Given this definition, androgyny affords the greatest adaptability, and leads to the highest levels of relationship functioning (Kaplan & Sedney, 1980). Some research has supported this contention (Narus & Fischer, 1982; Flaherty & Dusek, 1980; Spence & Helmreich, 1978). Androgynous college students of both sexes rate their close friends as more trustworthy, and rate the characteristics of their friends more positively than do sex-typed college students (Jones, Bloys, & Wood, 1990). College students also rate their dating relationships as more satisfying when both they and their partners are androgynous (Siavelis & Lamke, 1992). In other studies both masculinity and femininity were positively related to marital adjustment, suggesting that androgynous partners may be especially capable of building and maintaining a satisfactory marital relationship (Bradbury, Campbell, & Fincham, 1995; Sayers & Baucom, 1991).

Wright and Scanlon (1991) found that feminine and masculine personality characteristics do not predict adults' ratings of satisfaction with friendships but that their descriptions of their friends' femininity and masculinity did. In Wright and Scanlon's study participants rated androgynous partners as the most rewarding friends, undifferentiated partners (i.e., those who endorse few feminine or masculine characteristics) as the least rewarding, and masculine- and feminine-sex-typed partners in between. These partner effects were independent of the raters' feminine and masculine characteristics.

Some scholars have suggested that femininity alone is sufficient for predicting better-functioning close relationships (Harry, 1984; Jones & Dembo, 1989; D. Williams, 1985). Supporting this notion are studies that show that feminine-sex typing predicts relationship functioning as well as androgyny does. For example, in one study, androgynous and feminine-sex-typed college students of both sexes gave similar ratings of the emotional intimacy in their friendships. Their ratings were higher than those assigned by masculine-sex-typed and undifferentiated students, whose ratings were indistinguishable from one another (D. Williams, 1985). Jones and Dembo (1989) obtained similar results with a sample of U.S. schoolchildren aged 9 to 14. They found that androgynous children of both sexes and feminine-sex-typed females rate the intimacy levels of their close friendships similarly while-sex-typed males have relationships that are significantly less intimate. Harry's (1984) study of 1,440 gay men suggests that feminine personality characteristics are predictive of men's interest in having an intimate romantic relationship. Feminine characteristics have predicted marital satisfaction as well (Antill, 1983; Bradbury et al., 1995; Kurdek & Schmitt, 1986a). Kurdek and Schmitt found that gay male, lesbian, and heterosexual cohabiting couples are most satisfied when either they or their partners have feminine-sex-typed characteristics. Antill (1983) found that both husbands and wives are happiest with a spouse who has feminine characteristics.

Results from one study led Parmelee (1987) to conclude that "it is not femininity per se, but a gender-role identity opposite to one's sex that promotes marital satisfaction, particularly among men" (p. 439). She found that androgynous and masculine-sex-typed wives are more satisfied in their marriages than feminine-sex-typed wives while androgynous and feminine-sex-typed men are more satisfied than masculine sex-typed men.

Masculine- and feminine-sex-typed traits may also contribute to different aspects of relationships. While feminine-sex-typed traits may enhance intimacy in relationships, they may contribute less than masculine-sex-typed traits to effective problem-solving communication. In their study of maritally distressed couples Sayers and Baucom (1991) found that masculinity in wives was related to lower levels of negativity during marital conflict while femininity in wives was related to higher levels. Further, husbands and wives with higher femininity (but not masculinity) scores were less likely to terminate negative sequences of interaction. The authors reported these findings in the context of no husband–wife differences in the likelihood or amount of negative communication. Mixed results regarding masculine-sex typing and relationship functioning, then, may be due to variability in its contribution to relationship functioning.

Finally, masculine and feminine personality traits may contribute to changes in relationship functioning over time. In a recent study, Bradbury, Campbell, and Fincham (1995) found that husbands' masculine personality traits were predictive of changes in wives' marital satisfaction. They found that assessments of husbands' desirable masculine characteristics predicted increases in wives' satisfaction, while husbands' undesirable masculine characteristics predicted decreases in wives' satisfaction. (Wives' sex-typed traits did not predict changes in husbands' satisfaction.) Bradbury et al. also found associations between husbands' masculine and feminine personality traits and their behavior during problem-solving discussions with their wives. These behaviors did not explain links between husbands' traits and wives' satisfaction, however.

Perhaps the most reliable conclusion that can be drawn from these studies is that masculine-and feminine-sex-typed personality characteristics explain some of the gender-related variance in intimate relationships. Individuals with the same gender role orientation (androgynous, feminine-sex-typed, masculine-sex-typed) tend to resemble one another in how they approach and experience their intimate relationships, regardless of their anatomical sex. Gender-related patterns in intimate relationships may be due, then, to the fact that people are more likely to have same-sex-typed traits than opposite-sex-typed traits.

There is also evidence that one partners' sex-typed personality characteristics affect the others' satisfaction with the relationship. Findings from Bradbury et al.'s study may indicate that there is a causal relationship between husbands' masculine traits and wives' marital satisfaction. Perhaps sex-typed personality traits are associated with behavior in intimate interactions and thereby affect relationship satisfaction.

Group and Sociocultural Values. Some writers have examined gender-specific group and sociocultural norms in the United States to further understanding of gender-related patterns in intimate relationships (e.g., Risman & Schwartz, 1989). These efforts have been aimed at illuminating two sets of findings: (1) higher levels of intimacy in women's than in men's same-sex friendships and (2) differences in men's and women's approaches to intimacy need fulfillment in romantic heterosexual relationships.

Gender-related approaches to intimate relationships may reflect responses to gendered norms for interpersoanl behavior. Most writers agree that gender is a social category that exposes females and males (in Western culture) to distinct (although overlapping) sets of cultural norms (Cohen, 1992; Cross & Markus, 1993; Maccoby, 1990; Risman & Schwartz, 1989; Swain, 1989; Tannen, 1990b; J. Wood, 1993). Some proponents of this view submit that different interpersonal styles get positive versus negative responses from others depending on whether one is male or female (e.g., Geis, 1993). In particular, a review by Maccoby (1990a) suggests that females and males may face divergent expectations for social behavior within their same-sex peer groups beginning very early in life, expectations they will continue to confront throughout life.

Gender-related norms in the United States recapitulate Bakan's (1966) distinction between agentic and communal values (or "agency" and "communion"). In Bakan's model, agentic values protect and nurture the self; they encourage people to further their own self-interest, growth, development, and achievement; foster their own status and recognition; and resist pressures to make sacrifices. Communal values, in contrast, involve contact with others that is equitable, trusting, warm, nurturing, and/or affectionate, and are based on a willingness to put one's own agentic strivings aside to foster the well-being of the larger community. In the United States females are traditionally expected to pursue communal values more than are males while males, more than females, are expected to pursue agentic values (Bakan, 1966; Bardwick & Douvan, 1971; Brown & Gilligan, 1992; Lott & Maluso, 1993; Maccoby, 1990a; McAdams, 1984). The sex typing of personality traits reflects these expectations.

U.S. culture seems to laud masculine, agentic values more than feminine, communal ones, which may discourage men's intimacy. Cultural norms not only dictate that men and women pursue different values but also more or less privilege one set of values (agentic vs. communal) over the other. Cultures differ from one another in the extent to which they value agentic or communal norms. There is evidence that United States culture, compared with other cultures, puts a high premium on agentic values (Dion & Dion, 1988; Guisinger & Blatt, 1994) and on individualism in particular.

Individualism, which has been the focus of debate among psychological theorists for 10–15 years (e.g., Cushman, 1990; Guisinger & Blatt, 1994; Hermans, Kempen, & van Loon, 1992; Spence, 1985), is a value that seems to reflect the simultaneous privileging of agency and denigrating of communion that characterizes North American culture. Individualism, according to Spence (1985, p. 1288) is "a sense of the self with a sharp boundary that stops at one's skin and clearly demarks self from nonself." This bounded self has "an internal locus of control, and a wish to manipulate the external world for its own personal ends" (Cushman, 1990, p. 600). Western culture's endorsement of individualism seems to be inextricably bound to its privileging of agency, of "autonomy, independence, achievement motivation, and identity as essential components of psychological maturity" (Guisinger & Blatt, 1994). Agency, in turn, is embodied in the Western ideal of masculinity (Pleck, 1981).

North American individualism probably inhibits relational intimacy in men's friendships. This inhibiting effect should arise from (1) the valorizing of agency in individualism, and (2) the equating of individualism, agency, and masculinity. Individualism encourages people to derive self-worth from individual achievement and accomplishment rather than from contributions to the common good. Because the pursuit of individualistic values is the pursuit of masculinity, men are pitted against one another in a competition for external recognition and individually based rewards (e.g., Seidler, 1992). Individualism also encourages self-reliance (Doyle, 1989). Valuing friends too highly, then, may suggest a failure of self-reliance (and of masculinity). Men may therefore fail to cultivate friendships because they see the effort as energy wasted—or even as a sign of weakness. If a man becomes more concerned with friendship than with competition and self-reliance, his entire masculine self can be called into question by everyone around him (Doyle, 1989; Pleck, 1981).

Women's friendships, in contrast, seem to exist within a female subculture that valorizes intimate contact, harmony, emotional support, and togetherness while it discourages women's agency (Brown & Gilligan, 1992; Maccoby, 1990b; Pogrebin, 1987). Brown and Gilligan argued that the emotional support, harmony and intimate contact that adolescent girls offer one another through friendship often come at the expense of girls' developing individuation. Pogrebin suggested that traditional women's friendships may fulfill women's needs for intimacy and emotional support while simultaneously maintaining women's relative powerlessness within the culture.

It is probably too simplistic, however, to assume that agentic values and individualism unilaterally discourage intimacy, while communal values encourage it (e.g., Sharabany & Wiseman, 1993). Individualism supports intimate relationships by privileging the private over the public and thereby prizes individual expression, gratification and growth (Dion & Dion, 1988; Oyserman, 1993; Paul & White, 1990). Bestowing worth on private relationships is an extension of this value of individual privacy. Collectivist cultures, in contrast, value the extended family and the broader culture over individual well-being and happiness; the good of the group takes precedent over individual good (Dion & Dion, 1988). In this context, efforts to fulfill individual needs for intimacy might be viewed as self-indulgent and therefore a source of shame. In sum, because individualism is a pervasive value in American culture, its equation with masculinity likely serves to limit men's opportunities for intimate contact while leaving women free to enjoy intimacy. This contributes to gender-related patterns in intimate relationships. At the same time, individualism's concern with individual privacy facilitates intimacy in U.S. culture as a whole.

A self-fulfilling prophecy process may also maintain gender-related patterns of behavior in close relationships (Fiske & Taylor, 1991). Self-fulfilling prophecies arise directly from the interaction between one person's expectations of another and the second person's responses to those expectations. Risman and Schwartz's (1989) "microstructural theory" proposes that patterns of social behavior are formed and sustained as a result of subtle yet powerful cues conveyed in the day-to-day interactions between people. Most likely, we all convey, in one way or another, our disappointment, confusion, and/or disapproval to others when they behave contrary to the ways we expect members of their gender to behave. Our expectations are derived from gender-typed sociocultural norms.

Behavioral cues in interactions shape people's behavior in the expected direction because people adjust their behavior to meet the expectations of others. They are especially likely to do so if others' approval and/or goodwill is important to them (Fiske, 1993; Geis, 1993). In close relationships the goodwill of the other person is usually important, particularly if the other person has more power in the relationship (Adams & Blieszner, 1994; J. Wood, 1993). Ironically, then, stereotypic expectations about others may perpetuate themselves in social interaction via self-fulfilling prophecies.

Gender-typed behavior, then, does not emerge as much from one's anatomy, physiology, personality, or socialization as it does from day-to-day, minute-to-minute behavior with other people (Risman & Schwartz, 1989; West & Zimmerman, 1991; J. Wood, 1993). Within daily interactions conventional gender-typed behavior is more frequently rewarded with attention, smiles, and expressions of approval than is unconventional behavior (Eagly, Makhijani, & Klonsky, 1990; Fagot, 1978, 1984b; Lytton & Romney, 1991).

If women more frequently than men find themselves in romantic relationships in which they want more intimate contact than their partners do, factors other than dispositional gender differences in intimacy needs may be responsible. Risman and Schwartz's theory advocates the simultaneous consideration of psychological and social structural forces as shapers of intimate relating. In that spirit, I suggest that some people, at least in North American culture, actively (though sometimes unconsciously) pursue relationships that allow them to enact gender-typed roles. People do not only respond to environmental input but seek out situations in which a preexisting self-concept is likely to be confirmed and supported (Magnussen, 1990). Because gender is a broadly influential aspect of the self-concept (Cross & Markus, 1993), people may, as a result, gravitate to situations that encourage gender-typed behavior (e.g., boxing matches, bridal showers, and the "right" intimate partner). Perhaps, to the extent that people seek opportunities to fulfill gender-related expectations, they seek interaction partners whose behavior facilitates that gendered behavior. Women paired with men who need less intimacy than they do can fulfill their gender-consistent role of intimacy seeking with their husbands. They may gravitate to such men (unconsciously) in order to do so.

If anxious and avoidant attachment styles can be construed as rough approximations of high versus minimal needs for intimacy, a recent study by Kirkpatrick and Davis (1994) supports my hypothesis that people seek out opportunities to enact gender-stereotypic roles in intimate relationships. Kirkpatrick and Davis asked 354 couples in a "serious dating relationship" to complete Hazan and Shaver's (1987) Attachment Style measure and Davis and Todd's (1985) Relationship Rating Form. Couple members were also contacted for two follow-ups (12–14 months later and 30–36 months later) to determine whether they were still together. The authors found that anxious women and avoidant men were disproportionately paired with one another at the initial contact. Further, relationships between anxious women and avoidant men showed remarkably high levels of stability at follow-up, especially considering the fact that both partners were likely to rate their relationship as unsatisfying. These relationships were stable even when prior duration was controlled for. The stability of these relationships suggests that they may be serving some as yet undetected purpose for the partners. Perhaps that purpose is to allow the participants to to enact gender-stereotypic roles and thereby maintain gender-stereotypic self-concepts. A more definitive test of this hypothesis requires further work.

Lest we all resign ourselves to a fate of undiluted gender stereotyping in our intimate relationships, it is important to note sources of individual differences in people's concerns with and responsiveness to gender-related behavior. Cross and Markus (1993) argued that for some individuals "gender becomes a basic identifying feature of the self and gender is chronically used in thinking about and describing and evaluating the self" (p. 76). For these gender-schematic individuals, then, gender becomes an intensely salient aspect of their self- schemas.

For people who have gender-schematic self-concepts, a mate whose behavior reinforces gender-typed behavior may be highly desirable. The people gender-schematic individuals are most attracted to, enjoy interacting with, and choose as mates should be those whose typical behavior elicits and reinforces gender-typed behavior in them. How might this work in romantic relationships? Consider the example of Carlos below:

> Carlos complains that his wife, Carmen, is continually nagging him about spending too much time at the office, on the golf course, on hunting trips, and in other pursuits that they cannot enjoy together. He feels stifled and smothered yet acknowledges that she feels lonely and neglected. However, when asked why he chose Carmen over another young woman he was dating at the time, he answers, "Carmen was prettier, of course. But it was more than that. She was warmer, more affectionate, loved to be with me. Most important of all, she seemed to need me. The other woman I was dating just didn't seem to need me as much. It was like she didn't really love me."

My own clinical experience working with couples has told me that stories like Carlos's are common. As much as Carlos may complain of being suffocated in his current relationship, it is questionable whether he could be comfortable with a woman he would have to pursue for intimate contact.

An explanation for Carlos's attraction to Carmen, and for why he ultimately chose to marry her, may lie in his gender schematicity. If Carlos' self-concept is gender schematic, he may fervently desire to see himself as the traditional self-reliant, independent male. Choosing a mate who seems to prefer more intimate contact than he is comfortable with could be the best way Carlos has to continuously confirm this gender-typed self-concept. In a relationship with such a mate the role of limiting intimate contact would fall to Carlos because he prefers less intimate contact than she does. Each time Carlos must limit intimate contact with Carmen, he witnesses himself behaving according to the masculine sex-typed traits he hopes characterize him: independent, self-reliant, in control, and strong, that is, with few interpersonal needs (Bem, 1983; Rosencrantz, Vogel, Bee, Broverman, & Broverman, 1968). If Carlos were to become involved with a partner whose needs for intimacy were less than his, he would have to pursue her (Napier, 1978) to get his intimacy needs met. This behavior might force him to revise his concept of himself as self-reliant.

If women and men seem to have different intimacy needs in their romantic relationships, it may be because heterosexual gender-schematic individuals tend to choose one another as partners. When they choose one another, both partners then get to enact familiar gender-related behaviors within the relationship. Researchers (and clinicians), however, only see the couple after the relationship is established, when gender-related patterns, such as the pursuer–distancer pattern, are already apparent.

Homophobia. It is impossible to discuss intimate homosexual relationships without considering the impact of Western culture's long history of homophobia (Bullough, 1990). According to Shildo (1994), the term *homophobia* was coined by Weinberg (1972) and refers to "the dread of being in close quarters with homosexuals" (p. 4). For several hundred years people in Europe and the New World who engaged in homosexual relationships could lose their jobs, their freedom, or, frequently, their lives (Blumstein & Schwartz, 1983; Bullough, 1990). Shildo reported that in 1991, 66% of Americans condemned homosexual behavior as morally wrong. In the same study nearly 10% of lesbians and 5% of gay men reported experiences of being physically assaulted because of their sexual orientation; among youth this figure is considerably higher (Hershberger & D'Augelli, 1995). Over half of lesbians and gay men report having experienced some form of verbal harassment (Hershberger & D'Augelli, 1995).

The need for secrecy among many gay couples may explain in part why there is so little research on gay and lesbian intimate relationships. Throughout history, people desiring intimate romantic relationships with others of the same sex have had to carry out their relationships in secrecy (Blumstein & Schwartz, 1983). As Harry (1984) put it, "To the extent that the form of deviance being examined is popularly considered serious or abhorrent the deviant will be hesitant to reveal her- or himself to the researcher, either out of personal embarrassment or out of fear of ensuing legal/economic or social sanctions" (p. 23). Changes in the way psychiatrists and psychologists view homosexuality have opened doors to research on individuals who identify primarily with a homosexual orientation (e.g., Greene & Herek, 1994), but research on relationships is still rare (Peplau & Cochran, 1990). This is despite the fact that between 40% and 60% of men and between and 45% and 80% of women who identify themselves as homosexual live with a same-sex romantic partner (Blumstein & Schwartz, 1983; Kurdek, 1994; Peplau & Cochran, 1990).

The few studies that have assessed satisfaction in gay and lesbian relationships indicate that, despite homophobia, the developmental course and sources of satisfaction in these relationships are quite similar to those in heterosexual relationships (Kurdek, 1994; Rosenbluth & Steil, 1995). McWhirter and Mattison (1984) found that gay couples, like their heterosexual counterparts, describe relationships that begin with high levels of passion and intimacy and then decline in intensity as couples face issues of conflict and power. Feelings of security and attachment increase as relationships persist over time. Gay and lesbian couples report levels of satisfaction in their relationships that are similar to those for heterosexual couples (Kurdek, 1994; Kurdek & Schmitt, 1986b). What is notable about results from research comparing homosexual and heterosexual relationships is the similarity between them, suggesting that cultural homophobia and secrecy exert minimal effects on the internal workings of romantic relationships.

Homophobia has also been recognized as a sociocultural force discouraging intimate friendships between heterosexual men (R. Lewis, 1978). Support for the constraining effect of cultural homophobia exists in studies that compare men's relationships in present-day North America with those 100 years ago. This period is significant because the dualistic notion of sexual orientation so familiar to present-day Americans did not take hold until the 20th century (Bullough, 1990). It would not have occurred to heterosexual male friends in the 19th century that their affection for one another might imply the possibility of sexual attraction. In antebellum New England, for example, it was possible and reasonable for men to openly express their positive feelings about each other either verbally or in writing (Bullough, 1990; Hansen, 1992) —as it was for women as well (see Smith-Rosenberg, 1986). Physical expressions of affection (such as hugging, kissing, and sleeping in the same bed) were quite acceptable between young, unmarried men (Hansen, 1992b). Intimate friendships between men were most commonly documented for middle-class men, but there is limited evidence that they were common among the working classes as well (Nardi, 1992b). In earlier centuries Western European culture closely associated "manly" virtues such as chivalry and heroism with intimate male friendship (Nardi, 1992b). These patterns changed, however, when the dualistic notion of heterosexuality versus homosexuality became widely endorsed.

SUMMARY AND CONCLUSIONS

In this chapter I have proposed that relational intimacy enhances the functioning of intimate relationships. Frequent intimate interactions should contribute to the satisfaction, harmony, and stability of intimate relationships. They should also contribute to other relationship characteristics that foster relationship functioning, such as affection, trust, and cohesiveness. In this chapter I also reiterate my emphasis on contextual factors. Contextual factors directly influence intimate relationship functioning. They also determine how important relational intimacy will be to relationship functioning.

This chapter first develops some notions about how relational intimacy influences and is influenced by other, overlapping, aspects of relationships. Reviews show ample support for the notion that intimacy and love (e.g., Critelli, Myers, & Loos, 1986), trust (Murray & Holmes, 1993; Rawlins & Holl, 1987), and cohesion (Hays, 1989; Reissman et al., 1993) are closely linked in personal relationships.

Because of the extensive theorizing about love and intimacy that already exists in the literature, I was able to identify several ways that love and intimacy might be linked. Loving emotions are likely concomitants of intimate interactions and are likely to prompt intimate behavior. Intimate interactions in turn seem to have positive effects on love relationships (e.g., Tolstedt & Stokes, 1983). The circumstances that allow loving emotions to evoke intimate behavior have yet to be clearly identified. While the notion that people who love are likely to express positive feelings through words or affectionate physical contact is hardly revolutionary, researchers know little about individual differences and situational factors that might encourage or inhibit such expressions. Given how likely it is that these intimate behaviors extend considerable benefits to their recipients, further exploration of the circumstances that allow for them seems warranted.

A better understanding of the conditions under which intimate relationships are likely to flourish requires consideration of contextual factors. All relationships exist in personal, relational, group, and sociocultural contexts. There is reason to believe that variables at each level impinge on and enhance the partners' opportunities to create a rewarding relationship.

The majority of the work on contextual factors has thus far concentrated on the impact of personal/relational factors on intimate relationships. Personality characteristics can affect the initiation (Canary & Cupach, 1988), development (Snyder & Simpson, 1984), and ongoing quality (Franzoi, Davis, & Young, 1985) of intimate relationships. Attitudes, expectations, and beliefs also affect relationship functioning. Research indicates that people are less satisfied with their marital relationships when their expectations are violated (Belsky & Rovine, 1990) and when they attribute negative intent to their partner's actions (Fincham, 1989). Specific beliefs about marriage (e.g., believing that each partner should know what the other is thinking without either having to say any-thing) also predict poor marital functioning (Pretzer et al., 1991).

At the group level, intimate relationship functioning is affected by the demands made and support given by other relationships in the net-work. For good or ill, each intimate relationship is embedded in a social network that can affect relationship functioning. The position of any giv-en relationship in the network and the impact of other relationships on it differ from one point in the life span to the next. Beginning in ado-lescence there is evidence that the presence of a romantic relationship in the network results in less time for friends (e.g., Milardo et al., 1983). Further, people seem to monitor their friendships to ensure that those friendships do not threaten or interfere with their romantic rela-tionship (Tschann, 1988). Married adults who are able to maintain inti-mate friendships seem to have more satisfying marriages (Stein et al., 1992). Future research would do well to discover how some couples are able to maintain networks of intimate friends and kin while others are not.

Many of the contextual factors discussed in this chapter affect the importance relationship partners place on intimacy. McAdams and his colleagues have identified individual differences in the strength of peo-ple's intimacy motives (e.g., McAdams, 1986, 1988a; McAdams, Healy, & Krause, 1984), which might contribute to relationship partners placing different amounts of emphasis on intimacy. Relational factors also seem to affect the importance people place on different types of intimacy in a particular relationship. Which partner places more emphasis on sexual intimacy—the male or the female—seems to depend on how long the couple has been together (W. Adams, 1988). Partners' sexual orientation is predictive of how frequently they engage in sexual activity at different points in their relationship (Blumstein & Schwartz, 1983). A combina-tion of gender and sexual orientation predicts how people think about sexual intimacy in relationships that are defined primarily as friendships (e.g., Nardi & Sherrod, 1994). Partners' definition of their relationship as close or casual also seemed to affect how important nonsexual forms of intimacy, such as self-disclosure, are to the relationship (Reisman, 1990).

Research has identified reliable, if modest, differences between women's and men's intimate relationships. Women's same-sex friendships seem to be more intimate than men's on several dimensions, including self-disclosure (Wright, 1982), expression of feelings (Caldwell & Peplau, 1982), and affectionate physical contact (Monsour, 1992). Evidence that men and women prefer different amounts of relational intimacy within romantic relationships is still quite limited (L. Rubin, 1983). There is a modest trend indicating that men may value sexual intimacy more than verbal intimacy, whereas women value verbal intimacy more (e.g., Hatfield et al., 1988).

Initial efforts to explain gender-related patterns in intimate relationships principally concerned themselves with variables at the personal/relational contextual level. There is evidence, for example, that women value intimacy more highly in their friendships, relative to other relationship characteristics, than do men (Camarena et al., 1990). Perhaps as a result, women use fewer criteria for choosing friends than men do, relying more on whether intimate contact is possible in those friendships. Their friendships may be more intimate, then, because they weed out or discount friendships that are less intimate (Duck & Wright, 1993).

Researchers have also looked to sex differences in sex-typed personality traits as a possible explanation for gender-related patterns in intimate relationships. Personality characteristics seem to be better predictors of relationship functioning than is anatomical sex. Research consistently indicates that feminine-sex-typed traits are more predominant in people with satisfying intimate relationships (e.g., D. Williams, 1985). Results are mixed, however, regarding the contribution of masculine-sex-typed traits.

Documented sex differences in intimate relationships have arguably done more to stimulate scholars' interest in sociocultural factors than any other aspect of intimate relationships. Because sociocultural factors are difficult to operationalize, explanations of the impact of these variables on gender-related patterns are mostly speculative. Some writers have proposed that gender-related expectations are communicated both directly and indirectly in people's interactions with others, beginning very early in life (e.g., Maccoby, 1990a; Risman & Schwartz, 1989). These sociocultural factors should be evident in people's expectations about one another, in the subtle ways they reinforce one another's behavior in interactions, and in their values and beliefs about proper behavior.

Gender-related expectations purportedly come from culture-based associations between women and communal values, and between men and agentic values (Bakan, 1966). People seem to expect these values to be evident in both their own and others' interpersonal behavior (Geis, 1993), and they shape their own behavior to reflect these values. Associations between masculinity and agentic values, for example, may result in norms precluding certain kinds of intimate contact between male friends (Seidler, 1992). To the extent that intimate contact falls into the communal realm, it will be defined as feminine and therefore inappropriate for men (Cancian, 1986). Many men, as a result, will spurn intimate contact with other men.

Perhaps because cultural images of masculinity and femininity incorporate prescriptions for behavior in intimate relationships, some individuals may wish to enact these prescribed behaviors as a way of bolstering their own gender identities. For this reason, people may select romantic partners whose behavior helps to sustain and accentuate gender-related behavior and characteristics in themselves. A wife's feminine behavior, for example, stands out more dramatically if it is contrasted with her husband's masculine behavior. Each partner thereby provides the other with a contrast effect which highlights and substantiates each partner's gender identity (i.e., their security and comfort in their own gender).

Despite the persistent focus on differences that pervades the literature on gender and intimate relationships, however, it is important to remember that there are more similarities than differences between women's and men's intimate relationships (Duck & Wright, 1993). Women's and men's criteria for a close relationship are more similar than different (Waring et al., 1981), and both men and women differentiate between best friends and other friends when deciding how much to disclose (Reis et al., 1985). The ability to self-disclose is the primary characteristic of intimate relationships for both males and females (Camarena et al., 1990), and both women and men desire approximately the same amount of caring and closeness in their romantic relationships (Hatfield et al., 1988). Further, both females and males are more satisfied with their interactions with friends when there is some intimacy involved (Reis et al., 1985), although they may nevertheless give relational intimacy a different rating of importance relative to other relationship rewards (Camarena et al., 1990; Rose, 1985; Duck & Wright, 1993). Finally and most importantly, while gender differences are quite reliable, they explain only a small fraction of the variance in relationship functioning and intimacy.

Future research would do well to discover whether intimate interactions early in the development of relationships foreshadow later relationship functioning. A growing body of work has already demonstrated that certain characteristics of early marital and parent–child relationships predict relationship quality several years later (e.g., Gottman, 1993; Main et al., 1985). Little is known about intimacy in this regard, however.

There are several aspects of intimacy that may be predictive of relationship quality later on. First, the total amount of intimate contact shared by the partners may be predictive. For example, beginning a relationship with high levels of intimacy may bode well for the relationship's stability. Second, and more likely, discrepancies between partners' desired amounts of intimacy and the intimacy they perceive in the relationship predict later relationship functioning. Partners who are unable to resolve

such discrepancies may either dissolve their relationships or be less satisfied if they stay together. Finally, the problem-solving skills partners are
able to bring to intimacy-related conflicts should predict later relationship functioning. Better skills should also predict smaller discrepancies
between partners' desired and perceived levels of intimacy in their relationship. The final chapter addresses the latter two issues in detail.

Need Fulfillment in Intimate Relationships

Love, lord, ay, husband, friend! I must hear from thee every
day in the hour, For in a minute there are many days."
—WILLIAM SHAKESPEARE, *Romeo and Juliet*, act 3, scene 5

An important function of intimate relationships, from the point of view
of individual well-being, is to fulfill the needs of the partners involved.
This chapter's specific focus is on partners' needs for intimacy. As discussed in Chapter 9, needs for intimacy refer to people's desires for intimate experiences. More precisely, they refer to individual differences in
people's tendencies to feel gratified by intimate experiences and to feel
deprived in their absence.

Intimacy needs represent one subset of a larger group of human
needs. Personality theorists have argued for several decades (e.g., Leary,
1957; Maslow, 1968; Murray, 1938; Rotter, 1982) that people have a variety of psychological needs. These include needs for achievement, power,
affiliation with others, recognition and status, and autonomy. Theorists
have argued further that fulfillment of these needs is associated with well-
being and good adjustment (e.g., Maslow, 1968; Wilson, 1967) while
frustration and deprivation of needs are linked to adjustment problems
and symptomatology (e.g., Deiner, 1984).

Intimacy needs may be best understood as needs for intimate experience (see Figure 1.2). That is, when people need intimacy, they likely
need to perceive themselves as fully and accurately understood by another person and regarded with positive affect.[1] It is also likely that needs for
intimacy include a reciprocal desire to know the other person well. For
example, not only may Jason need Jean to understand him but he may

need Jean to let herself be known to him. The fulfillment of Jason's needs for intimacy is likely to depend on mutual understanding between Jason and Jean.

Figure 1.2 also suggests that needs for intimacy are met through intimate behavior. That is, needs for intimacy are fulfilled when partners' behavior involves sharing that which is personal and private about themselves. Since no single intimate interaction is likely to fulfill an ongoing need for intimacy, it makes sense to talk about fulfilling needs within the context of an intimate relationship. Repeated intimate interactions are more likely to be a source of intimacy need fulfillment. I am suggesting, then, that relational intimacy is the principle source of intimacy need fulfillment in a relationship.

Partners' intimacy needs should be fulfilled to the extent that the amount of relational intimacy in their relationship approximates their optimum or desired amount of relational intimacy (e.g., see Rogers-Doll et al., 1992). The amount of relational intimacy refers to the frequency with which partners share themselves with one another, the depth or affective intensity of sharing, and the extensiveness or amount of sharing that occurs between partners over time. Because there are likely individual differences in the strength of intimacy needs (see discussion below), I am not proposing that more relational intimacy is automatically more likely to fulfill partners' needs. Instead, I suggest that relational intimacy should approach partners' optimum amount, which may vary considerably from one relationship to the next.

Given that need fulfillment and relational intimacy are both associated with individual well-being, it is surprising that more attempts have not been made to investigate need fulfillment within intimate relationships. Partners in relationships that fulfill their needs should have higher levels of well-being and should report higher levels of relationship satisfaction (Prager & Buhrmester, 1992). Clinebell and Clinebell (1970), for example, argued that mutual need fulfillment is a hallmark of an intimate, satisfying relationship. Drigotas and Rusbult's (1992) study of college students' romantic relationships suggests that when the relationship meets a couple's needs, the partners are less likely to seek an alternative.

The study of intimacy need fulfillment is important for at least two reasons. First, it is a neglected area of research. Most studies on the inner workings of romantic relationships, for example, have addressed destructive conflict in marriage (see review by Gottman, 1994). Some marital researchers and clinicians have noted, however, that helping a couple change destructive communication processes may curb conflict but does not necessarily bring joy or pleasure into the relationship (e.g., Babcock & Jacobson, 1993). Helping relationship partners create opportunities for intimate contact may increase their enjoyment of one another. Second, there is reason to believe that incompatibility of intimacy needs is especially destructive to intimate relationships (e.g., Christensen & Shenk, 1991). Incompatibility seems to elicit dysfunctional communication patterns in marital relationships (Christensen & Shenk, 1991). It may also increase the likelihood that dating partners will seek alternative relationships (Drigotas & Rusbult, 1992). Finally, the exploration of intimacy need fulfillment in relationships presents an opportunity to consider afresh the oft-cited concern intimate partners have with incorporating both intimacy and separateness into their relationship (e.g., see Baxter, 1990; Baxter & Simon, 1993; Boon, 1994; Bowen, 1966; Bowlby, 1969; Guisinger & Blatt, 1994). In the following sections, I explore links between partners' negotiations for the fulfillment of intimacy and separateness needs. While friendships and parent–child relationships are briefly addressed here, most of this section deals with romantic relationships.

Three dimensions of relational intimacy should contribute to the fulfillment of intimacy needs: (1) the frequency of intimate interactions (i.e., how often partners share personal experiences), (2) the depth (i.e., level of personalness or affective intensity) of the sharing, and (3) the amount of intimate sharing that occurs over time. For purposes of this discussion these three dimensions together constitute the amount of relational intimacy in an intimate relationship. The smaller the discrepancy between the amount of relational intimacy the partners each want and expect, and the amount they experience in the relationship, the more satisfied they should be.

This chapter addresses two aspects of intimate relationships that are likely to affect how well a particular relationship fulfills the partners' needs for intimacy. The first is the partners' compatibility regarding important relational needs. Intimacy need compatibility is defined here as similarity between partners on one or more of the following: (1) the amount of relational intimacy experienced as optimum in the relationship, (2) the minimum amount of relational intimacy found acceptable in the relationship, and (3) the maximum amount of relational intimacy tolerated in that relationship. Compatibility of intimacy needs, then, refers to whether partners' needs are sufficiently similar to maintain a functional intimate relationship.

The fulfillment of partners' intimacy needs within a particular relationship may depend not only on compatibility of intimacy needs but also on compatibility of other needs whose fulfillment partners may perceive as conflicting with the fulfillment of intimacy needs. For example, when partners have differing needs for privacy, these incompatibilities may interfere with relational intimacy. Possibly, partners have compatible intimacy needs but are unable to sustain their relationship because bids for intimacy are interpreted as invasions of privacy. This chapter discusses four needs that are likely to affect and be affected by relational intimacy: needs for individuation, needs for separateness, needs for privacy, and needs for distance.

A functional relationship may also depend on negotiations about how much relational intimacy partners will share and how and when they will be intimate. There are at least two reasons why negotiations about intimacy are so important to relationships. First, since two people's needs for intimacy are rarely perfectly matched, partners should find a way to address their different preferences. Second, negotiations about intimacy are important because they are ongoing, the incompatibility between partners' intimacy needs being never completely resolved (Baxter & Simon, 1993). Baxter and Simon have argued that all relationships have conflicts about intimacy built into them because intimacy exists in "dialectical tension" with important individual needs (p. 227). Simply by establishing a relationship, partners "sacrifice some of their individual autonomy" and become answerable to each other (p. 227). There are many ways to handle negotiations (e.g., see Baxter, 1988). Partners' ability to (1) effectively communicate their own needs, (2) listen to and understand the other's needs, and (3) generate creative solutions to problems likely affect whether either partner's needs can be met. For example, a husband may seek to get his intimacy needs met through sexual contact while his wife more often seeks fulfillment through verbal interaction. Arranging to combine both kinds of intimate contact within a single experience or negotiating for trade-offs (e.g., sex tonight and conversation tomorrow night) is likely to provide for the intimacy needs of both partners. Partners who turn incompatibilities into power struggles (each withholds, waiting for the other to give in) are unlikely to provide for the fulfillment of either partner's needs.

Christensen and Shenk (1991) have argued that partners' abilities to negotiate satisfactory arrangements concerning the fulfillment of intimacy needs are not wholly independent of their compatibilities. Their argument suggests that the more similar partners' needs for intimacy are, the more likely they are to make arrangements satisfying to both. Theoretically, if one partner's minimally acceptable level of intimacy does not exceed the other partner's maximally tolerable levels of intimacy, there is some amount of intimacy acceptable to both partners. The likelihood of successful negotiations is thereby increased by partner compatibility.

The impact of partner compatibility and partners' negotiation processes on relationship functioning is likely dependent on the type of relationship the partners have. Parents and children do not choose one another and therefore may rely heavily on skillful negotiation to fulfill intimacy needs within their relationships (although intimacy may rarely be the explicit focus of discussion). Friends, in contrast, who face fewer constraints on choice and can elect partners who are highly compatible, may depend only minimally on negotiation processes. Romantic partners, particularly spouses, rely heavily on their negotiation skills to fulfill important needs within their relationship.

I am proposing, then, that intimate relationships fulfill partners' needs for intimacy when people choose compatible partners and then engage in skillful, ongoing negotiations to ensure that each partner's needs are met. The sections below review literature that suggests that compatible intimacy needs are important to relationship functioning. They also address compatibility concerning the four needs mentioned earlier (individuation, separateness, privacy, and distance), whose fulfillment may at times be incompatible with the fulfillment of intimacy needs. Finally, I suggest that the processes by which relationship partners negotiate need fulfillment in these areas can themselves influence compatibility.

PARTNER COMPATIBILITY

There is research to support the notion that incompatibility of intimacy needs is detrimental to relationship functioning. This research has largely been confined to marital relationships. Christensen and Shenk (1991) found that the greater the discrepancies between wives' and husbands' desired levels of intimacy and independence, the greater their marital distress. Kelley and Burgoon (1991) found that the greater the discrepancy between partners' expected levels of intimacy and their perceptions of their spouse's actual behavior, the greater their marital dissatisfaction. The presence of conflict regarding the amount of intimacy in the relationship is predictive of dysfunctional communication in marriage (Babcock & Jacobson, 1993; Christensen, 1988) and is one of the most common reasons why couples enter marital therapy (Jacobson, 1989).

There is less information available about the impact of incompatible intimacy needs on other kinds of relationships. Friendships have been described as the most compatible kinds of relationships, presumably because they would be terminated if they were not (Furman, 1985). Compatible friendships in general are more stable (Griffin & Sparks, 1990; Knapp & Harwood, 1977), but little is known about the impact of compatible intimacy needs per se.

Research has just begun to document the normal range of intimate contact for parents and their children (Buhrmester & Furman, 1987;

Hunter & Youniss, 1982; Spencer, 1994; Youniss & Smollar, 1985), but we know little about the consequences of incompatibility. In part, this is because researchers presume that parents set the outer boundaries of intimate contact (Dunn, 1993) to which children then adapt. As children get older, however, their own preferences are likely to play an increasingly important role in determining parent–child compatibility. Lamb and Gilbride's (1985) review of the literature on child maltreatment suggests that incompatibility between parents and children can have devastating effects on children under certain circumstances. The extent to which intimacy need incompatibilities are hard on parent–child relationships is unknown.

Compared to the research findings available on heterosexual romantic relationships, there is little information on intimacy incompatibilities in gay and lesbian relationships. The bulk of the available data, however, shows that lesbian and gay relationships are similar to heterosexual relationships. Results of one study suggest that lesbian partners may be the most compatible. Kurdek and Schmitt (1986b) found that lesbian romantic partners are more similar to one another on several personality traits and relationship values than are partners in heterosexual or gay male relationships. While Kurdek and Schmitt suggested that this might reflect a greater emphasis on intimate contact in lesbian relationships, this has not yet been determined.

Sources of Partner Compatibility

There are two ways that partners may come to have compatible or incompatible needs for intimacy. First, partners enter their relationship with predetermined expectations and desires for intimacy (Bradbury & Fincham, 1988). These individual differences may have their foundation in innate temperamental characteristics, and/or they may reflect the accumulated effects of prior experiences with intimate relationships (Bowlby, 1969). If these expectations and desires are well matched between the partners, the relationship should have a better chance of developing successfully.

Baxter (1991) and others (e.g., Cooley, 1902; Duck, 1994a; LaFollette & Graham, 1986; Stern, 1985; and Youniss, 1980, to name a few) have criticized the notion that individuals bring ready-made sets of need strengths into their relationships that then affect them for good or ill. In Baxter's view, selves are not discovered but are continually recreated within the context of intimate interaction.

This continuous creation and recreation of selves may result in a second source of incompatibility (Reis, 1984b). Partners' need strengths may emerge as a function of their interactions with each other. Carmen, from the example in Chapter 9 may find that the subjective strength of her need for intimacy becomes increasingly palpable the longer she is married to Carlos, who is relatively unavailable for intimate contact. This is because the nature of the partners' negotiations about relational intimacy probably influences each partner's perception of his or her own need for intimacy. At their best, relational communication patterns help partners discover needs within themselves that may have previously been outside their awareness, perhaps by enhancing partners' identifications with one another (L. Rubin, 1985). Consider the following example:

> In the early part of their relationship, Lisa and Janice argued frequently about how much time to spend together on the weekends. Because both had demanding professional jobs and worked long hours, they had little leisure time. Janice was content if she and Lisa spent an evening or two together, but Lisa wanted very much to spend more time with Janice. Once they realized that this conflict was repeating itself from one weekend to the next, Lisa and Janice decided to discuss it. Lisa's view was that she wanted to savor as much time as possible during the weekend to make up for the weekdays. She needed the time, she said, to "reconnect" with Janice and to feel close to her again. Janice stressed her strong need to spend time alone to get "reenergized" for the week ahead. Janice and Lisa agreed to spend the next few weekends with a combination of time alone and together. Over the next month Lisa and Janice experimented with various combinations. When they brought the subject up again, Lisa acknowledged that she, like Janice benefited from the time she spent alone. Janice then revealed to Lisa that she realized how much she valued their time together and how much she counted on it.

Through their interactions with each other Lisa and Janice both became more aware of needs that had previously been outside their awareness. This would represent a functional outcome in which partners come to recognize the full range of their own needs and, as a result, can better understand the other's needs.

Dysfunctional negotiation processes, on the other hand, may either mask or intensify partners' needs within their relationship. They do this by increasing polarization between the partners. Polarization refers to a communication process in which one partner voices one need while the other voices an opposite need (Jacobson, 1989; Napier, 1978). While one partner asks for more relational intimacy (as Lisa did in the example above), the other partner may resist by arguing that she or he needs more separateness (as Janice did above). By definition, the partners experience their own communication efforts as motivated by a particular unfulfilled need (Napier, 1978). If allowed to continue, polarized communication may result in masking the strength of one need while creating an exaggerated awareness of another. In polarized communication, by definition, partners attempt to influence one another. When they are unable to do so, they make increasingly exaggerated claims about their opposing needs (perhaps akin to "self-summarizing," as described by Gottman, Notarius, Gonso, & Markman, 1976). If, in the example above, Janice had continued to push for separateness, Lisa might have become more intensely aware of her own "opposing" and unmet need for intimacy. Moreover, if it had become increasingly difficult for Lisa to get intimate contact with Janice, she would have been less likely to recognize her own needs for separateness; instead, she might have increasingly experienced separateness as something imposed on her by Janice. Polarization may be self-perpetuating because partners become painfully aware of their own unmet needs while remaining unaware, in themselves, of the opposite need the other is expressing.

In sum, incompatibilities between partners' intimacy needs may originate with individual characteristics that partners bring with them into the relationship. Partners' interactions with one another may reduce or exaggerate these characteristics, however. It seems likely that partners' ability to negotiate the amount of intimacy in their relationship will depend in part on how similar their needs are when they enter the relationship. Their negotiating skills should in turn determine how compatible or incompatible the relationship partners are.

INCOMPATIBILITY BETWEEN PARTNERS' NEEDS AND RELATIONAL INTIMACY

Partners' conflicts about relational intimacy may stem from incompatibilities in needs other than intimacy if fulfillment of these needs is viewed as interfering with the fulfillment of intimacy needs. The literature mentions four needs whose fulfillment could potentially conflict with intimacy: individuation, separateness, privacy and distance. It is these that I will address next.

Individuation, separateness, privacy, and distance needs have frequently been treated as synonymous in the literature, which has allowed mutually contradictory theories about the relation of each need to intimacy to flourish. In brief, the main theories are as follows:

- Intimacy inevitably competes with (one or more of) these needs. Intimacy must therefore be balanced against these needs to achieve good relationship functioning (Kerr & Bowen, 1988).
- These needs neither conflict with nor promote intimacy, but are neutral to it and can peacefully coexist along with it (Baxter & Wilmot, 1985; Dindia, 1994).
- Not only do these needs not compete with intimacy but (one or more of) these needs can be fulfilled within intimate interactions (e.g., Bowlby, 1969; Fairbairn, 1954; Grotevant & Cooper, 1985; Mahler, 1975).
- Not only do (one or more of) these needs not compete with intimacy but intimacy needs cannot be fulfilled unless these needs are fulfilled as well (Beavers & Hampson, 1990; Hatfield, 1988; Israelstam, 1989; White et al., 1983).

In reality, the process of clarifying and distinguishing these concepts from one another reveals merit in each of these apparently mutually contradictory arguments. Drawing from the literature on each of these needs, I propose the following definitions:[2]

First, *individuation* refers to the individual's ability to maintain a subjective experience of distinctiveness and identity within a close relational context (e.g., see Karpel, 1976). An individuated person can maintain, pursue, and express opinions, beliefs, interests, goals, values, and tastes that are not necessarily the same as those of an important relationship partner yet still maintain an intimate relationship with that person (Grotevant & Cooper, 1986). Needs for individuation are needs for experiences that facilitate the development of a sense of distinctiveness and identity. Because the value of individuation varies widely from one culture to another, the salience of individuation needs should demonstrate intercultural variation (Dion & Dion, 1988).

Separateness (called "physical privacy" by Burgoon et al., 1989) refers to physical separation and the need partners have to be physically apart from one another (Larson, 1990). Separateness comes in a variety of forms: separate vacations, separate dwellings, separate rooms in the same house (for a young child and his or her parent, separateness could mean 10 meters apart but still in visual range.) Separateness is likely to be valued by those who want to collect their thoughts without interruption, to enjoy solitary pastimes, or to concentrate on solitary work. Some cultures value separateness more than others. In American culture those who can afford it purchase it—in the form of a multiroom dwelling, a house in the country, and so forth.

Privacy is "control over the amount of interaction we choose to maintain with others . . . how much or how little to divulge about oneself to another voluntarily" (Derlega & Chaikin, 1977, p. 102; see Margulis, 1977; also see Burgoon et al.'s [1989] definition of "social and psychological privacy"). Privacy is not completely synonymous with separateness in that privacy does not always require physical separateness (Altman, 1977). Privacy does require individual control over whether one engages in interaction and over what one chooses to tell or show of oneself to another.

The need for *distance* is a desire to withhold oneself from (i.e., to avoid sharing oneself with) a specific partner (or group) in order to limit contact and intimacy. A need for distance arises specifically in the context of another's desire or expectation of intimate contact and "arises from closeness or expected closeness and requires some prior connection that is noticeably strained" (Helgeson, Shaver, & Dyer, 1987, p. 199). Distance is different from individuation, separateness, and privacy because distance is specifically aimed at obstructing intimacy.

On the basis of the above definitions, I argue here that partners' conflicts about how much intimacy they will have in their relationship may become intensified when needs for individuation, separateness, or privacy seem to be incompatible with the fulfillment of intimacy needs. Specifically, bids for individuation, separateness, and privacy can intensify partners' conflicts about intimacy when these bids are interpreted as a need for distance. A need for distance, by definition, aims to block intimate contact with the partner and may signal the presence of unexpressed or unresolved conflict. Bids for distance are easily disguised as bids for individuation, separateness, and privacy since the same behavior and/or activity may fulfill both needs. Partners may understandably, then, confuse these requests. They may also use requests for individuation, separateness, and privacy to disguise a need for distance, further muddying the waters. Even if a need for distance is not involved, conflict about fulfilling intimacy needs may occur when partners' needs for individuation, separateness, and privacy are different.

The issue of whether individuation, separateness, and privacy inevitably conflict with relational intimacy or promote and enhance it has been an ongoing debate in the literature on close relationships for many years. The nature of this debate and the issues that it raises are best captured by the extensive theoretical literature on intimacy and individuation.

The notion that intimate relationships might at times be incompatible with individuation has been a tenet of psychodynamic theory (Blos,

1967; Fairbairn, 1954; Guntrip, 1968; Mahler, 1986). Psychodynamic theorists have suggested that normal development requires a withdrawing, or separation, of the young child from the close relationship she or he had with the mother as an infant. Observations of young children with their parents led Mahler to suggest that separation (the ability to maintain physical distance and to play alone) is a necessary precursor to individuation. Individuation itself conceived of as a kind of intrapsychic separation requiring the gradual abandonment of an infantile, dependent orientation to internalized representations of important others.

Psychodynamic theorists have also postulated an incompatibility between intimacy and individuation needs in relationships occurring later in development. The adolescent's task in Western culture, according to these theorists, is to break away from parents and their influence and transfer needs for intimate contact to peers (Douvan & Adelson, 1966; Sullivan, 1953). This "breaking away" process is a necessary precondition to identity development. Later, in adulthood, romantic relationships are especially prone to elicit conflicts between needs for intimacy and individuation (Beavers & Hampson, 1990; Peplau, Cochran, Rook, & Padesky, 1978; Raush, Barry, Hertel, & Swain, 1974; Weiner, 1980). Weiner postulated a normal stage in the development of couple relationships in which intimacy inevitably declines in the service of fostering partner individuation.

The emphasis in psychodynamic theory on relinquishing intimate ties in the service of individuation has been sharply criticized (Franz & White, 1985; J. B. Miller, 1991). Some say this view has identified independence and self-reliance as harbingers of mental health while ignoring the importance of functional intimate relationships (e.g., J. Miller, 1991). Erikson's (1963, 1968) vision of psychological development and maturity, for example, has been criticized for placing inordinate emphasis on self-differentiation processes and paying too little attention to how individuals come to form functional intimate relationships (Franz & White, 1985; J. Miller, 1991). Grotevant and Cooper (1986) have criticized Douvan and Adelson's (1966) emphasis on "severing childhood ties" and "relinquishing dependency" (p. 83) in parent–adolescent relationships. Grotevant and Cooper reviewed research showing that "autonomy was not gained by means of disengagement from . . . parents . . . [and that] adolescents who felt the greatest autonomy were more likely to view their parents as close, to turn to their parents for guidance" (p. 84). J. B. Miller (1991) argued that "to see all of development as a process of separating oneself out from the matrix of others . . . is to advocate a model that has little to do with the way most people live their lives" (p. 11). These critics have suggested, then, that the relinquishing of intimate relationships (or relational intimacy within relationships) is not a necessary accompaniment to individuation.

While critics insist that psychodynamic theory has overemphasized "separation and individuation," they argue that the literature on intimacy pays inadequate attention to individuation processes. Baxter (1991; Baxter & Wilmot, 1985) argued that this literature has focused too much on closeness, communication, and self-disclosure and has ignored the value of individuation. Carpenter [1986] argued that the research on intimate relationships has encouraged an unrealistic image of close relationships as characterized by frequent bids for intense, self-revealing interaction.

Several writers have recently argued for a dialectical approach that emphasizes the simultaneous importance of intimate relating and individuation at all stages of human development (Baxter, 1988, 1991, 1993; Bowlby, 1982; Cooper, Grotevant, & Condon, 1983; Franz & White, 1985; J. Miller, 1991; Olson, 1993; Surrey, 1991; Williamson, 1991; see Chapters 3 of this volume). In this approach, relationship functioning increases to the extent that both intimacy and individuation are fostered within intimate relationships.

Grotevant and Cooper (1985), for example, have studied how individuation can be encouraged or discouraged depending on the kind of communication that occurs between partners in intimate relationships. In their model, communication fosters individuation when it includes "expressions of the distinctiveness of self from others" and "the expression of one's own point of view and . . . taking responsibility for communicating it clearly." Communication fosters connectedness when it expresses partners' "sensitivity to and respect for the views of others" and their openness to others' views without the fear of their own views being "absorbed."

Family systems theorists suggest that when intimate relationships do not foster individuation, partners may find themselves in a state of fusion (Bowen, 1978). In its most extreme form partners in a state of fusion may interpret one another's expressions of individuality as acts of betrayal threatening the survival of the relationship (Karpel, 1976). As a result of these interpretations, interactions may be dominated by strong, uncontrollable emotions and the accompanying behavior—attack, defensiveness, withdrawal, and recrimination (Kerr & Bowen, 1988; Williamson, 1991).

In sum, theorists from a variety of perspectives—psychodynamic, communication, and family systems—have argued in turn that relational intimacy interferes with, happily coexists with, or enhances individuation. Perhaps the debate has gone as far as it needs to. The next step may be to define and describe the conditions under which needs for intimacy interfere with or enhance needs for individuation, separateness, privacy, and even distance. The next section addresses this issue.

The Negotiation of Intimacy Need Fulfillment

In the next few sections, I argue that relational intimacy neither always obstructs nor always enhances fulfillment of needs for separateness, privacy, individuation, and distance. Rather, I argue that there are conditions under which the needs are likely to be in opposition and conditions under which they are likely to be in harmony. I further suggest that effective negotiation can minimize their mutual opposition.

Separateness: Conflicts with Fulfillment of Intimacy Needs

Separateness needs may conflict with intimacy needs indirectly because they conflict with partners' needs for togetherness or physical proximity. Although intimacy can be enjoyed via telephone or letter, most frequently it requires togetherness. Separateness and togetherness may be mutually exclusive for any given moment in time, and partners may require negotiations to decide whether a particular time slot (e.g., Saturday afternoon, while the children are napping) will be spent together or separately. Desires for different amounts of separateness should not be confused with different intimacy needs, however. Paradoxically, the partner who desires more togetherness may also want less relational intimacy than the partner who desires more separateness. For example, one of L. Rubin's (1983) interviewees often wanted his wife to be physically present but he did not necessarily want to talk.

Separateness: Enhancement of Intimacy Need Fulfillment

Separateness and relational intimacy are not necessarily in direct conflict. They can promote one another. Separateness should enhance intimacy to the extent that it provides partners with new experiences they can then bring to the relationship and share. Temporary separation from one intimate partner may also permit more intimate contact with another intimate partner by creating privacy for the second dyad (Burgoon et al., 1989; Derlega & Chaikin, 1977; Oliker, 1989).

Contact with others and separateness can foster one another because each provides relief from the other (Olsen & Zubek, 1970). People seem to require a certain amount of respite from a partner's company to feel renewed and ready to interact again (R. Larson, 1990). Pedersen

(1988) argued that being with others requires a certain amount of being "on stage," which increases arousal (Berscheid, 1977) and cannot be sustained indefinitely. Separateness seems to provide "off stage" time. Separateness in excess, however, can be lonely and boring (R. Larson, 1990). Partners may, consequently, especially appreciate and enjoy intimacy following periods of separateness (Larson, Csikszentmihalyi, & Graef, 1982).

Privacy: Conflicts with Fulfillment of Intimacy Needs

Privacy needs may appear to conflict with intimacy needs when individuals are secretive (A. Weiss, 1987). On the surface, keeping secrets may appear to be one way of maintaining privacy. Secrets, after all, allow people to keep information to themselves and avoid the prying of others.

It is more useful, however, to think of secrecy as different from privacy. While privacy involves having control over access to information about oneself (Altman, 1977), secrecy involves the deliberate withholding of information that is clearly of concern to one's partner. Secrets may create emotional tensions in relationships, the source of which will be unknown to one partner (LaFollette & Graham, 1986; H. Lerner, 1993). LaFollette and Graham suggested that "denying an intimate [crucial] information . . . [creates] a guarded atmosphere [that] will encompass the relationship and inevitably limit the closeness" and questioned how partners could "regain intimacy with a pregnant secret between them polluting the atmosphere of trust?" (p. 12). The secretive partner may meet the other partner's efforts to understand the intimacy gap with lies or other distracting maneuvers. In this case the secret may have a further destructive effect on intimacy, relationship functioning, and, perhaps, the other partner's faith in his or her own reality testing (H. Lerner, 1993; Vangelisti, 1994).

Even when needs for privacy have nothing to do with secrecy or distancing, these may interfere with the fulfillment of intimacy needs under certain circumstances. Consider the following example:

> Ken has a high need for privacy. He feels strongly that he does not want people, including his wife, Gwen, to know personal things about him, such as the problems he is having at work. Gwen would prefer that Ken share more about himself but has learned to respect his strong needs for privacy and does not ask him about his feelings. As a result, Ken and Gwen often find themselves talking about trivial matters, although Ken's facial expressions and body movements register unexpressed emotion. At these times Gwen does not know what is really going on with

Ken and does not feel free to ask. In certain important ways, she does not understand or know him.

In this example, the husband has a strong need for privacy, which should not be confused with a need for distance from his wife for he allows no one access to his thoughts and feelings. His wife respects his need by not intruding with questions and solicitations for information. Although the couple has learned to avoid destructive conflict about their differing privacy needs, the husband's strong needs for privacy have created a barrier to intimacy in this relationship.

Privacy: Enhancement of Intimacy Need Fulfillment

The fulfillment of privacy needs can also promote intimate experience, in large part because of the association between privacy and personal control, or consent to share. Theoretically, privacy is what allows individuals to experience sharing as freely chosen and freely given (Berscheid, 1977). Interference with the fulfillment of privacy needs is intrusion, which is the experience of being checked on or having to interact or reveal oneself without consent, as, for example, when someone snoops or pries (Burgoon et al., 1989). Requests for intimate interaction (e.g., "A penny for your thoughts") will not be experienced as intrusive when partners feel free to share or not without jeopardizing their relationship. This freedom, by definition, requires privacy.

If privacy is control over access to the self (Margulis, 1977), perhaps intimacy and privacy must peacefully coexist within an intimate relationship in order for either to thrive within it (A. Weiss, 1987). The sharing involved in intimate interactions must be voluntary or it is unlikely that positive affect and perceptions of understanding will follow from it. That is, coerced intimacy is no intimacy at all. Intrusiveness, then, is antithetical to intimacy, while respect for privacy should ultimately enhance it.

Individuation: Conflicts with Fulfillment of Intimacy Needs

Conflicts between intimate partners' needs may stem in part from differences in their preferred modes of nourishing their own individuation. Individuation is a need that can be fulfilled through separateness, privacy, and distance, but it can also be fulfilled through intimate interaction. Partners may have conflict not because intimacy and individuation needs inevitably clash but because of individual differences in their preferred, or most frequent, mode of fulfilling individuation needs.

The most extreme case of opposition between intimacy and individuation needs is exemplified by people who believe that individuation can only be achieved while distant from others (Erikson, 1963). Karpel (1976) called this "unrelatedness" or the "schizoid position" (p. 70). The position of unrelatedness is one of being out of relationship and theoretically serves to preserve individuality for those who would otherwise feel engulfed in close relationships (Erikson, 1963). These individuals may experience the pressures to merge identities (become a "we") that normally accompany close relationships as overwhelming because of their own fragile sense of identity.

Some people may find that separateness is particularly conducive to meeting their individuation needs (Larson, 1990). Moustakas (1975) has been an especially articulate proponent of the connection between separateness and individuation. In describing a child who spent a lot of time alone, he wrote, "Often, it became clear that isolated activity was not a problem for the child, as teachers and parents often claimed. Rather it was a particular way of being, a way of responding to inner life, a satisfying process that expressed itself in fantasy, imagination, day dreaming and meditation" (pp. 4–5). Moustakas described his own experience of self-discovery in the context of separation:

> Though I am certain it has sometimes been painful for others to permit me to wander away alone when I was plagued by a problem or living with shattered moments, tragedies, and broken communications, most people respected my solitude and saw it as my way of communion with myself and not as a rejection of them or an indication of loss or absence. Going off alone . . . became my way of self-renewal . . . continues to be the central source of self-growth" (pp. 6–7)

Empirical research on separateness over the life span shows that separateness can nurture individuation. On the basis of a review of the literature on solitude and well-being Larson (1990) concluded that teenagers who spent more time alone "reported future plans that were justified in terms of internal personal values and standards, while adolescents with less solitude were more likely to justify their plans in terms of external conventional values" (p. 171).

Berscheid (1977) discussed two aspects of privacy and suggested that it too may foster individuation. She noted that anonymity sometimes provides a kind of privacy (control over revealing one's identity) that seems to allow people to try on and possibly incorporate behaviors they might not otherwise consider. Moreover, when certain personal beliefs and values are private, people have the option to behave in public as though they believe differently. In each of these cases, privacy allows people to hold some aspect of themselves apart and distinct from the interactional context.

It seems possible that people for whom distance, separateness, or privacy enhance individuation might be less inclined to seek individuation through communication with their intimate partners (Moustakas argued that this was a problem in his relationship with his wife). Their partners, in turn, depending on the strength of their own intimacy needs, may experience intimacy deprivation within the relationship.

Individuation: Enhancement of Intimacy Need Fulfillment

As discussed in Chapter 6, individuation can be enhanced within intimate partners' interactions. Cooper, Grotevant, and their colleagues (Cooper & Ayers-Lopez, 1985; Cooper & Grotevant, 1987; Cooper, Grotevant, & Condon, 1982, 1983; Grotevant & Cooper, 1985, 1986) have an especially well-articulated model of individuation enhancement within intimate interaction. Their research has documented links between adolescent identity development and the presence of four characteristics of parent–adolescent communication: (1) self-assertion, which indicates awareness of one's own point of view and acceptance of the responsibility for communicating it clearly; (2) permeability, which expresses a responsiveness to the views of others; (3) mutuality, which shows sensitivity and respect for others' views; and (4) separateness, which expresses distinctiveness of self from others (Grotevant & Cooper, 1986; Cooper et al., 1983). The work of other investigators has supported this hypothesized relationship between identity development and intimate relationships while using different models of each (e.g., Campbell et al., 1984; Dyk & Adams, 1990; Hauser, 1978; Leaper et al., 1989). Leaper et al. found that adolescents, particularly sons, who were higher in ego development participated with their fathers in more reciprocated enabling, or interaction that "reflect[s] speakers' positive involvement with others by facilitating their participation in interaction (e.g., showing curiosity)" (p. 337). In contrast, constraining speeches, which "reflect speakers' negative involvement . . . by impeding their participation in the interaction (e.g., distracting) . . ." (p. 337), had a neutral or negative association with adolescent ego development.

Some writers have proposed that intimate relationships facilitate individual development through the incorporation of the other into the self (Aron et al., 1992; Solomon, 1988). Campbell and Tesser (1985) suggested that fluctuations in self-regard can occur as a function of our close relationship partners' performance on tasks requiring competence. When a relationship partner does well, we can either bask in the reflected glory, thus enhancing self-evaluation through association, or we can make invidious comparisons between ourselves and our partner and feel diminished because we do not perform as well (Campbell & Tesser, 1985; Pilkington & Tesser, 1991).

Partners in intimate relationships may promote their own individuation when they compare themselves with their partners (Pilkington, Tesser, & Stephens, 1991). Comparisons may delineate distinct identities for each partner (e.g., one may be the athlete, while the other is the artist). There is evidence that friends, siblings, and romantic partners mold distinct identities within the context of their relationship by carving out different areas of self-relevant expertise (Pilkington et al., 1991; Pilkington & Tesser, 1991; Tesser, 1980), perhaps thereby avoiding demoralizing competitions.

Distance: Conflicts with Fulfillment of Intimacy Needs

When might distance be sought? Distance is defined here as the avoidance of intimate contact. Those who wish to end a relationship (Rusbult et al., 1982) or who wish to avoid developing a relationship (Baumeister, Wotman, & Stillwell, 1993) may seek distance. Distance may serve those well who experience intimacy as an untenable psychological risk (Jack & Dill, 1992; Pilkington & Richardson, 1988). In established intimate relationships, partners may seek distance because they are angry or hurt or afraid of rejection. They may also seek distance when positive feelings feel overwhelming in the face of fears of being known or engulfed. Distance for any of these reasons could come into direct conflict with the fulfillment of intimacy needs. There is evidence that sustained distance is destructive to the maintenance of intimate relationships (Rusbult et al., 1986).

Sometimes partners may simultaneously want intimacy and distance. Although there is little research data available in this area, simultaneous moves toward distance and intimacy have received considerable attention by clinicians (Karpel, 1976; L'Abate & L'Abate, 1979). Simultaneous intimacy–distance moves allow a partner to claim that he or she is seeking intimacy even as his or her behavior predictably effects distance with the partner. Napier (1978) described an interaction pattern, observable between spouses and between parents and children in clinical interviews, in which bids for intimacy are couched in criticism, demands, and efforts to control the partner. Christensen and Shenk (1991) discovered a similar pattern of behavior ("demand behavior") in their research on distressed marital partners. Karpel (1976) described a pattern in marriage in which partners, over time, alternate between pursuing intimacy and preserving distance. What remains constant is that one partner is always running away from the other partner's bid for more intimacy, so that the partners never really have a chance to be intimate. What does not happen in any of these patterns of behavior is successful negotiation regarding when and how much partners will be intimate. Some writers have viewed behavior patterns like these as implicit contracts to keep the amount of relational intimacy and distance in the relationship at a comfortable level for both (Bowen, 1978).

Why would relationship partners experience ambivalence about intimacy with one another? Some writers argue that fear of intimacy is normal, given the risks that intimacy entails (Dindia, 1994; Kieffer, 1977). Intimate interaction, after all, simultaneously promises rewarding human interaction (Berscheid, 1988) and contains the threat of exposure, ridicule, and rejection (Hatfield, 1984; L'Abate & L'Abate, 1979).

Distance: Enhancement of Intimacy

Although distance is active avoidance of intimate contact, it may foster intimacy in relationships under certain conditions. Behavior therapists, for example, advocate a procedure called "time-out" for people who are coping with strong negative emotions toward one another. Strong negative emotions can prompt destructive communicative exchanges that are better left unsaid (e.g., Gottman, 1979). During time-out, intimate partners deliberately avoid contact until the emotional intensity of a particular encounter dissipates and problem solving becomes possible.

This deliberate and time-limited use of distancing may promote relational intimacy eventually if not immediately. It serves to interrupt a common dysfunctional pattern of handling intense negative emotions within the marital relationship. Spouses in a distressed marriage often match negative, coercive statements made by their partner with an equally negative, coercive statement of their own, thus creating an escalating cycle of negativity in their communication (Gottman, 1979, 1994; Gottman & Levenson, 1992; Levenson & Gottman, 1983; Margolin & Wampold, 1981). This escalating cycle of negativity is likely both cause and effect of intense frustration, anger, and other negative affect for both partners (Lindahl & Markman, 1990). There is evidence that when this negative escalation is allowed to continue without interruption, it leaves a residue of unresolved problems and festering anger between spouses. Both unresolved problems and festering anger would significantly compromise a couple's ability to be intimate (Basco et al., 1992; Lindahl & Markman, 1990; Markman & Notarius 1987). Short periods of distance may provide needed interruption.

There is evidence that the positive impact of distance on relationship intimacy can only exist under limited conditions (Raush, Barry, Hertel, & Swain, 1974). First, distance must be a short-term solution to managing intense feelings, not a means of avoiding problems. Second, and related, distance must be followed up with efforts to discuss and negotiate the issues at hand. Third, relationships seem to thrive best when partners who have been distant for a time make a point of spending some cohesive and/or intimate time together.

The preceding sections have discussed intimacy in relation to four needs—separateness, privacy, individuation, and distance—that can exist in opposition to intimacy. I have resisted taking sides in a debate about the role these needs play in enhancing or interfering with intimacy. I suggest instead that fulfillment of these needs can be synergistic with intimacy need fulfillment or can result in intimacy deprivation, depending on how the relationship partners think about and negotiate the fulfillment of each need.

In order to negotiate successfully, partners must start with the premise that loving and enjoying intimacy with someone does not eliminate needs for separateness, privacy, and so on. Further, they must presume that needs for separateness and privacy do not obviate needs for intimacy. Partners who understand that the presence of needs for separateness and privacy does not automatically signal a lack of love are more likely to negotiate effective solutions to their conflicts.

Social scientists have yet to explore empirically the extent to which needs for separateness, privacy, individuation, and distance are inconsistent with or encourage intimacy need fulfillment. Within a Western cultural context, however, it seems likely that the more relational intimacy, individuation, separateness, and privacy promote each other, the more rewarding, harmonious, and enduring an intimate relationship is likely to be.

Intimacy-Related Goals and Negotiation Processes

To enjoy smoothly functioning relationships, most relationship partners must eventually negotiate how much intimate contact they will have. This is because partners are rarely perfectly matched regarding the amount of intimacy in the relationship that would be optimum for each.

People have four main avenues by which they can attempt to influence the level of intimacy in their relationship. First, they can encourage more intimacy from their partners by engaging in intimate behavior themselves (McAdams, Healy, & Krause, 1984). (See Chapter 8 for a discussion of intimate behavior.) Second, they can encourage intimacy from their partner by creating an atmosphere or climate in the relationship that increases the likelihood of intimate interaction. Examples of this approach are (1) promoting positive affect through pleasing behaviors such as giving gifts, relieving the other of chores, giving compliments, and planning or engaging in a shared recreational activity (Stuart, 1980) and (2) creating an atmosphere in which the dyad has privacy (e.g., locked doors, a table for two, a baby-sitter). Third, partners can discourage intimate contact by withholding these behaviors or by eliciting emotional states, such as anger, that are incompatible with intimacy. Frequent dysfunctional conflict may allow partners to maintain intense contact with one another without having to take the risks that accompany intimacy. There is evidence that the demand–withdraw pattern of communication may function in this way (Rogers-Doll et al., 1992). Fourth, intimate partners can attempt to influence their partners directly by asking for more (or insisting on less) relational intimacy. These discussions may come as requests for more togetherness, more sexual contact, or more conversation, depending on the type of relationship the partners have and on how they each prefer to fulfill their intimacy needs.

When the means by which other relational needs, such as separateness or privacy, are fulfilled seem to conflict with fulfillment of intimacy needs, partners can take one of several routes to resolving these conflicts. Baxter (1988) described the following options: (1) selection, by which partners abandon one need as unfulfillable and focus only on the other; (2) segmentation, by which partners fulfill different needs at different times or in different places; (3) neutralization, by which partners seek a compromise so that there is neither too much intimacy nor, for example, too much separateness; (4) disqualification, by which partners use language to express what they want while obscuring their meaning, thus avoiding direct confrontation; and (5) reframing, in which apparent conflicts between fulfilling needs are redefined so that there no longer seems to be a conflict (such as when intimate conversation serves to assist partners with individuation efforts).

Implicit in the notion that people engage in negotiations to fulfill their intimacy needs is a goal-based model of behavior in intimate relationships (Cantor & Malley, 1991; McAdams & Constantian, 1983; Miller & Read, 1991). Traditionally, the study of needs and goals has been directed toward understanding individual personality (Cantor, Norem, Langston, Fleeson, & Cook-Flannagan, 1993; Murray, 1938; Palys & Little, 1983; Pervin, 1989). More recently, theorists have suggested that social interaction can be "analyzed in terms of people's goals and the plans and strategies necessary to achieve those goals" (Read & Miller, 1989, p. 416). Cantor and Malley (1991) suggested that needs, which are primarily affective states, are translated into goals, which are "recipes" for "how that person will address that need in his or her current life" (p. 102). Once attained, goal states fulfill a particular need. People then develop behavioral strategies organized toward accomplishing their goals (Read & Miller, 1989).

Each of the four influence strategies described above is behavior de-signed to accomplish a particular goal. Perhaps people's goals vary on the basis of their understanding of the best ways of getting intimacy needs met (or of limiting intimacy). For example, one person's goal may be to spend more time in shared recreational activity with a partner. Whether people are consciously aware that they have made the association or not, they may hope that shared recreation with their partner will provide a setting for intimate contact.

One way to identify commonalities among the disparate goals that people set for their intimate relationships is to connect those goals with the needs that goal attainment will supposedly fulfill, such as needs for intimacy or needs for individuation. Once researchers identify some of people's need–goal links, they may understand better the diversity of strategies people use to get their needs met. These strategies can then be evaluated according to how effective they are in specific relationship contexts.

SUMMARY AND CONCLUSIONS

Needs for intimacy and efforts to fulfill them coexist with a broad range of other psychological needs. Intimate relationships are likely primary arenas in which people seek to fulfill important needs. Through fulfill-ment of needs, intimate relationships may enhance individual well-being.

In this chapter I focus on how intimacy needs are fulfilled in con-junction with other needs whose fulfillment seems, on the surface, to be antagonistic to intimacy. I simultaneously emphasize, however, that ful-fillment of other needs may enhance and be enhanced by the fulfillment of intimacy needs (Baxter, 1988, 1993).

A couple of factors are likely to play an important role in determin-ing whether and to what extent relationship partners' needs for intimacy are met. First, although no two people have intimacy needs of exactly equal strength, for a successful relationship partners should come into the relationship with needs that are sufficiently compatible. Needs are sufficiently compatible, in this context, when partners can agree on an amount of relational intimacy that can adequately fulfill the needs of each. The amount of relational intimacy refers to the frequency, depth, and amount of intimate interactions over time.

Second, partners' communication and negotiation about intimacy need fulfillment can affect whether intimacy needs are met. When partners are flexible and can generate several ways of interacting intimately, they may be more likely to fulfill one another's needs. In contrast, when partners turn their incompatibilities into power struggles, polarization is likely, with an exaggeration of the partners' apparent incompatibilities. Under these circumstances they are unlikely to meet one another's needs.

The processes by which partners fulfill each other's intimacy needs will likely be best understood within the context of partners' efforts to fulfill other important psychological needs. This chapter reviews theoretical and research approaches to understanding how intimacy needs are met along with needs for separateness, privacy, individuation, and distance. Because the latter four needs are often viewed as existing in opposition to needs for intimacy, intimacy scholars have attended mostly to these. I have argued that investigations into how relationships fulfill these needs should take a fresh approach. Rather than asking whether separateness, privacy, individuation, and distance are at odds with or in harmony with intimacy, I have suggested that we explore circumstances under which they can be in harmony. These initial explorations might fruitfully begin with an examination of personal/relational factors such as partner compatibility.

A promising place to begin a study of partner compatibility might be in the area of intimacy motivation. While the effect of intimacy motivation on intimate interactions has been established (e.g., McAdams, Healy, & Krause, 1984), there is little work investigating its impact in ongoing relationships. Scholars do not know, for example, whether people choose as mates those who have similar levels of intimacy motivation. Further, little is known about the effects of partners having different levels of intimacy motivation. Compatibility of partners' intimacy needs might effectively be assessed by means of McAdams's (1980, 1982a) TAT-based measure of intimacy motivation.

The needs discussed in this chapter are only a subset of the broader set of psychological needs people seek to fulfill in their personal relationships. In a factor analytic study of adults' psychological needs, Prager and Buhrmester (1992) found that needs for nurturance, acceptance, affection, and intimacy together loaded on a communal needs factor. What these communal needs had in common were strivings toward integration, connection, cooperation, and working toward a common good with others. These are the needs traditionally believed to be fulfilled in the con-text of intimate relationships (e.g., Davis & Oathout, 1992; R. S. Weiss, 1986).

Fulfillment of needs that are not necessarily communal may also de-pend, directly or indirectly, on intimate relationship processes. For exam-ple, Prager and Buhrmester's (1992) factor analytic study revealed a sec-ond dimension of psychological needs: *agentic needs*. Needs loading on this dimension included identity, self-esteem, power and influence, au-tonomy, and achievement. Prager and Buhrmester found that adults' lev-el of agentic need fulfillment was positively correlated with their reports of relationship satisfaction, as were their reports of communal need ful-fillment. Relationship functioning may depend, therefore, on partners' fulfilling both agentic and communal needs within their current life space.

Relational intimacy may make a critical contribution not only to the fulfillment of intimacy needs but to the fulfillment of other commu-nal and agentic needs as well. One way it may do so is through the higher levels of mutual understanding that partners may share as a result of their intimate interactions. Theoretically, the better partners understand one another's needs and how each wishes to see those needs fulfilled, the bet-ter equipped they are to provide the resources to fulfill the needs.

Future investigations of intimate relationship functioning would do well to explore more fully the processes by which relationships fulfill the psychological needs of the partners. Quite possibly, intimate interactions and relationships exert their beneficial effects on the people who partici-pate in them by directly or indirectly fulfilling people's needs.

EPILOGUE

Reflections on Intimacy

> Love is possible only if two persons communicate with
> each other from the center of their existence. . . . Only in
> this "central experience" is human reality, only here is
> aliveness, only here is the basis of love.
>   —ERICH FROMM, *The Art of Loving*

Intimate relationships play a central role in people's health, well-being,
and happiness. They provide the setting in which people learn how to
enjoy life and how to adapt to stress. The interest that social scientists are
taking in the study of intimate relationships promises to significantly increase our understanding of how to promote human well-being. What
follows are issues concerning intimacy that deserve further consideration.

THE STUDY OF INTIMACY SHOULD BE REPLACED WITH THE STUDY OF SPECIFIC INTIMATE INTERACTIONS AND RELATIONSHIPS

The currently diverse approaches to studying intimacy are the strength
and weakness of the field (Berscheid, 1994). We have rich insights into
healthy and dysfunctional relationships from clinicians, a solid theory
and a life span perspective from developmentalists, and methodological
elegance from experimentalists. Although each of these perspectives
could benefit from the strengths of the others, cross-fertilization among
these traditions is scanty. One reason is that theorists from different perspectives often refer to different phenomena when they talk about intimacy.

Chapter 1 of this book proposes a multitiered structure for the intimacy concept that should integrate the many contributions to the study

of intimacy into a meaningful whole. Paradoxically, scholars may best achieve this integration when we stop studying intimacy as a general abstraction. Chapter 1 argues that the most useful definition of intimacy begins with intimate interactions. This is because, in my view, intimate relationships are built in part on the enduring cognitive and emotional sequelae of repeated intimate interactions (e.g., loving feelings, expectations of further intimacy).

The multitiered intimacy concept in Figure 1.2 suggests two fruitful emphases for research on intimate interactions. First, we should study the components of intimate interaction (behavior and experience) and their impact on one another (see Figure 8.1). Intimate experiences (e.g., experiences of being accepted and understood) may arise directly from intimate behavior. Further, intimate experiences are likely an important source of individual well-being. Certain kinds of intimate behavior, such as self-disclosure, can exert beneficial effects on the health and well-being of the discloser (Pennebaker et al., 1989). It seems reasonable to presume that intimate behavior is beneficial in part because of the affective and cognitive experiences that accompany it. The better scholars understand how intimate behaviors generate intimate experiences, the more we may learn about how intimate interactions exert their beneficial effects.

Second, we should study the impact of intimate interactions on relationships. The definition in Chapter 1 distinguishes intimate relationships from other personal relationships by the frequency of relational intimacy (intimate interactions between relationship partners). Possibly, relational intimacy fosters other characteristics of relationships (such as affection, trust, and cohesiveness) that give intimate relationships their special flavor. These characteristics in turn should result in intimate relationships that are more satisfying, stable, and harmonious (see Figure 9.1).

Research on intimate relationships might arguably have three purposes. First, because satisfying intimate relationships are so crucial to people's well-being, we should identify the factors that impinge on or enhance their functioning. One way to do this is to examine the characteristics of relationships themselves and investigate how these contribute to relationship functioning. This approach has wide support in the literature on personal relationships. It has amassed a substantial amount of data about how relationships work and what makes them work well (e.g., see Duck, 1994a, on meaningful communication; Derlega et al., 1993, on self-disclosure; Gottman, 1994, on conflict management; Rusbult et al., 1982, 1986, on commitment; Holmes, 1991, on trust; and Hatfield & Sprecher, 1986, on love).

Second, we should identify processes by which intimate relationships enhance (or are detrimental to) the well-being of the partners. Chapter 10 proposes that intimate relationships enhance partners' well-being in part by fulfilling important needs. Intimacy researchers might be most interested in the processes by which relationships fulfill intimacy needs. I have argued that compatibility of partners' needs and skillful negotiation are both likely to contribute to intimacy need fulfillment. They may also predict whether in the process of fulfilling some needs partners fail to help (or even permit) one another to fulfill others.

We should, finally, examine the circumstances under which intimate relationships are likely to be effective in meeting people's needs. Research in this area might address questions such as the following: When does more relational intimacy (i.e., more frequent, intense, or extended intimate interactions) enhance versus detract from a relationship's functioning? What kinds of individuals and relationships are most likely to benefit from training or other assistance in intimate relating? What kinds of discriminations should people learn to make among situations regarding when intimate relating is most likely to meet their needs? The study of intimacy has advanced sufficiently so that we can move beyond asking whether more intimacy is better than less. Now we can learn when, how, and under what circumstances relational intimacy enhances relationship functioning.

THE SYSTEMATIC INCLUSION OF CONTEXTUAL FACTORS IN RESEARCH ON INTIMACY IS NECESSARY FOR THE FIELD TO PROGRESS

None of the aforementioned purposes can be realized without systematic consideration of contextual factors. As Figures 8.1 and 9.1 show, intimate interactions, intimate relationships, and the associations between the two always exist in context. Research to date confirms the important influence of contextual factors (e.g., Duck, 1993b).

Chapters 8 and 9 discuss four ways that context likely affects intimacy. First, contextual factors can directly affect intimate behavior. For example, the strength of partners' intimacy motives affects how frequently they will engage in intimate behavior (McAdams & Constantian, 1983). Second, contextual factors can modify the impact of intimate behavior on intimate experience. The gender composition of a dyad, for example, determines whether people will judge certain self-disclosures to be appropriate (e.g., Banikiotes, Kubinski, & Pursell, 1981). Third, context can exert direct effects on intimate relationship functioning. For example,

Miller et al. (1983) found that relationships are more likely to become intimate when one partner is an "opener" (i.e., has skills and characteristics that encourage others to share personal material). Finally, contextual factors seem to determine how important relational intimacy is to intimate relationship functioning. The importance of sexual intimacy, for example, varies depending on whether partners are involved in a gay, lesbian, or heterosexual romantic relationship (Blumstein & Schwartz, 1983).

Figure 8.1 identifies four levels of context, each of which appears to exert effects on intimacy. There is reason to believe, however, that some contexts exert more powerful effects than others. The type of relationship the partners have is an influential context. Perhaps in recognition of this, programs of research on various relationship types (parent–child relationships, romantic relationships, friendships) have largely remained separate from each other (Berscheid, 1994). Once the study of relationships within a particular context becomes isolated, however, the contextual factor itself can escape examination. Direct comparisons among relationship types on processes common to all would better illuminate the effects of this contextual factor. Research on relationship networks has made progress in this area (e.g., Buhrmester & Furman, 1987).

Life stage also exerts a strong influence on intimate interactions and relationships. In recognition of this influence, I give extensive attention to life stage effects in Part II of this book. In the chapters in Part II I argue that each life stage has its own set of needs, concerns, and stresses that preoccupy people and shape their behavior. I propose that people's efforts to fulfill, respond, and adapt to these needs and concerns affect their behavior in intimate interactions and relationships (see Figure 3.1). In turn, their intimate relationship partners can, through intimate (and other) interactions, affect how people fulfill their needs and adapt to stresses. Life stage affects intimate relationships, then, through the effects of needs, concerns, and stresses on people's behavior in intimate interactions and relationships.

Despite an extensive literature on personal relationships through the life span, much work remains to be done on intimacy. Figure 3.1 suggests three important directions this work should take. First, it should aim to illuminate processes by which intimate interactions and relationships fulfill needs and address concerns that emerge at each life stage. For example, existing work has addressed the role of intimate relationships in fulfilling infants' needs for security and safety (e.g., Bretherton, 1988). By broadening the boundaries of this work, we could learn more about how intimate relationships fulfill needs associated with later stages, such as toddlers' needs for autonomy, school-age children's needs for approval, and young adults' needs for support during life transitions. Second, research efforts should seek to identify effects of individual life-stage-related concerns on the functioning of intimate relationships. For example, a growing body of work has documented important effects of the transition to parenthood on marital relationships (e.g., C. Fischer, 1982). We might also wish to devote more attention to the impact other life-stage-related concerns have on intimate relating, such as concerns with gender role conformity, bodily changes, or work and achievement. Finally, research efforts should explore longitudinal links between adaptations from earlier stages and intimate interactions and relationships in later ones. Work on the long-term sequelae of secure and insecure parent-infant attachments has been under way for some time (e.g., Eliker et al., 1992). However, longitudinal research is expensive and time-consuming and is therefore difficult to come by. There are few areas in the study of intimacy that would not benefit from more longitudinal investigations.

The current work points to several additional steps that would bring us closer to these goals. First, a systematic effort to chart developmental changes in what constitutes (or is reasonably defined as) intimate interaction would advance our understanding of intimate interactions throughout the life span. For example, on the basis of reviews mentioned in Part II, I suggest that the sensitive responses called "affective attunement" in parents' interactions with their young children are one form of intimate interaction. Affectionate physical contact between parents and school-age children may represent a second form, about which we know very little. Further, the development of increasingly sophisticated communication and reasoning skills in children should coincide with more complex ways of intimate relating. We have much to learn about these processes.

Second, though there is general agreement that some behaviors are intimate (e.g., self-disclosure), we know more about their effects on intimate experience during some life stages (e.g., adolescence and young adulthood) than others (e.g., middle childhood and middle adulthood). If, as some theorists have suggested (e.g., Erikson, 1963), intimate interaction has less influence on need fulfillment and well-being during some life stages than others, we might learn much about the concerns and stresses of those life stages by understanding why this is so. It is possible that the importance of intimate interactions for fulfilling people's needs changes as life-stage-related concerns change. It is also possible, however, that social and economic pressures in U.S. culture make intimate interaction more accessible to people during some life stages than in others. R. Adams's (1987) work, for example, suggests that intimate relationships with friends are more easily maintained after retirement than before.

Gender is a contextual factor also receiving extensive attention in this book. Gender-related effects are pervasive in the literature on intimacy. There are indications that gender-related sociocultural norms, group norms, and individual personality characteristics can mildly or even severely limit the range of intimate interactions and relationships people seek or have access to. If we underestimate the effects of gender-related contextual factors, perhaps it is because we have tended to measure them one at a time. For example, of the gender-related phenomena discussed throughout this book, personality factors (masculine and feminine personality characteristics) have received the most detailed study. As one might expect when the effects of a variable stem from multiple sources, the results of research investigating sex-typed personality traits alone are inconsistent. Increasingly, scholars are recognizing that gender is a systemic as well as an individual variable.

The impact of gender on intimate relating will not be fully apparent until scholars systematically investigate the effects of those variables known to co-occur with gender. More systematic investigation may mean, in Blieszner and Adams' (1992) terms, that we must stop using gender as a proxy for other variables. Instead, we must directly investigate phenomena that covary with gender. Some examples of those phenomema are: (1) intimate partners' relative power (e.g., which one has the highest income? who adapts her/his schedule for the other's convenience?); (2) intimate partners' role restrictions (e.g., does either partner spurn certain household chores or leisure activities?), or (3) intimate partners' group memberships (e.g., what are partners' hobbies and interests? who do they share these with? do these compete with family responsibilities, etc.?) Gender-related effects most likely reflect the effects of these and many other variables on intimate relating. In sum, I am urging researchers to avoid treating gender as a simple biological or individual-difference variable! Gender-related phenomena impinge upon us at all contextual levels; for this reason, gender can serve as a window onto the processes by which sociocultural, group, interpersonal, and situational phenomena affect intimate relating (e.g., see Bleiszner & Adams, 1992; Wood, 1994).

The study of gay and lesbian relationships, still in its infancy, has the potential to shed additional light on gender-related behaviors and experiences in romantic relationships and friendships. This is because comparisons between gay, lesbian, and heterosexual relationships allow us to compare how men and women relate to female and male romantic partners (Huston & Schwartz, 1991). Further, as intimacy research includes lesbian and gay relationships more systematically, the pervasive and unexamined influence of heterosexuality should become more visible as well.

This list of contextual factors, which addresses those that have received the most attention in the personal relationships literature, leaves out some conspicuous aspects of context. The literature on intimacy rarely addresses race and social class, which are nearly isomorphic in U.S. society. Little is known, for example, about whether economic pressures result in more or less need for intimacy. On the one hand, Maslow's (1968) theory suggests that when needs for survival are not met, people pay less attention to higher needs like intimacy. On the other hand, there is evidence that people who work in jobs with little reward and those who, for a variety of reasons, are under stress turn to intimate relationships for support and rewarding experiences. More attention to race and social class might also raise questions about the impact of different family forms on intimate interactions and relationships. Members of certain U.S. ethnic groups, for example, are more likely than others to live as nuclear families, relatively isolated from extended kin. Members of other ethnic groups, in contrast, maintain close geographic proximity and often share living quarters with extended kin (Rhodes et al., 1994). People's networks of intimate relationships, for example, would likely look quite different in these two groups, yet little is known about the effects of these different kinds of intimate relationship networks on life-stage-related needs and concerns.

Cultural background has also been neglected in the study of intimacy. A full understanding of the impact of cultural norms and values on intimate relationships and their beneficial effects awaits further work as a result. North American psychologists are beginning to consider the influence of individualism (Guisinger & Blatt, 1994) and the privileging of agency (Seidler, 1992) on personal relationships. Accumulating evidence for intimacy's beneficial effects may encourage culture-wide efforts to foster value systems that facilitate intimate contact between people. For example, some forward-looking companies are paying increasing attention to the effect of work environments on people's intimate relationships (e.g., Gilbert, 1993).

The organization of contextual factors that I have proposed in this book reveals (1) how few main effects there really are in the field of intimacy, (2) the hierarchical, multilayered nature of context, and (3) the continuity between intrapsychic, interpersonal, and sociocultural phenomena. There are few main effects because contextual factors so often interact with one another and with intimate behavior to determine how people view, understand, and experience intimate interactions.

If contextual factors pervasively interact, perhaps it is because they coexist in a hierarchical, multilayered structure. For example, gender-related cultural norms, gender-related social pressures in groups, individual gender-related attitudes and schemas, and gender differences in behavior represent similar phenomena at different contextual levels. Each likely augments the effects of the others.

Finally, because of the continuity that exists among different levels of context, individual personality and relationship factors are as much a part of context as social and group norms or physical environment characteristics. This is because factors outside the dyad get represented in people's expectations, attitudes, and hopes within their relationships. Research documenting the internalization of cultural gender-related norms reveals this continuity (Beall & Sternberg, 1993).

Categorizations of contextual factors are valuable because they organize our thinking and ensure that research addresses these different levels. It is best to assume, however, that the categories are arbitrary divisions in a context that is continuous from individual to culture.

MODELS OF SOCIAL COGNITION MAY HELP DEFINE THE LINKS BETWEEN BEHAVIOR AND EXPERIENCE IN PERSONAL RELATIONSHIPS

Schemas representing self, other, relationship, and situation may serve as guides to interpretation, affect, and behavior within a particular interaction or set of interactions. Relationship schemas contain representations of people's expectations about themselves, their relationship partner, and the interaction that is likely to take place between them. Research on social cognition has suggested that schemas exist for specific relationship partners (Andersen & Cole, 1990) and for contextual factors, such as relationship type (Sedikides, Olsen, & Reis, 1993), partner's gender (Cross & Markus, 1993), and ethnic background (Thiedeman, 1991), and for the social situation (Mischel, 1993). People may also form partner-in-situation schemas for long-term relationship partners, each of which reflects their expectations of themselves, their partners, and their interaction in a particular type of situation (Baldwin, 1992).

There are individual differences and within-culture similarities in the nature of people's schemas. Both should be relevant to our understanding of how people interpret their interactions and come to experience intimacy. For example, normative culture-specific schemas may help to explain why both females and males are more likely to confide in female interaction partners. Within U.S. culture, people may expect females to be more verbally responsive. Individual differences in schemas may help to explain why some individuals have several confidantes while others have none. A person's expectations that people are trustworthy and likable (and that others will like him or her) may shape behavior that increases or decreases the likelihood that he or she will find a confidante.

It seems reasonable to presume that if an interaction is to be experienced as intimate by the participants, it must be understood and interpreted through schemas that contain positive expectations about intimacy. The attachment styles described by Hazan and Shaver (1987) and by subsequent research (e.g., Bartholomew, 1993) may reflect one such set of expectations. Work on dysfunctional relationship beliefs (Epstein et al., 1987) may have identified another set. Future work may identify additional sets of schemas about relationships, some of which may be more likely to promote intimate relationships than others. Further, future work may identify behavior likely to be associated with particular schema contents. For example, there is already evidence that people who are high in intimacy motivation more frequently behave in such a way as to encourage intimate interaction (McAdams, Healy, & Krause, 1984).

THE STUDY OF INTIMACY SHOULD BE MORE INCLUSIVE

Two areas that have been strangely absent from the study of intimacy are sexuality and parent–child relationships. The omission of sexuality is unfortunate, given how central sexual activity is to people's conceptions of intimacy (Helgeson et al., 1987). It is surprising how little researchers know about the interplay between sexuality and other forms of intimacy and, in particular, how little we know about how sexual activities are experienced and thought of by teens. The void in our knowledge of adolescents' dating relationships is striking when compared with the extensive work done on adolescent friendship, yet there is evidence that the quality of adolescent dating relationships is predictive of adolescent sexual activity (Christopher & Cate, 1988). Although more research has examined sexual activity in adults' relationships, information about adults' experiences with sex is still scarce. Recent efforts to connect information about sexuality to the expanding literature on intimate interactions and relationships (e.g., Henderson-King & Veroff, 1994; Sprecher & McKinney, 1993) seem a step in the right direction.

Parent–child relationships have also been left out of the literature on intimacy. Beyond the preschool years, researchers know little about change or stability in intimate contact between parents and children. There is little information available on what forms of intimate contact are normative at different stages of a child's (and parent's) development and on what impact children's new skills and capabilities have on parent–child intimacy. Similarly, it would be worthwhile to investigate whether patterns of intimate contact between parents and their children generalize to children's peer relationships. The literature on adults' relationships with parents leaves just as many unanswered questions. While parents may not be primary intimate partners for many adults, there is reason to believe that good relationships with parents can facilitate adjustment to life transitions (Lopez et al., 1988). Clinicians have suggested that relationships with parents may continue to affect relational schemas in adulthood, shaping adults' expectations of their spouses, friends, and their own children (e.g., H. Lerner, 1989). Much may be gained, therefore, from further exploration of parent–child intimacy beyond infancy and preschool.

INTIMACY PROMOTES INDIVIDUAL WELL-BEING BY FULFILLING IMPORTANT PSYCHOLOGICAL NEEDS

It is important to learn more about intimacy because (1) intimate contact is rewarding, (2) it enhances satisfaction in relationships, and (3) it fosters individual well-being. I have proposed that intimacy enhances individual well-being by fulfilling important psychological needs. By definition, it fulfills people's needs for intimacy, that is, their needs to be attended to, understood, and, ultimately, known deeply by another while still being accepted and valued (Reis & Shaver, 1988). Intimate interactions and relationships can also fulfill a variety of other needs throughout the life span, as the chapters in Part II make clear. Through intimate interactions infants may learn to expect experiences of shared joy and excitement with others. Toddlers may learn that their increasing autonomy does not interfere with their feelings of security with important intimate partners (Mahler, 1975). Young adolescents may learn that feelings of uncertainty accompanying pubertal changes are shared by others and that they are not alone (Buhrmester & Prager, 1995). Older adults may find that intimate interactions help them explore afresh their experiences of religious devotion (Jerrome, 1992).

Intimate interactions may fulfill any of these needs in the moment. Minimally, they do this through intimate experiences, that is, through positive feelings about oneself and the other person and through perceptions of being understood by another. They can also do much more. As Derlega and Grzelak (1979) said, intimate interactions can provide validation, self-clarification, relationship enhancement, and opportunities for catharsis. They can be vehicles for enhanced self-understanding and personal growth (Rogers, 1951; Youniss, 1980).

Intimate relationships can become reliable sources of need fulfillment over time. Not only can people fulfill current needs within intimate relationships, but they can expect their needs to be fulfilled in the future. Intimate relationships, then, likely fulfill enduring needs for a secure attachment and a sense of belonging as well as momentary needs for validation and catharsis (Ainsworth & Bowlby, 1991). Moreover, by serving as a secure base, they may enhance individual efforts to fulfill agentic needs, that is, for achievement and mastery, recognition, meaning and purpose, and self-esteem (Hazan & Shaver, 1990).

Ultimately, the beneficial effects of intimacy must be understood in light of its risks. Because intimate partners share what is personal and private, they make themselves more emotionally vulnerable to one another. Because of intimate interaction, people may acquire information that they can use, deliberately or inadvertently, to hurt one another (Hatfield, 1988).

A risk of intimacy that behavioral scientists have debated at length is the risk of loss of self or identity. People may view intimate interactions and relationships as directly competing with, and compromising the fulfillment of, needs for individuation, separateness, and privacy (Kerr & Bowen, 1988). Others have argued that needs for intimacy and individuation can peacefully coexist (Baxter & Wilmot, 1985) or even depend on each other (Beavers & Hampson, 1990).

I am suggesting that instead of continuing this debate we should identify the conditions that allow intimacy needs to be compatible with (or enhance fulfillment of) other needs. This approach to studying intimacy and individuation has already proved fruitful in research on adolescents' relationships with their parents (Cooper & Grotevant, 1987) and their friends (Thorbecke & Grotevant, 1982). The conditions that promote compatibility among needs may lie in interaction processes, such as partners' efforts to avoid power struggles in their negotiations about intimate contact. They may also be found in contextual factors. For example, a partner's belief that intimacy requires continual togetherness is likely to result in behavior that sabotages negotiations about private time.

I have advocated an approach to understanding intimacy that emphasizes the interplay between intimate interactions and relationships on the one hand and individual needs and concerns on the other. This approach could provide a broad base of information about the impact of intimate relating on individual health and well-being. It could answer questions regarding (1) the immediate impact of intimate interactions and (2) the more global impact of intimate relationships. Further, it might encourage a closer look at the factors that nourish intimate relationships themselves, because these relationships are so important to the individual.

An important outcome of intimacy research is a set of targeted interventions to aid people's efforts to sustain intimate relationships. The psychotherapist's office is one place where such interventions could be used. However, interventions that target individuals can have only limited influence. We must also propose and help implement interventions within broader social institutions (e.g., the workplace) that traditionally compromise people's efforts to sustain intimate relationships. By targeting interventions at multiple contextual levels, we stand the best chance of creating an environment in which satisfying intimate relationships are likely to flourish.

Notes

INTRODUCTION

1. Recent research by Reis and Franks (1994) suggests that social support may account for a significant percentage of the health benefits derived from intimate relationships.

2. Hobfoll and Lieberman (1989) found that new mothers who confided in family members and looked to them for affection, warmth, and appreciation reported *higher* levels of anxiety following their child's birth. Intimacy with spouses, however, predicted lower levels of anxiety.

CHAPTER ONE

1. See Duck (1994a) for a broader but parallel notion in which *personal* interactions consist of sharing that which is *meaningful*.

2. The frequency partners find acceptable likely varies from one relationship to the next.

3. Recent evidence from a study by Guldner and Swensen (1995) suggests that telephone and written contact can provide opportunities for intimacy comparable to physical togetherness. Results from this study revealed no differences in reported intimacy levels between college-aged couples in long-distance relationships and those who lived close by.

CHAPTER TWO

1. The focus of this book is dyadic intimacy. It is reasonable to presume, however, that three or more people can engage in intimate interactions.

2. A Guttman scale arranges items in a hierarchy so that a person who endorses items high up in the scale should also endorse items lower down in the scale.

3. For example, the present definition might include research interviews as intimate interactions! In my research with the intimacy status interview (e.g., Prager, 1991), interviewees sometimes reported feeling accepted and understood as a result of sharing personal material with a skilled interviewer. This definition would not automatically exclude such interviews from consideration, and therefore may err in the direction of overinclusiveness.

Chapter Three

1. Recall from Chapter 1 that *relational intimacy* in this book is a shorthand term for partners' history of and expectations for ongoing, frequently occurring intimate interactions.

Chapter Four

1. Research comparing infants' attachments to mothers and fathers has indicated that infants may have as many attachment styles as they have caregivers (e.g., Cox, Owen, Henderson, & Margang, 1992; Main, Kaplan, & Cassidy, 1985).

2. Throughout the book references to mothers only will be made when specific research results are available for mothers but not for fathers.

3. Attachments may also be formed with siblings.

Chapter Five

1. Although children enjoy competing during this period, competitive games likely require as much cooperation as competition. After all, one must follow the rules and play fair or genuine competition is not really possible (Sroufe & Cooper, 1988).

2. Bem (1989) found evidence that children can probably learn gender constancy sooner if they are taught that "genitalia constitute the defining attributes of male and female" (Bem, 1993, p. 115). Those toddlers who do have this knowledge are able to conserve the gender of a child pictured in a series of photographs even when the external signs of gender, such as hairstyle and dress, are altered.

Chapter Six

1. If familiarity bred contempt, of course, more conflict and disharmony might be expected in mother–adolescent than in father–adolescent relation-

ships. There is no evidence that this is the case, however (Youniss & Smollar, 1985).

CHAPTER SEVEN

1. There is some evidence that this decline is in part an artifact of averaging in (1) unhappy marriages that stay intact until children leave home and (2) only the happier marriages that remain among post-launching couples (Whitbourne, 1986).

2. Under ordinary circumstances, however, whether wives work inside or outside the home exerts little impact on marital satisfaction for husbands or wives (England & Farkas, 1986; J. Wilkie, 1988).

CHAPTER EIGHT

1. Because of its brevity, Grant and Katie's intimate interaction could also be called an "intimate moment." This term might usefully distinguish brief intimate interactions from more extended exchanges.

2. People may also smile in anticipation of an unpleasant interaction and may have negative feelings about the person they are smiling at (M. Patterson, 1982).

3. The reader is referred to Robbins and Haase (1985) for other dimensions of nonverbal behavior that may account for its salience in communication.

4. Bateson, Jackson, Haley, and Weakland (1956) called it a "double bind" when someone feels unable to comment on the incongruence between the verbal message in a communication and the accompanying affect.

CHAPTER NINE

1. Rauch, Barry, Hertel, and Swain (1974) make a useful distinction between constructive and destructive conflict: Constructive conflict "is characterized by a concentration on the issue . . . use of mutual problem-solving tactics . . . and mutal enhancement with a minumum of threat and defensiveness. "Destructive conflict" is characterized by a tendency to expand and escalate so that it [conflict] . . . becomes independent of the initial issue" (pp. 32–33).

2. In the literature on love, references to love relationships nearly always mean romantic love (Aron & Aron, 1993).

3. Beach and Tesser (1988) also distinguish these two activities on emotional intensity, a less useful distinction in my view (see my discussion in Chapter 1).

4. Observational studies of marital conflict, however, show wives generat-

ing more negative affect and behavior than husbands (Margolin & Wampold, 1981; Rausch, Barry, Hertel, & Swain, 1974). (See Sayers & Baucom, 1991, for different findings.)

CHAPTER TEN

1. It is quite possible that when we perceive ourselves to be understood and simultaneously feel positively about ourselves and our partner, it is because our partner is successfully communicating acceptance. The importance of acceptance is receiving increasing attention from relationships researchers (Hayes, Jacobson, Follette, & Dougher, 1994).

2. Readers are referred to others' efforts to clarify similar concepts: Steinberg and Silverberg (1986) identified several types of autonomy, and Burgoon et al. (1989) defined five types of privacy.

References

Abbott, D. A., & Brody, G. H. (1985). The relation of child age, gender, and number of children to the marital adjustment of wives. *Journal of Marriage and the Family, 47,* 77–84.

Abele, A. (1986). Functions of gaze in social interaction: Communication and monitoring. *Journal of Nonverbal Behavior, 10,* 83–101.

Acitelli, L. K. (1988). When spouses talk to each other about their relationship. *Journal of Social and Personal Relationships, 5,* 185–199.

Acitelli, L. K. (1993). You, me and us: Perspectives on relationship awareness. In S. Duck (Ed.), *Individuals in Relationships* (pp. 144–174). Newbury Park, CA: Sage.

Acitelli, L. K., & Antonucci, T. C. (1994). Social support in older couples. *Journal of Personality and Social Psychology, 67,* 688–698.

Acitelli, L. K., Douvan, E., & Veroff, J. (1993). Perceptions of conflict in the first year of marriage: How important are similarity and understanding? *Journal of Social and Personal Relationships, 10,* 5–19.

Acitelli, L. K., & Duck, S. (1987). Intimacy as the proverbial elephant. In D. Perlman & S. Duck (Eds.), *Intimate Relationships* (pp. 297–308). Beverly Hills, CA: Sage.

Acker, M., & Davis, M. H. (1992). Intimacy, passion, and commitment in adult romantic relationships: A test of the triangular theory of love. *Journal of Social and Personal Relationships, 9,* 21–50.

Adams, D. L. (1971). Correlates of satisfaction among the elderly. *The Gerontologist, 11,* 64–68.

Adams, G. R., & Gullotta, T. (1989). *Adolescent Life Experiences.* Pacific Grove, CA: Brooks/Cole.

Adams, R. G. (1987). Patterns of network change: A longitudinal study of friendships of elderly women. *The Gerontologist, 27,* 222–227.

Adams, R. G. (1989). Conceptual and methodological issues in studying friendships of older adults. In R. G. Adams & R. Blieszner (Eds.), *Older Adult Friendship: Structure and Process* (pp. 17–41). Newbury Park, CA: Sage.

Adams, R. G., & Blieszner, R. (1994). An integrative conceptual framework for friendship research. *Journal of Social and Personal Relationships, 11*, 163–184.

Adams, W. J. (1988). Sexuality and happiness ratings of husbands and wives in relation to first and second pregnancies. *Journal of Family Psychology, 2*, 67–81.

Adler, A. (1964). *Superiority and Social Interest: A Collection of Later Writings* (H. L. Ansbacher & R. R. Ansbacher, Eds.). Evanston, IL: Northwestern University Press.

Ainsworth, M. D. S. (1967). *Infancy in Uganda: Child Care and the Growth of Love*. Baltimore: Johns Hopkins University Press.

Ainsworth, M. D. S. (1989). Attachments beyond infancy. *American Psychologist, 44*, 709–716.

Ainsworth, M. D. S., Blehar, M. S., Waters, E., & Wall, S. (1978). *Patterns of Attachment: A Psychological Study of the Strange Situation*. Hillsdale, NJ: Erlbaum.

Ainsworth, M. D. S., & Bowlby, J. (1991). An ethological approach to personality development. *American Psychologist, 46*, 333–341.

Albert, S. M., & Moss, M. (1990). Consensus and the domain of personal relations among older adults. *Journal of Social and Personal Relationships, 7*, 353–369.

Allan, G. (1993). Social structure and relationships. In S. Duck (Ed.), *Social Context and Relationships* (pp. 1–25). London: Sage.

Altman, I. (1977). Privacy regulation: Culturally universal or culturally specific? *Journal of Social Issues, 33*, 66–84.

Altman, I., & Taylor, D. A. (1978). *Social Penetration: The Development of Interpersonal Relationships*. New York: Holt, Rinehart & Winston.

Ambert, A. M. (1992). *The Effect of Children on Parents*. New York: Haworth Press.

Andersen, P. A. (1993). Cognitive schemata in personal relationships. In S. Duck (Ed.), *Individual in Relationships* (pp. 1–29). Newbury Park, CA: Sage.

Andersen, P. A., & Leibowitz, K. (1978). The development and nature of the construct touch avoidance. *Environmental Psychology and Nonverbal Behavior, 3*, 89–106.

Andersen, P. A., & Sull, K. K. (1985). Out of touch, out of reach: Tactile predispositions as predictors of interpersonal distance. *Western Journal of Speech Communication, 49*, 57–72.

Andersen, S. M., & Cole, S. W. (1990). "Do I know you?": The role of significant others in general social perception. *Journal of Personality and Social Psychology, 59*, 384–399.

Antill, J. K. (1983). Sex-role complementarity versus similarity in married couples. *Journal of Personality and Social Psychology, 45*, 145–155.

Antill, J. K., & Cotton, S. (1987). Self-disclosure between husbands and wives: Its relationship to sex roles and marital happiness. *Australian Journal of Psychology, 39*, 11–24.

Applegate, J. L., Burleson, B. R., & Delia, J. G. (1992). Reflection-enhancing parenting as an antecedent to children's social-cognitive and communicative development. In I. E. Sigel, A. V. McGullicuddy-DeLisi, & J. J. Goodnow (Eds.), *Parent Belief Systems: The Psychological Consequences for Children* (Vol. 2, pp. 3–39). Hillsdale, NJ: Erlbaum.

Archer, R. L. (1979). Role of personality and the social situation. In G. J. Chelune (Ed.), *Self-Disclosure: Origins, Patterns, and Implications of Openness in Interpersonal Relationships* (pp. 28–58). San Francisco: Jossey-Bass.

Archer, R. L. (1987). Commentary: Self-disclosure, a very useful behavior. In V. J. Derlega & J. H. Berg (Eds.), *Self-Disclosure: Theory, Research, and Therapy* (pp. 329–342). New York: Plenum.

Arend, R., Gove, F., & Sroufe, L. A. (1979). Continuity of individual adaptation from infancy to kindergarten: A predictive study of ego-resiliency and curiosity in preschoolers. *Child Development, 50*, 950–959.

Argyle, M., & Dean, J. (1965). Eye-contact, distance and affiliation. *Sociometry, 28*, 289–304.

Argyle, M., & Furnham, A. (1983). Sources of satisfaction and conflict in long-term relationships. *Journal of Marriage and the Family, 45*, 481–493.

Argyle, M., Ingham, R., Alkema, R., & McCallin, M. (1973). The different functions of gaze. *Semiotica, 7*, 19–32.

Aries, E. J., & Johnson, F. L. (1983). Close friendship in adulthood: Conversational content between same-sex friends. *Sex Roles, 9*, 1183–1196.

Arling, G. (1976). The elderly widow and her family, neighbors and friends. *Journal of Marriage and the Family, 38*, 757–868.

Arnold, M. B. (1960). *Emotion and Personality*. New York: Columbia University Press.

Aron, A., Aron, E. N., & Smollan, D. (1992). Inclusion of Other in the Self Scale and the structure of interpersonal closeness. *Journal of Personality and Social Psychology, 63*, 596–612.

Aron, E., & Aron, A. (1994). Love. In A. L. Weber & J. H. Harvey (Eds.), *Perspectives on Close Relationships* (pp. 131–152). Boston: Allyn & Bacon.

Atchley, R. C. (1985). *Social Forces and Aging: An Introduction to Social Gerontology*. Belmont, CA: Wadsworth.

Attili, G. (1989). Social competence versus emotional security: The link between home relationships and behavior problems at school. In B. H. Schneider, G. Attili, J. Nadel, & R. P. Weissberg (Eds.), *Social Competence in Developmental Perspective* (pp. 293–311). London: Kluwer.

Aukett, R., Ritchie, J., & Mill, K. (1988). Gender differences in friendship patterns. *Sex Roles, 19*, 57–66.

Babcock, J., & Jacobson, N. S. (1993). A program of research on behavioral marital therapy: Hot spots and smoldering embers in marital therapy research. *Journal of Social and Personal Relationships, 10*, 119–135.

Bakan, D. (1966). *The Duality of Human Existence*. Chicago: Rand McNally.

Baldwin, M. W. (1992). Relational schemas and the processing of social information. *Psychological Bulletin, 112*, 461–484.

Bandura, A. (1982). Self-efficacy mechanism in human agency. *American Psychologist, 37*, 122–147.

Banikiotes, P. G., Kubinski, J. A., & Pursell, S. A. (1981). Sex-role orientation, self-disclosure and gender-related perceptions. *Journal of Counseling Psychology, 28,* 140–146.

Bardwick, J., & Douvan, E. (1971). Ambivalence: The socialization of women. In V. Gornick & B. K. Moran (Eds.), *Woman in Sexist Society* (pp. 147–159). New York: Basic Books.

Barkham, M., & Shapiro, D. A. (1986). Counselor verbal response modes and experienced empathy. *Journal of Counseling Psychology, 33,* 3–10.

Barnett, R. C., & Marshall, N. L. (1991). The relationship between women's work and family roles and their subjective well-being and psychological distress. In M. Frankenhaeuser, U. Lundberg, & M. Chesney (Eds.), *Women, Work and Health: Stress and Opportunities* (pp. 111–136). New York: Plenum.

Barnett, R. C., Marshall, N. L., Raudenbush, S. W., & Brennan, R. T. (1993). Gender and the relationship between job experiences and psychological distress: A study of dual-earner couples. *Journal of Personality and Social Psychology, 64,* 794–806.

Barnett, R. C., Marshall, N. L., & Singer, J. D. (1992). Job experiences over time, multiple roles, and women's mental health: A longitudinal study. *Journal of Personality and Social Psychology, 62,* 634–644.

Bartholomew, K. (1993). From childhood to adult relationships: Attachment theory and research. In S. Duck (Ed.), *Learning About Relationships* (pp. 30–62). Newbury Park, CA: Sage.

Basco, M. A., Prager, K. J., Pita, J. M., Tamir, L. M., & Stephens, J. J. (1992). Depression and marital discord. *Journal of Family Psychology, 6,* 184–194.

Bateson, G., Jackson, D., Haley, J., & Weakland, J. (1956). Toward a theory of schizophrenia. *Behavioral Science, 1,* 251–264.

Baucom, D. H., & Epstein, N. (1990). *Cognitive-Behavioral Marital Therapy.* New York: Brunner/Mazel.

Baumeister, R. F., Wotman, S. R., & Stillwell, A. M. (1993). Unrequited love: On heartbreak, anger, guilt, scriptlessness, and humiliation. *Journal of Personality and Social Psychology, 64,* 377–394.

Baumrind, D. (1967). Child care practices anteceding three patterns of preschool behavior. *Genetic Psychology Monographs, 75,* 43–83.

Baumrind, D. (1971). Current patterns of parental authority. *Developmental Psychology Monographs, 4,* 1–101.

Baxter, L. A. (1986). Gender differences in the heterosexual relationship rules embedded in break-up accounts. *Journal of Social and Personal Relationships, 3,* 289–306.

Baxter, L. (1993). Relationship maintenance strategies and dialectical contradictions in personal relationships. *Journal of Social and Personal Relationships, 10,* 225–242.

Baxter, L. A. (1988). A dialectical perspective on communication strategies in relationship development. In S. W. Duck (Ed.), *Handbook of Personal Relationships* (pp. 257–273). New York: Wiley.

Baxter, L. A. (1990). Dialectical contradictions in relationship development. *Journal of Social and Personal Relationships, 7*, 69–88.

Baxter, L. A. (1991, June). *Thinking dialogically about personal relationships*. Invited address to the Conference of the International Network on Personal Relationships, Normal, IL.

Baxter, L. A., & Dindia, K. (1990). Marital partners' perceptions of marital maintenance strategies. *Journal of Social and Personal Relationships, 7*, 187–208.

Baxter, L. A., & Simon, E. P. (1993). Relationship maintenance strategies and dialectical contradictions in personal relationships. *Journal of Social and Personal Relationships, 10*, 225–242.

Baxter, L. A., & Wilmot, W. W. (1985). Taboo topics in close relationships. *Journal of Social and Personal Relationships, 2*, 253–269.

Beach, S. R. H., Mendolia, M., & Tesser, A. (1992, November). *Self-esteem maintenance and relationship closeness*. Paper presented at the Annual Meeting, Association for Advancement of Behavior Therapy, New York.

Beach, S. R. H., Nelson, G. M., & O'Leary, K. D. (1988). Cognitive and marital factors in depression. *Journal of Psychopathology and Behavioral Assessment, 10*, 93–105.

Beach, S. R. H., Sandeen, E. E., & O'Leary, K. D. (1990). *Depression in Marriage: A Model for Etiology and Treatment*. New York: Guilford Press.

Beach, S. R. H., & Tesser, A. (1988). Love in marriage: A cognitive account. In R. J. Sternberg & M. L. Barnes (Eds.), *The Psychology of Love* (pp. 330-358). New Haven, CT: Yale.

Beall, A. E. (1993). A social constructionist view of gender. In A. E. Beall & R. J. Sternberg (Eds.), *The Psychology of Gender* (pp. 127–147). New York: Guilford Press.

Beall, A. E., & Sternberg, R. J. (Eds.). (1993). *The Psychology of Gender*. New York: Guilford Press.

Beavers, W. R., & Hampson, R. B. (1990). *Successful Families: Assessment and Intervention*. New York: Norton.

Bee, H. L. (1992). *The Journey of Adulthood*. New York: Macmillan.

Beier, E. G., & Sternberg, D. P. (1977). Marital communication: Subtle cues between newly-weds. *Journal of Communication, 27*, 92–103.

Bell, R. A., Buerkel-Rothfuss, N. L., & Gore, K. E. (1987). "Did you bring the yarmulke for the cabbage patch kid?" The idiomatic communication of young lovers. *Human Communication Research, 14*, 47–67.

Bell, R. R. (1981). *Worlds of Friendship*. Beverly Hills, CA: Sage.

Belsky, J. (1979). The interrelation of parental and spousal behavior during infancy in traditional nuclear families: An exploratory analysis. *Journal of Marriage and the Family, 41*, 62–68.

Belsky, J. (1984). The determinants of parenting: A process model. *Child Development, 55*, 83–96.

Belsky, J., Fish, M., & Isabella, R. (1991). Continuity and discontinuity in infant negative and positive emotionality: Family antecedents and attachment consequences. *Developmental Psychology, 27,* 421–431.

Belsky, J., Lang, M. E., & Rovine, M. (1985). Stability and change in marriage across the transition to parenthood: A second study. *Journal of Marriage and the Family, 47,* 855–865.

Belsky, J., & Nezworski, T. (1988). Clinical implications of attachment. In J. Belsky & T. Nezworksi (Eds.), *Clinical Implications of Attachment* (pp. 3–17). Hillsdale, NJ: Erlbaum.

Belsky, J., & Rovine, M. (1990). Q-sort security and first-year nonmaternal care. *New Directions for Child Development, 49,* 7–22.

Belsky, J., Youngblade, L., Rovine, M., & Volling, B. (1991). Patterns of marital change and parent–child interaction. *Journal of Marriage and the Family, 53,* 487–498.

Bem, S. L. (1974). The measurement of psychological androgyny. *Journal of Consulting and Clinical Psychology, 42,* 155–162.

Bem, S. L. (1977). On the utility of alternative procedures for assessing psychological androgyny. *Journal of Clinical and Consulting Psychology, 45,* 196–205.

Bem, S. L. (1983). Gender schema theory and its implications for child development: Raising gender-aschematic children in a gender-schematic society. *Signs: Journal of Women in Culture and Society, 8,* 598–616. (Reprinted in Walsh, M. R. (Ed.). (1987). *The Psychology of Women: Ongoing Debates* (pp. 226–245). New Haven, CT: Yale University Press.)

Bem, S. L. (1989). Genital knowledge and gender constancy in preschool children. *Child Development, 60,* 649–662.

Bem, S.L. (1993). *The Lenses of Gender: Transforming the Debate on Sexual Inequality.* New Haven, CT: Yale University Press.

Benin, M. H., & Edwards, D. A. (1990). Adolescents' chores: The difference between dual- and single-earner families. *Journal of Marriage and the Family, 52,* 361–373.

Bentler, P. M., & Newcomb, M. D. (1978). Longitudinal study of marital success and failure. *Journal of Consulting and Clinical Psychology, 46,* 1053–1070.

Berg, J. H. (1984). Development of friendship between roommates. *Journal of Personality and Social Psychology, 46,* 346–356.

Berg, J. H. (1987). Responsiveness and self-disclosure. In V. J. Derlega & J. H. Berg (Eds.), *Self-Disclosure: Theory, Research and Therapy* (pp. 101–130). New York: Plenum.

Berg, J. H., & Archer, R. L. (1980). Disclosure or concern: A second look at liking for the norm breaker. *Journal of Personality, 48,* 245–257.

Berg, J. H., & McQuinn, R. D. (1986). Attraction and exchange in continuing and noncontinuing dating relationships. *Journal of Personality and Social Psychology, 50,* 942–952.

Berman, B., & Margolin, G. (1992). Analysis of the association between marital relationships and health problems: An interactional perspective. *Psychological Bulletin, 112,* 39–63.

Berman, J. J., Murphy-Berman, V., & Pachauri, A. (1988). Sex differences in friendship patterns in India and in the United States. *Basic and Applied Social Psychology, 9,* 61–71.

Bernard, J. (1972). *The Future of Marriage.* New York: World.

Berndt, T. J. (1979). Developmental changes in conformity to peers and parents. *Developmental Psychology, 15,* 608–616.

Berndt, T. J. (1982). The features and effects of friendship in early adolescence. *Child Development, 53,* 1447–1460.

Berndt, T. J., & Perry, T. B. (1986). Children's perceptions of friendships as supportive relationships. *Developmental Psychology, 22,* 640–648.

Berscheid, E. (1977). Privacy: A hidden variable in experimental social psychology. *Journal of Social Issues, 33,* 85–101.

Berscheid, E. (1983). Emotion. In H. H. Kelley, E. Berscheid, A. Christensen, J. H. Harvey, T. L. Huston, G. Levinger, E. McClintock, L. A. Peplau, & D. R. Peterson (Eds.), *Close Relationships: Development and Change* (pp. 110–168). New York: Freeman.

Berscheid, E. (1994). Interpersonal relationships. *Annual Review of Psychology, 45,* 79–129.

Berscheid, E., Snyder, M., & Omoto, A. M. (1989). The Relationship Closeness Inventory: Assessing the closeness of interpersonal relationships. *Journal of Personality and Social Psychology, 57,* 792–807.

Berscheid, E., & Walster, E. (1971). Adrenalin makes the heart grow fonder. *Psychology Today, 5,* 47–50.

Berscheid, E., & Walster, E. (1978). *Interpersonal Attraction* (2nd ed.). Reading, MA: Addison-Wesley.

Bigelow, B. J., & LaGaipa, J. J. (1975). Children's written descriptions of friendship: A multidimensional analysis. *Developmental Psychology, 11,* 857–858.

Biller, H. B. (1993). *Fathers and Families: Paternal Factors in Child Development.* Westport, CT: Auburn House.

Birchler, G. R., & Webb, L. J. (1977). Discriminating interaction behavior in happy and unhappy marriages. *Journal of Consulting and Clinical Psychology, 45,* 494–495.

Blau, Z. S. (1973). *Old Age in a Changing Society.* New York: Franklin Watts.

Blehar, M. C., Lieberman, A. F., & Ainsworth, M. D. S. (1977). Early face-to-face interaction and its relation to later infant-mother attachment. *Child Development, 48,* 182–194.

Blier, M. J., & Blier-Wilson, L. A. (1989). Gender differences in self-rated emotional expressiveness. *Sex Roles, 21,* 287–295.

Blieszner, R., & Adams, R. G. (1992). *Adult Friendship.* Newbury Park, CA: Sage.

Blos, P. (1967). The second individuation process of adolescence. *Psychoanalytic Study of the Child, 22,* 162–186.

Blumstein, P., & Schwartz, P. (1983). *American Couples: Money, Work, Sex.* New York: Morrow.

Blyth, D. A., & Foster-Clark, F. (1987). Gender differences in perceived intimacy with different members of adolescents' social networks. *Sex Roles, 17,* 687–718.

Blyth, D. A., & Traeger, C. (1988). Adolescent self-esteem and perceived relationships with parents and peers. In S. Salzinger, J. Antrobers, & M. Hammer (Eds.), *Social Networks of Children, Adolescents, and College Students* (pp. 171–194). Hillsdale, NJ: Erlbaum.

Bolger, N., DeLongis, A., Kessler, R. C., & Schilling, E. A. (1989). Effects of daily stress on mood. *Journal of Personality and Social Psychology, 57,* 808–818.

Boon, S. D. (1994). Dispelling doubt and uncertainty: Trust in romantic relationships. In S. Duck (Ed.), *Dynamics of Relationships* (pp. 86–111). Thousand Oaks, CA: Sage.

Booth, A., & Hess, E. (1974). Cross-sex friendship. *Journal of Marriage and the Family, 36,* 38–47.

Bott, E. (1971). *Family and Social Network.* London: Tavistock.

Bowen, M. (1966). The use of family therapy in clinical practice. *Comprehensive Psychiatry, 7,* 345–374.

Bowen, M. (1978). *Family Therapy in Clinical Practice.* Northvale, NJ: Aronson.

Bowlby, J. (1969). *Attachment.* New York: Basic Books.

Bowlby, J. (1973). *Attachment and Loss: Vol. 2. Separation.* New York: Basic Books.

Bowlby, J. (1982). Attachment and loss: Retrospect and prospect. *American Journal of Orthopsychiatry, 52,* 664–678.

Bradbury, T. N., Campbell, S. M., & Fincham, F. D. (1995). Longitudinal and behavioral analysis of masculinity and feminity in marriage. *Journal of Personality and Social Psychology, 68,* 328–341.

Bradbury, T. N., & Fincham, F. D. (1987). Affect and cognition in close relationships: Towards an integrative model. *Cognition and Emotion, 1,* 59–87.

Bradbury, T. N., & Fincham, F. D. (1988). Individual difference variables in close relationships: A contextual model of marriage as an integrative framework. *Journal of Personality and Social Psychology, 54,* 713–721.

Bradbury, T. N., & Fincham, F. D. (1990). Dimensions of marital and family interaction. In J. Touliatos, B. F. Perlmutter, & M. A. Straus (Eds.), *Handbook of Family Measurement Techniques* (pp. 36–61). Newbury Park, CA: Sage.

Bradbury, T. N., & Fincham, F. D. (1992). Assessing dysfunctional cognition in marriage: A reconsideration of the Relationship Belief Inventory. *Psychological Assessment, 5,* 92–101.

Brazelton, T. B., Koslowski, B., & Main, M. (1974). The origins of reciprocity: The early mother-infant interaction. In M. Lewis & L. A. Rosenblum (Eds.), *The Effects of the Infant on Its Caregiver* (pp. 49-76). New York: Wiley.

Bretherton, I. (1988). Open communication and internal working models: Their role in the development of attachment relationships. *Nebraska Symposium on Motivation, 36,* 57–133.

Bretherton, I. (1990). Communication patterns, internal working models, and the intergenerational transmission of attachment relationships. *Infant Mental Health Journal, 11,* 237–252.

Bretherton, I. (1991). The roots and growing points of attachment theory. In C.

M. Parkes, J. Stevenson-Hinde, & P. Marris (Eds.), *Attachment Across the Life Cycle* (pp. 9–32). London: Routledge.

Bretherton, I., Biringen, Z., Ridgeway, D., Maslin, C., & Sherman, M. (1989). Attachment: The parental perspective. *Infant Mental Health Journal, 10,* 203–221.

Broderick, J. E., & O'Leary, K. D. (1986). Contributions of affect, attitudes, and behavior to marital satisfaction. *Journal of Consulting and Clinical Psychology, 54,* 514–517.

Brooks-Gunn, J., & Ruble, D. N. (1983). Dysmenorrhea in adolescence. In S. Golub (Ed.), *Menarche: The Transition from Girl to Woman* (pp. 251–261). Lexington, MA: Lexington Books.

Broude, G. J. (1987). The relationship of marital intimacy and aloofness to social environment: A hologeistic study. *Behavioral Science Research, 21,* 50–69.

Brown, B. B. (1981). A lifespan approach to friendship: Age-related dimensions of an ageless relationship. In H. Z. Lopata & D. Maines (Eds.), *Research on the Interweave of Social Roles and Friendship* (Vol. 2). Greenwich, CT: JAI Press.

Brown, G. W., Bhrolchain, M., & Harris, T. (1975). Social class and psychiatric disturbance among women in an urban population. *Sociology, 9,* 225–254.

Brown, G. W., & Harris, T. (1978). Social origins of depression: A reply. *Psychological Medicine, 8,* 577–588.

Brown, G. W., & Harris, T. O. (1986). Stressor, vulnerability and depression: A question of replication. *Psychological Medicine, 16,* 739–744.

Brown, L. M., & Gilligan, C. (1992). *Meeting at the Crossroads: Women's Psychology and Girls' Development.* Cambridge, MA: Harvard University Press.

Brown, M. T. (1989). A cross-sectional analysis of self-disclosure patterns. *Journal of Mental Health Counseling, 11,* 384–395.

Bruch, M. A., Kaflowitz, N. G., & Pearl, L. (1988). Mediated and nonmediated relationships of personality components to loneliness. *Journal of Social and Clinical Psychology, 6,* 346–355.

Buck, R. (1989). Emotional communication in personal relationships: A developmental-interactionist view. In C. Hendrick (Ed.), *Close Relationships: Review of Personality and Social Psychology* (Vol. 10, pp.144–163). Newbury Park, CA: Sage.

Buhrke, R. A., & Fuqua, D. R. (1987). Sex differences in same- and cross-sex supportive relationships. *Sex Roles, 17,* 339–352.

Buhrmester, D. (1990). Intimacy of friendship, interpersonal competence, and adjustment during preadolescence and adolescence. *Child Development, 61,* 1101–1111.

Buhrmester, D. (in press). Need fulfillment, interpersonal competence, and the developmental contexts of friendship. In W. N. Bukowski, A. F. Newcomb, & W. W. Hartup (Eds.), *The Company They Keep: Friendship in Childhood and Adolescence.* New York: Cambridge University Press.

Buhrmester, D., & Carbery, J. (1992, March). *Daily patterns of self-disclosure and adolescent adjustment.* Paper presented at the Biennial Meeting of the Society for Research on Adolescence, Washington, DC.

Buhrmester, D., & Furman, W. (1986). The changing functions of friends in childhood: A neo-Sullivanian perspective. In V. J. Derlega & B. A. Winstead (Eds.), *Friendship and Social Interaction* (pp. 43–62). New York: Springer-Verlag.

Buhrmester, D., & Furman, W. (1987). The development of companionship and intimacy. *Child Development, 58,* 1101–1113.

Buhrmester, D., Goldfarb, J., & Cantrell, D. (1992). Self-presentation when sharing with friends and non-friends. *Journal of Early Adolescence, 12,* 61–79.

Buhrmester, D., & Prager, K. J. (1995). Patterns and functions of self-disclosure during childhood and adolescence. In K. J. Rotenberg (Ed.), *Disclosure Processes in Children and Adolescents* (pp. 10–56). New York: Cambridge University Press.

Bukowski, W. M., Gauze, C., Hoza, B., & Newcomb, A. F. (1993). Differences and consistency between same-sex and other-sex peer relationships during early adolescence. *Developmental Psychology, 67,* 56–68.

Bullough, V. (1990). The Kinsey Scale in historical perspective. In D. P. McWhirter, S. A. Sanders, & J. M. Reinisch (Eds.), *Homosexuality/Heterosexuality: Concepts of Sexual Orientation* (pp. 3–14). New York: Oxford University Press.

Burgoon, J. K. (1991). Relational message interpretations of touch, conversational distance and posture. *Journal of Nonverbal Behavior, 15,* 233–259.

Burgoon, J. K., Buller, D. B., Hale, J. L., & deTurck, M. A. (1984). Relational messages associated with nonverbal behaviors. *Human Communication Research, 10,* 351–378.

Burgoon, J. K., & Hale, J. L. (1988). Nonverbal expectancy violations: Model elaboration and application to immediacy behaviors. *Communication Monographs, 55,* 58–79.

Burgoon, J. K., & Koper, R. J. (1984). Nonverbal and relatonal communication associated with reticence. *Human Communication Research, 2,* 131–146.

Burgoon, J. K., Parrott, R., LePoire, B. A., Kelley, D. L., Walter, J. B., & Perry, D. (1989). Maintaining and restoring privacy through communication in different types of relationships. *Journal of Social and Personal Relationships, 6,* 131–158.

Burhenne, D., & Mirels, H. L. (1970). Self-disclosure in self-descriptive essays. *Journal of Consulting and Clinical Psychology, 35,* 409–413.

Burke, R. J., Weir, T., & Harrison, D. (1976). Disclosure of problems and tensions experienced by marital partners. *Psychological Reports, 38,* 531–542.

Buss, D. M. (1988). Love acts: The evolutionary biology of love. In R. J. Sternberg & M. L. Barnes (Eds.), *The Psychology of Love* (pp. 100–118). New Haven, CT: Yale University Press.

Butler, R. N. (1974). Successful aging and the role of the life review. *Journal of the American Geriatrics Society, 22,* 529–535.

Caldwell, M. A., & Peplau, L. A. (1982). Sex differences in same-sex friendship. *Sex Roles, 8,* 721–732.

Camarena, P. M., Sarigiani, P. A., & Petersen, A. C. (1990). Gender-specific pathways to intimacy in early adolescence. *Journal of Youth and Adolescence, 19,* 19–32.

Campbell, E., Adams, G. R., & Dobson, W. R. (1984). Familial correlations of identity formation in late adolescence: A study of the predictive utility of connectedness and individuality in family relations. *Journal of Youth and Adolescence, 13,* 509–525.

Campbell, J. D., & Tesser, A. (1985). Self-evaluation maintenance processes in relationships. In S. Duck & D. Perlman (Eds.), *Understanding Personal Relationships: An Interdisciplinary Approach* (pp. 107–135). London: Sage.

Campos, J., Barrett, K., Lamb, M., Goldsmith, H., & Sternberg, C. (1983). Socioemotional development. In P. H. Mussen (Ed.), *Handbook of Child Psychology: Vol 2. Infancy and Developmental Psychology* (pp. 783–915). New York: Wiley.

Canary, D. J., & Cupach, W. R. (1988). Relational and episodic characteristics associated with conflict tactics. *Journal of Social and Personal Relationships, 5,* 305–325.

Cancian, F. M. (1986). The feminization of love. *Signs: Journal of Women in Culture and Society, 11,* 692–709.

Cantor, N., Acker, M., & Cook-Flannagan, C. (1992). Conflict and preoccupation in the intimacy life task. *Journal of Personality and Social Psychology, 63,* 644–655.

Cantor, N., & Malley, J. (1991). Life tasks, personal needs, and close relationships. In G. O. Fletcher & F. D. Fincham (Eds.), *Cognition in Close Relationships* (pp. 101–125). Hillsdale, NJ: Erlbaum.

Cantor, N., & Mischel, W. (1979). Prototypes in person perception. *Advances in Experimental Social Psychology, 12,* 3–52.

Carbery, J. (1993). *The changing significance of friendship across three young adult phases.* Unpublished doctoral dissertation, University of Texas at Dallas.

Carkhuff, R. R. (1972). *The Art of Helping.* Amherst, MA: Human Resource Development Press.

Carkhuff, R. R. (1973). *The Art of Problem-Solving.* Amherst, MA: Human Resource Press.

Carpenter, J. (1986). And so they lived happily ever after: Intimacy and the idealization of marriage. A comment on Birtchnell. *Journal of Family Therapy, 8,* 173–177.

Carpenter, J. D. C., & Freese, J. J. (1979). Three aspects of self-disclosure as they relate to quality of adjustment. *Journal of Personality Assessment, 43,* 78–85.

Carr, S. J., Dabbs, J. M., & Carr, T. S. (1975). Mother–infant attachment: The importance of the mother's visual field. *Child Development, 46,* 331–338.

Carson, R. C., & Butcher, J. N. (1992). *Abnormal Psychology and Modern Life* (9th ed.). New York: HarperCollins.

Cassidy, J. (1988). Child–mother attachment and the self in six-year-olds. *Child Development, 59,* 121–134.

Cassidy, J., & Asher, S. R. (1992). Loneliness and peer relations in young children. *Child Development, 63,* 350–365.

Catalbiano, M. L., & Smithson, M. (1983). Variables affecting the perception of self-disclosure appropriateness. *Journal of Social Psychology, 120,* 119–128.

Chaikin, A. L., Derlega, V. J., Bayma, B., & Shaw, J. (1975). Neuroticism and disclosure reciprocity. *Journal of Consulting and Clinical Psychology, 43,* 13–19.

Chamberlaine, C., Barnes, S., Waring, E. M., Wood, G., & Fry, R. J. (1989). The role of marital intimacy in psychiatric help-seeking. *Canadian Journal of Psychiatry, 34,* 3–7.

Chelune, G. J. (1976). The self-disclosure situations survey: A new approach to measuring self-disclosure. *JSAS Catalog of Selected Documents in Psychology,* 6, 111.

Chelune, G. J., & Figueroa, J. L. (1981). Self-disclosure, neuroticism, and effective interpersonal communication. *Western Journal of Speech Communication, 45,* 27–37.

Chelune, G. J., Robison, J. T., & Krommor, M. J. (1984). A cognitive interactional model of intimate relationships. In V. J. Derlega (Ed.), *Communication, Intimacy, and Close Relationships* (pp. 11–40). Orlando, FL: Academic Press.

Chelune, G. J., Rosenfeld, L. B., & Waring, E. M. (1985). Spouse disclosure patterns in distressed and nondistressed couples. *American Journal of Family Therapy, 13,* 24–32.

Chelune, G. J., Skiffington, S., & Williams, C. (1981). Multidimensionsal analysis of observers' perceptions of self-disclosing behavior. *Journal of Personality and Social Psychology, 41,* 599–606.

Chelune, G. J., Sultan, F. E., Vosk, B. N., & Ogden, K. (1984). Self-disclosure and its relationship to marital intimacy. *Journal of Clinical Psychology, 40,* 216–219.

Chodorow, N. (1979). Feminism and difference: Gender, relation, and difference in psychoanalytic perspective. *Socialist Review, 46,* 42–64. (Reprinted in Walsh, M. R. (Ed.). (1987). *The Psychology of Women.* New Haven, CT: Yale University Press).

Chojnacki, J. T., & Walsh, W. B. (1990). Reliability and concurrent validity of the Sternberg Triangular Love Scale (1990). *Psychological Reports, 67,* 219–224.

Christensen, A. (1987). Assessment of behavior. In K. D. O'Leary (Ed.), *Assessment of Marital Discord* (pp. 13–57). Hillsdale, NJ: Erlbaum.

Christensen, A. (1988). Dysfunctional interaction patterns in couples. In P. Noller & M. A. Fitzpatrick (Eds.), *Perspectives on Marital Interaction* (pp. 31–52). Clevedon, UK: Multilingual Matters.

Christensen, A., & Heavy, C. L. (1990). Gender and social structure in the demand/withdraw pattern of marital conflict. *Journal of Personality and Social Psychology, 59,* 73–81.

Christensen, A., & Shenk, J. L. (1991). Communication, conflict, and psychological distance in nondistressed, clinic, and divorcing couples. *Journal of Consulting and Clinical Psychology, 59,* 458–463.

Christensen, A., & Sullaway, M. (1984). *Relationship Issues Questionnaire*. Unpublished questionnaire.

Christopher, F. S., & Cate, R. M. (1984). Factors involved in premarital sexual decision-making. *Journal of Sex Research, 20*, 363–376.

Christopher, F. S., & Cate, R. M. (1988). Premarital sexual involvement: A developmental investigation of relational correlates. *Adolescence, 23*, 793–803.

Christopher, F. S., & Roosa, M. W. (1991). Factors affecting sexual decisions in the premarital relationships of adolescents and young adults. In K. McKinney & S. Sprecher (Eds.), *Sexuality in Close Relationships* (pp. 111–133). Hillsdale, NJ: Erlbaum.

Cicirelli, V. G. (1983). Adult children and their elderly parents. In T. H. Brubaker (Ed.), *Family Relationships in Later Life*. Beverly Hills, CA: Sage.

Clark, M. S., & Reis, H. T. (1988). Interpersonal processes in close relationships. *Annual Review of Psychology, 39*, 609–672.

Clarke-Stewart, K. A. (1989). Infant day care: Maligned or malignant? *American Psychologist, 44*, 266–273.

Clinebell, H. J., & Clinebell, C. H. (1970). *The Intimate Marriage*. New York: Harper & Row.

Coffman, S., Levitt, M. J., Deets, C., & Quigley, K. L. (1991). Close relationships in mothers of distressed and normal newborns. *Journal of Family Psychology, 5*, 93–107.

Cohen, S., & Hoberman, H. M. (1983). Positive events and social supports as buffers of life change stress. *Journal of Applied Social Psychology, 13*, 99–125.

Cohen, T. F. (1992). Men's families, men's friends: A structural analysis of constraints on men's social ties. In P. Nardi (Ed.), *Men's Friendships* (pp. 115–131). Newbury Park, CA: Sage.

Cohn, D. A. (1990). Child–mother attachment in six-year-olds and social competence at school. *Child Development, 61*, 152–162.

Cohn, D. A., Patterson, C. J., & Christopoulos, C. (1991). The family and children's peer relations. *Journal of Social and Personal Relationships, 8*, 315–346.

Cole, C. L., & Goettsch, S. L. (1981). Self-disclosure and relationship quality: A study among nonmarital cohabiting couples. *Alternative Lifestyles, 4*, 428–466.

Cole, R. E., Baldwin, A. L., Baldwin, C. P., & Fisher, L. (1982). Family interaction in free play and children's social competence. *Monographs of the Society for Research in Child Development, 47*, 60–71.

Collins, N. L., Dunkel-Schetter, C., Lobel, M., & Scrimshaw, C. M. (1993). Social support in pregnancy: Psychosocial correlates of birth outcomes and postpartum depression. *Journal of Personality and Social Psychology, 65*, 1243–1258.

Collins, N. L., & Read, S. J. (1990). Adult attachment, working models, and relationship quality in dating couples. *Journal of Personality and Social Psychology, 58*, 644–663.

Condie, S. J. (1989). Older married couples. In S. J. Bahr & E. T. Peterson (Eds.), *Aging and the Family* (pp. 143–158). Lexington, MA: Heath.

Connidis, I. A., & Davies, L. (1990). Confidants and companions in later life: The place of family and friends. *Journal of Gerontology: Social Sciences, 45,* S141–S149.

Constantinople, A. (1969). An Eriksonian measure of personality development in college students. *Developmental Psychology, 1,* 357–371.

Cook, W. L. (1994). A structural equation model of dyadic relationships within the family system. *Journal of Consulting and Clinical Psychology, 62,* 500–509.

Cooley, C. H. (1902). *Human Nature and the Social Order..* New York: Scribner's.

Cooper, C. H., Baker, H., Polichar, D., & Welsh, M. (1993). Values and communication of Chinese, Filipino, European, Mexican, and Vietnamese-American adolescents with their families and friends. *New Directions for Child Development, 62,* 73–89.

Cooper, C. R., & Ayers-Lopez, S. (1985). Family and peer systems in early adolescence: New models of the role of relationships in development. *Journal of Early Adolescence, 5,* 9–21.

Cooper, C. R., & Cooper, R. G. (1992). Links between adolescents' relationships with their parents and peers: Models, evidence, and mechanisms. In R. D. Parke & G. W. Ladd (Eds.), *Family–Peer Relationships: Modes of Linkage* (pp. 135–159). Hillsdale, NJ: Erlbaum.

Cooper, C.R., & Grotevant, H. D. (1987). Gender issues in the interface of family experience and adolescents' friendship and dating identity. *Journal of Youth and Adolescence, 16,* 247–264.

Cooper, C. R., Grotevant, H. D., & Condon, S. M. (1982). Methodological challenges of selectivity in family interaction: Assessing temporal patterns of individuation. *Journal of Marriage and the Family,* 749–754.

Cooper, K., & Gutmann, D. (1987). Gender identity and ego mastery style in middle-aged, pre- and post-empty nest women. *The Gerontologist, 27,* 347–352.

Cornwall, M. (1989). Faith development of men and women over the life span. In S. J. Bahr & E. T. Peterson (Eds.), *Aging and the Family* (pp. 115–142). Lexington, MA: Heath.

Cotterell, N., Eisenberger, R., & Speicher, H. (1992). Inhibiting effects of reciprocation wariness of interpersonal relationships. *Journal of Personality and Social Psychology, 62,* 658–668.

Cox, M. J., Owen, M. T., Henderson, V. K., & Margand, N. A. (1992). Prediction of infant–father and infant–mother attachment. *Developmental Psychology, 28,* 474–483.

Coyne, J. C. (1976). Depression and the response of others. *Journal of Abnormal Psychology, 85,* 186–193.

Coyne, J. C. (1991). Social factors and psychopathology: Stress, social support, and coping processes. *Annual Review of Psychology, 42,* 401–425.

Coyne, J. C., & Smith, D. A. F. (1991). Couples coping with myocardial infarction: A contextual perspective on wives' distress. *Journal of Personality and Social Psychology, 61,* 404–412.

Coyne, J. C., & Smith, D. A. F. (1994). Couples coping with a myocardial infarction: Contextual perspective on patient self-efficacy. *Journal of Family Psychology, 8,* 43–54.

Cozby, P. C. (1973). Self-disclosure: A literature review. *Psychological Bulletin, 79,* 73–91.

Craig, J. A., Koestner, R., & Zuroff, D. C. (1994). Implicit and self-attributed intimacy motivation. *Journal of Social and Personal Relationships, 11,* 491–507.

Cramer, D. (1990). Disclosure of personal problems, self-esteem, and the facilitativeness of friends and lovers. *British Journal of Guidance and Counseling, 18,* 186–196.

Critelli, J. W., Myers, E. J., & Loos, V. (1986). The components of love: Romantic attraction and sex-role orientation. *Journal of Personality, 54,* 354–370.

Crittenden, P. M. (1990). Internal representation models of attachment relationships. *Infant Mental Health Journal, 11,* 259–277.

Crockett, L. J., & Peterson, A. C. (1987). Pubertal status and psychosocial development: Findings from the early adolescent study. In R. M. Lerner & T. T. Foch (Eds.), *Biological–Psychosocial Interactions in Early Adolescence* (pp. 173–188). Hillsdale, NJ: Erlbaum.

Cross, S. E., & Markus, H. R. (1993). Gender in thought, belief, and action: A social-cognitive approach. In A. E. Beall & R. J. Sternberg (Eds.), *The Psychology of Gender* (pp. 55–98). New York: Guilford Press.

Crowther, J. H. (1985). The relationship between depression and marital maladjustment: A descriptive study. *Journal of Nervous and Mental Disease, 173,* 227–231.

Cuber, J., & Haroff, P. (1965). *The Significant Americans: A study of sexual behavior among the affluent.* New York: Appleton-Century-Crofts.

Cummings, E. M., & Davies, P. T. (1994). *Children and Marital Conflict: The Impact of Family Dispute and Resolution.* New York: Guilford Press.

Cunningham, J. A., Strassberg, D. S., & Haan, B. (1986). Effects of intimacy and sex-role congruency of self-disclosure. *Journal of Social and Clinical Psychology, 4,* 393–401.

Cunningham, J. D., & Antill, J. K. (1981). Love in developing romantic relationships. In S. Duck & R. Gilmour (Eds.), *Personal Relationships, Vol. 2. Developing Personal Relationships* (pp. 27–51). London: Academic Press.

Cunningham, M. R. (1988). Does happiness mean friendliness? Induced mood and heterosexual self-disclosure. *Personality and Social Psychology Bulletin, 14,* 283–297.

Cushman, P. (1990). Why the self is empty: Toward a historically situated psychology. *American Psychologist, 45,* 599–611.

Cutrona, C. E. (1982). Transition to college: Loneliness and the process of social adjustment. In L. A. Peplau & D. Perlman (Eds.), *Loneliness: A Sourcebook of Current Theory, Research, and Therapy* (pp. 291–309). New York: Wiley.

Cutrona, C. E., Cole, V., Colangelo, N., Assouline, S. G., & Russell, D. W.

(1994). Perceived parental social support and academic achievement: An attachment theory perspective. *Journal of Personality and Social Psychology, 66,* 369–378.

Dahms, A. M. (1972). *Emotional Intimacy.* Boulder, CO: Pruett.

Damon, W., & Hart, D. (1982). The development of self-understanding from infancy through adolescence. *Child Development, 53,* 841–864.

Davidson, L. R., & Duberman, L. (1982). Friendship: Communication and interactional patterns in same-sex dyads. *Sex Roles, 8,* 809–822.

Davis, J. D. (1978). When boy meets girl: Sex-roles and the negotiation of intimacy in an acquaintance exercise. *Journal of Personality and Social Psychology, 7,* 684–692.

Davis, K. E., & Latty-Mann, H. (1987). Love styles and relationship quality: A contribution to validation. *Journal of Social and Personal Relationships, 4,* 409–428.

Davis, K. E., & Todd, M. J. (1985). Assessing friendship: Prototypes, paradigm cases and relationship description. In S. Duck & D. Perlman (Eds.), *Understanding Personal Relationships: An Interdisciplinary Approach* (pp. 17–38). London: Sage.

Davis, M. H., & Franzoi, S. L. (1987). Private self-consciousness and self-disclosure. In V. J. Derlega & J. H. Berg (Eds.), *Self-disclosure: Theory, Research and Therapy* (pp. 59–79). New York: Plenum.

Davis, M. H., & Kraus, L. A. (1991). Dispositional empathy and social relationships. In W. H. Jones & D. Perlman (Eds.), *Advances in Personal Relationships* (Vol.3, pp.75–115). London: Kingsley.

Davis, M. H., & Oathout, H. A. (1992). The effect of dispositional empathy on romantic relationship behaviors: Heterosocial anxiety as a moderating influence. *Personality and Social Psychology Bulletin, 18,* 76–83.

Davis, M. S. (1973). *Intimate Relations.* London: Free Press.

Dean, A., Kolody, B., Wood, P., & Ensel, W. M. (1989). The effects of types of social support from adult children on depression in elderly persons. *Journal of Community Psychology, 17,* 349–355.

Deiner, E. (1984). Subjective well-being. *Psychological Bulletin, 95,* 542–575.

Derlega, V. J., & Chaikin, A. L. (1975). *Sharing Intimacy.* Englewood Cliffs, NJ: Prentice-Hall.

Derlega, V. J., & Chaikin, A. L. (1977). Privacy and self-disclosure in social relationships. *Journal of Social Issues, 33,* 102–115.

Derlega, V. J., & Grzelak, J. (1979). Appropriateness of self-disclosure. In G. J. Chelune (Ed.), *Self-Disclosure: Origins, Patterns, and Implications of Openness in Interpersonal Relationships* (pp. 151–176) San Francisco: Jossey-Bass.

Derlega, V. J., Metts, S., Petronio, S., & Margulis, S. T. (1993). *Self-Disclosure.* Newbury Park, CA: Sage.

Derlega, V. J., Wilson, M., & Chaikin, A. L. (1976). Friendship and disclosure reciprocity. *Journal of Personality and Social Psychology, 34,* 578–582.

Derlega, V. J., Winstead, B. A., Wong, P. T. P., & Hunter, S. (1985). Gender effects in an initial encounter: A case where men exceed women in disclosure. *Journal of Social and Personal Relationships, 2,* 25–44.

DeRosier, M. E., & Kupersmidt, J. B. (1991). Costa Rican children's perceptions of their social networks. *Developmental Psychology, 27*, 656–662.

Descutner, C. J., & Thelen, M. H. (1991). Development and validation of a fear-of-intimacy scale. *Psychological Assessment, 3*, 218–225.

Deutsch, M. (1973). *The Resolution of Conflict: Constructive and Destructive Processes.* New Haven, CT: Yale University Press.

Deutscher, I. (1968). The quality of postparental life. In B. Neugarten (Ed.), *Middle Age and Aging.* Chicago: University of Chicago Press.

Diaz, R. M., & Berndt, T. J. (1982). Children's knowledge of a best friend: Fact or fancy? *Developmental Psychology, 18*, 787–794.

Dickens, W. J., & Perlman, D. (1981). Friendship over the life-cyle. In S. Duck & R. Gilmour (Eds.), *Personal Relationships: Vol. 2. Developing Personal Relationships* (pp. 91–122). London: Academic Press.

Dimitrovsky, L., Perez-Hirshberg, M., & Itskowitz, R. (1987). Depression during and following pregnancy: Quality of family relationships. *Journal of Psychology, 121*, 213–218.

Dimond, M., Lund, D. A., & Caserta, M. S. (1987). The role of social support in the first two years of bereavement in an elderly sample. *Gerontologist, 27*, 599–604.

Dindia, K. (1994). The intrapersonal–interpersonal dialectical process of self-disclosure. In S. Duck (Ed.), *Dynamics of Relationships* (pp. 27–57). Thousand Oaks, CA: Sage.

Dindia, K., & Allan, M. (1992). Sex differences in self-disclosure: A meta analysis. *Psychological Bulletin, 112*, 106–124.

Dindia, K., & Baxter, L. (1987). Strategies for maintaining and repairing marital relationships. *Journal of Social and Personal Relationships, 4*, 143–158.

Dindia, K., & Fitzpatrick, M. A. (1985). Marital communication: Three approaches compared. In S. Duck & D. Perlman (Eds.), *Understanding Personal Relationships: An Interdisciplinary Approach* (pp. 137–157). London: Sage.

Dingler-Duhon, M., & Brown, B. B. (1987). Self-disclosure as an influence strategy: Effects of Machiavellianism, androgyny and sex. *Sex Roles, 16*, 109–123.

Dion, K. L., & Dion, K. K. (1988). Romantic love: Individual and cultural perspectives. In R. J. Sternberg & M. L. Barnes (Eds.), *The Psychology of Love* (pp. 264–289). New Haven, CT: Yale University Press.

Dishion, T. J. (1990). The family ecology of boys' peer relations in middle childhood. *Child Development, 61*, 874–892.

Doi, S. C., & Thelen, M. H. (1992, November). *A fear-of-intimacy scale: Replication and extension.* Paper presented at the Annual Meeting, Association for Advancement of Behavior Therapy, Boston.

Dornbusch, S. M., Carlsmith, J. M., Duncan, P. D., Gross, R. T., Martin, J. A., Ritter, P. L., & Siegel-Gorelick, B. (1984). Sexual maturation, social class, and the desire to be thin among adolescent females. *Developmental and Behavioral Pediatrics, 5*, 308–314.

Dosser, D. A., Balswick, J. O., & Halverson, C. F. (1983). Situational context of emotional expressiveness. *Journal of Counseling Psychology, 30*, 375–387.

Douglas, K., & Arenberg, D. (1978). Age changes, cohort differences, and cultural change on the Guilford-Zimmerman Temperament Survey. *Journal of Gerontology, 33*, 737–747.

Douvan, E., & Adelson, J. (1966). *The Adolescent Experience*. New York: Wiley.

Downey, G., & Coyne, J. C. (1990). Children of depressed parents: An integrative review. *Psychological Bulletin, 108*, 50–76.

Doyle, J. A. (1989). *The Male Experience* (2nd ed.). Dubuque, IA: Brown.

Dressel, P. L., & Avant, W. R. (1983). Range of alternatives. In R. B. Weg (Ed.), *Sexuality in the Later Years: Roles and Behavior* (pp. 185–207). New York: Academic Press.

Drigotas, S., & Rusbult, C. (1992). Should I stay or should I go? *Journal of Personality and Social Psychology, 62*, 62–87.

Duck, S. W. (1986). *Human Relationships*. London: Sage.

Duck, S. W. (1990). Preface. In S. W. Duck (Ed.), *Personal Relationships and Social Support* (pp. x–xiv). London: Sage.

Duck, S. W. (1993a). Preface. In S. W. Duck (Ed.), *Social Context and Relationships* (pp. ix—xiv). Newbury Park, CA: Sage.

Duck, S. W. (Ed.). (1993b). *Learning About Relationships*. Newbury Park, CA: Sage.

Duck, S. W. (1994a). *Meaningful Relationships: Talking, Sense, and Relating*. Thousand Oaks, CA: Sage.

Duck, S. W. (Ed.). (1994b). *Dynamics of Relationships*. Thousand Oaks, CA: Sage.

Duck, S. W., & Miell, D. E. (1986). Charting the development of personal relationships. In R. Gilmour & S. W. Duck (Eds.), *The Emerging Field of Personal Relationships* (pp. 133–143). Hillsdale, NJ: Erlbaum.

Duck, S., Rutt, D. J., Hurst, M. H., & Strejc, H. (1991). Some evident truths about conversation in everyday relationships: All communications are not created equal. *Human Communication Research, 18*, 228–267.

Duck, S. W., & Sants, H. (1983). On the origin of the specious: Are personal relationships really interpersonal states? *Journal of Social and Clinical Psychology, 1*, 27–41.

Duck, S. W., & Wright, P. H. (1993). Re-examining sex differences in same-sex friendships: A closer look at two kinds of data. *Sex Roles, 28*, 709–727.

Duckro, R., Duckro, P., & Beal, D. (1976). Relationship of self-disclosure and mental health in black females. *Journal of Consulting and Clinical Psychology, 44*, 940–944.

Dunn, J. (1993). *Young Children's Close Relationships*. Newbury Park, CA: Sage.

Dunn, J., Bretherton, I., & Munn, P. (1987). Conversations about feeling states between mothers and their young children. *Developmental Psychology, 23*, 132–139.

Dyk, P. H., & Adams, G. R. (1990). Identity and intimacy: An initial investigation of three theoretical models using cross-lag panel correlations. *Journal of Youth and Adolescence, 19*, 91–110.

Eagly, A. H., Makhijani, M. G., & Klonsky, B. G. (1990). Gender and the evaluation of leaders: A meta-analysis. *Psychological Bulletin, 111*, 3–22.

Eagly, A. H., & Wood, W. (1991). Explaining sex differences in social behavior: A meta-analytic perspective. *Personality and Social Psychology Bulletin, 17,* 306–315.

Egan, G. (1975). *The Skilled Helper.* Monterey, CA: Brooks/Cole.

Egeland, B., & Farber, E. A. (1984). Infant–mother attachment: Factors related to its development and changes over time. *Child Development, 55,* 753–771.

Egeland, B., & Sroufe, A. (1981). Developmental sequelae of maltreatment in infancy. *New Directions for Child Development, 11,* 77–92.

Eidelson, R. J., & Epstein, N. (1982). Cognition and relationship maladjustment: Development of a measure of dysfunctional relationship beliefs. *Journal of Consulting and Clinical Psychology, 50,* 715–720.

Eisenberg, A. R. (1992). Conflicts between mothers and their young children. *Merrill-Palmer Quarterly, 38,* 21–43.

Eisenberg, N., Fabes, R. A., Murphy, B., Karbon, M., Maszk, P., Smith, M., O'Boyle, C., & Suh, K. (1994). The relations of emotionality and regulation to dispositional and situational empathy-related responding. *Journal of Personality and Social Psychology, 66,* 776–797.

Eisenberg, N., & Strayer, J. (1987). *Empathy and Its Development.* New York: Cambridge University Press.

Elicker, J., Englund, M., & Sroufe, L. A. (1992). Predicting peer competence and peer relationships in childhood from early parent–child relationships. In R. D. Parke & G. W. Ladd (Eds.), *Family–Peer Relationships: Modes of Linkage* (pp. 77–106). Hillsdale, NJ: Erlbaum.

Ellsworth, P., & Ross, L. (1975). Intimacy in response to direct gaze. *Journal of Experimental Social Psychology, 11,* 592–613.

Emmelkamp, P. M. G., Krol, B., Sanderman, S., & Ruphan, M. (1987). The assessment of relationship beliefs in a marital context. *Personality and Individual Differences, 8,* 775–780.

Engel, J. W., & Saracino, M. (1986). Love preferences and ideals: A comparison of homosexual, bisexual, and heterosexual groups. *Contemporary Family Therapy, 8,* 241–250.

England, P., & Farkas, G. (1986). *Households, Employment and Gender: A Social, Economic, and Demographic View.* New York: Aldine de Gruyter.

Epstein, N. (1986). Cognitive marital therapy: Multi-level assessment and intervention. *Journal of Rational-Emotive Therapy, 4,* 68–81.

Epstein, N., Pretzer, J. L., & Fleming, B. (1987). The role of cognitive appraisal in self-reports of marital communication. *Behavior Therapy, 18,* 51–69.

Erickson, M. F., Sroufe, L. A., & Egeland, B. (1985). The relationship between quality of attachment and behavior problems in preschool in a high-risk sample. In I. Bretherton & E. Waters (Eds.), Growing points of attachment theory and research. *Monographs of the Society for Research in Child Development, 50,* 147–256.

Erikson, E. H. (1959). Identity and the lifecycle. *Psychological Issues, 1,* 1–171.

Erikson, E. H. (1963). *Childhood and Society.* New York: Norton.

Erikson, E. H. (1968). *Identity: Youth and Crisis.* New York: Norton.

Ernster, V. L. (1975). American menstrual expressions. *Sex Roles, 1,* 3–13.

Esterling, B. A., Antoni, M. H., Fletcher, M. A., Margulies, S., & Schneiderman, N. (1994). Emotional disclosure through writing or speaking modulates latent Epstein-Barr virus antibody titers. *Journal of Consulting and Clinical Psychology, 62,* 130–140.

Etaugh, C. (1980). Effects of nonmaternal care on children. *American Psychologist, 35,* 309–319.

Fagot, B. I. (1978). The influence of sex of child on parental reactions to toddler children. *Child Development, 49,* 459–465.

Fagot, B. I. (1984a). The consequence of problem behavior in toddler children. *Journal of Abnormal Child Psychology, 12,* 385–396.

Fagot, B. I. (1984b). Teacher and peer reactions to boys' and girls' play styles. *Sex Roles, 11,* 691–702.

Fairbairn, W. R. D. (1954). *An Object Relations Theory of the Personality.* New York: Basic Books.

Falk, D. R., & Wagner, P. N. (1985). Intimacy of self-disclosure and response processes as factors affecting the development of interpersonal relationships. *Journal of Social Psychology, 125,* 557–570.

Fehr, B. (1988). Prototype analysis of the concepts of love and commitment. *Journal of Personality and Social Psychology, 55,* 557–579.

Fehr, B. (1993). How do I love thee? Let me consult my prototype. In S. Duck (Ed.), *Individuals in Relationships* (pp. 87–120). Newbury Park, CA: Sage.

Fehr, B., & Russell, J. A. (1991). The concept of love viewed from a prototype perspective. *Journal of Personality and Social Psychology, 60,* 425–438.

Feldman, S. S. (1987). Predicting strain in mothers and fathers of 6-month old infants: A short-term longitudinal study. In P. W. Berman & F. A. Pederson (Eds.), *Men's Transitions to Parenthood* (pp. 13–35). Hillsdale, NJ: Erlbaum.

Festinger, L., Schachter, S., & Back, K. (1950). *Social Pressures in Informal Groups.* New York: Harper.

Fields, N. S. (1983). Satisfaction in long-term marriage. *Social Work, 28,* 37–41.

Fincham, F. D. (1989). Understanding close relationships: An attributional perspective. In S. Zelen (Ed.), *New Models: New Extensions of Attribution Theory.* New York: Springer-Verlag.

Fincham, F. D., & Bradbury, T. N. (1988). The impact of attributions in marriage: Empirical and conceptual foundations. *British Journal of Clinical Psychology, 27,* 77–90.

Fincham, F. D., Bradbury, T. N., & Scott, C. K. (1990). Cognition in marriage: Retrospect and prospect. In F. D. Fincham & T. N. Bradbury (Eds.), *The Psychology of Marriage: Basic Issues and Applications* (pp. 118–149). New York: Guilford Press.

Fischer, C. S. (1982). *To Dwell Among Friends: Personal Networks in Town and City.* Chicago: University of Chicago Press.

Fischer, J. L., & Narus, L. R. (1981). Sex roles and intimacy in same and other sex relationships. *Psychology of Women Quarterly, 5,* 385–401.

Fischer, J. L., & Sollie, D. L. (1993). The transition to marriage: Network supports and coping. In T. H. Brubaker (Ed.), *Family Relations: Challenges for the Future*, (pp. 61-78). Newbury Park, CA: Sage.

Fischer, J. L., Sollie, D. L., Sorell, G. T., & Green, S. K. (1989). Marital status and career stage influences on social networks of young adults. *Journal of Marriage and the Family*, *51*, 521–534.

Fischer, L. (1981). Transitions in the mother–daughter relationship. *Journal of Marriage and the Family*, *43*, 613–622.

Fisher, M., & Stricker, G. (Eds.). (1982). *Intimacy*. New York: Plenum.

Fiske, M., & Chiriboga, D. A. (1990). *Change and Continuity in Adult Life*. San Francisco: Jossey-Bass.

Fiske, S. T. (1993). Controlling other people: The impact of power on stereotyping. *American Psychologist*, *48*, 621–628.

Fiske, S. T., & Taylor, S. E. (1991). *Social Cognition*. New York: McGraw-Hill.

Fiske, V., Coyne, J. C., & Smith, D. A. (1991). Couples coping with myocardial infarction: An empirical reconsideration of the role of overprotectiveness. *Journal of Family Psychology*, *5*, 4–20.

Fitzpatrick, M. A. (1988). *Between Husbands and Wives*. Newbury Park, NJ: Sage.

Fletcher, G. J. O., Fincham, F. D., Cramer, L., & Heron, N. (1987). The role of attributions in the development of dating relationships. *Journal of Personality and Social Psychology*, *53*, 481–489.

Fowers, B. J., Tredinnick, M., Pomerantz, B., & McIntosh, S. (1992, August). *Marital quality and its social context*. Paper presented at the Annual Convention, American Psychological Association, Washington, DC.

Fox, M. F., & Hesse-Biber, S. (1984). *Women at Work*. New York: Mayfield.

Frank, S. J., Avery, C. B., & Laman, M. S. (1988). Young adults' perceptions of their relationships with their parents: Individual differences in connectedness, competence, and emotional autonomy. *Developmental Psychology*, *24*, 729–737.

Franken, R. E., Gibson, K. J., & Mohan, P. (1990). Sensation-seeking and disclosure to close and casual friends. *Personality and Individual Differences*, *11*, 829–832.

Franz, C. E., & White, K. M. (1985). Individuation and attachment in personality development: Extending Erikson's theory. In A. J. Steward & M. B. Lykes (Eds.), *Gender and Personality: Current Perspectives on Theory and Research* (pp. 136–168). Durham, NC: Duke University Press.

Franzoi, S. L., Davis, M. H., & Young, R. D. (1985). The effects of private self-consciousness and perspective taking on satisfaction in close relationships. *Journal of Personality and Social Psychology*, *48*, 1584–1594.

French, M. (1977). *The Women's Room*. New York: Summit.

Freud, S. (1933). *New Introductory Lectures on Psychoanalysis*. New York: Norton.

Friedman, D. E. (1991) *Linking Work–Family Issues to the Bottom Line*. New York: The Conference Board.

Fruzzetti, A. E., & Jacobson, N. S. (1990). Toward a behavioral conceptualization of adult intimacy: Implications for marital therapy. In E. A. Blechman (Ed.), *Emotions and the Family* (pp. 117–136). Hillsdale, NJ: Erlbaum.

Furman, W. (1985). Compatibility and incompatibility in children's peer and sibling relationships. In W. Ickes (Ed.), *Compatible and Incompatible Relationships* (pp. 61–79). New York: Springer Verlag.

Furman, W., & Buhrmester, D. (1985). Children's perceptions of the personal relationships in their social networks. *Developmental Psychology, 21,* 1016–1024.

Furman, W., & Buhrmester, D. (1992). Age and sex differences in perceptions of networks of personal relationships. *Child Development, 63,* 103–115.

Gaelick, L., Bodenhausen, G. V., & Wyer, R. S. (1985). Emotional communication in close relationships. *Journal of Personality and Social Psychology, 49,* 1246–1265.

Geis, F. L. (1993). Self-fulfilling prophecies: A social-psychological view of gender. In A. E. Beall & R. J. Sternberg (Eds.), *The Psychology of Gender* (pp. 9–54). New York: Guilford Press.

Geller, P. A., & Hobfoll, S. E. (1994). Gender differences in job stress, tedium and social support in the workplace. *Journal of Social and Personal Relationships, 11,* 555–572.

George, C., & Main, M. (1979). Social interactions of young abused children: Approach, avoidance, and aggression. *Child Development, 50,* 306–318.

Gifford, R. (1991). Mapping nonverbal behavior on the interpersonal circle. *Journal of Personality and Social Psychology, 61,* 279–288.

Gifford, R., & O'Conner, B. (1986). Nonverbal intimacy: Clarifying the role of seating distance and orientation. *Journal of Nonverbal Behavior, 10,* 207–214.

Gilbert, L. A. (1993). *Two Careers/One Family: The Promise of Gender Equality.* Newbury Park, CA: Sage.

Gilbert, S. J. (1976). Self-disclosure, intimacy and communication in families. *The Family Coordinator, 25,* 221–231.

Gilbert, S. J., & Horenstein, D. (1975). The communication of self-disclosure: Level vs. valence. *Human Communication Research, 1,* 316–322.

Gitter, A. G., & Black, H. (1976). Is self-disclosure self-revealing? *Journal of Counseling Psychology, 23,* 327–332.

Gladstein, G. A. (1983). Understanding empathy: Integrating counseling, developmental, and social psychology perspectives. *Journal of Counseling Psychology, 30,* 467–482.

Gold, D. T. (1989). Generational solidarity. *American Behavioral Scientist, 33,* 19–32.

Goldner, H. (1987). Instrumentalism, feminism, and the limits of family therapy. *Journal of Family Psychology, 1,* 109–116.

Gottlieb, A. (1993, August). Are men obsolete? *Mirabella,* pp. 56–58.

Gottlieb, B. H., & Pancer, S. M. (1988). Social networks and the transition to parenthood. In G. Y. Michaels & W. A. Goldberg (Eds.), *The Transition to Parenthood: Current Theory and Research* (pp. 235–269). New York: Cambridge University Press.

Gottman, J. M. (1979). *Marital Interaction: Empirical Investigations*. New York: Academic Press.

Gottman, J. M. (1983). How children become friends. *Monographs of the Society for Research in Child Development, 48*, 1–81.

Gottman, J. M. (1991). Predicting the longitudinal course of marriage. *Journal of Marital and Family Therapy, 17*, 3–7.

Gottman, J. M. (1993). The roles of conflict engagement, escalation and avoidance in marital interaction: A longitudinal view of five types of couples. *Journal of Consulting and Clinical Psychology, 61*, 6–15.

Gottman, J. M. (1994). *What Predicts Divorce?* Hillsdale, NJ: Erlbaum.

Gottman, J. M., & Krokoff, L. J. (1989). Marital interaction and satisfaction: A longitudinal view. *Journal of Consulting and Clinical Psychology, 57*, 47–52.

Gottman, J. M., & Levenson, R. W. (1986). Assessing the role of emotion in marriage. *Behavioral Assessment, 8*, 31–48.

Gottman, J. M., & Levenson, R. W. (1992). Marital processes predictive of later dissolution: Behavior, physiology and health. *Journal of Personality and Social Psychology, 63*, 221–233.

Gottman, J. M., & Mettetal, G. (1986). Speculations about social and affective development: Friendship and acquaintanceship through adolescence. In J.M. Gottman & J.G. Parker (Eds.), *Conversations of Friends: Speculations on Affective Development* (pp. 192–240). New York: Cambridge University Press.

Gottman, J., Notarius, C., Gonso, J., & Markman, H. (1976). *A Couple's Guide to Communication*. Champaign, IL: Research Press.

Gould, R. L. (1978). *Transformations: Growth and Change in Adult Life*. New York: Simon & Schuster.

Greenberg, E., & O'Neil, R. (1990). Parents' concerns about their child's development: Implications for fathers' and mothers' well-being and attitudes toward work. *Journal of Marriage and the Family, 52*, 621–635.

Greenberg, M., & Morris, N. (1974). Engrossment: The newborn's impact upon the father. *American Journal of Orthopsychiatry, 44*, 520–531.

Greenberg, M. A., & Stone, A. A. (1992). Emotional disclosure about traumas and its relation to health: Effects of previous disclosure and trauma severity. *Journal of Personality and Social Psychology, 63*, 75–84.

Greenberg, M. T., Siegel, J. M., & Leitch, C. J. (1983). The nature and importance of attachment relationships to parents and peers during adolescence. *Journal of Youth and Adolescence, 12*, 373–386.

Greene, B., & Herek, G. M. (Eds.). (1994). *Lesbian and Gay Psychology: Theory, Research, and Clinical Applications*. Thousand Oaks, CA: Sage.

Greenspan, S. I., & Lourie, R. (1981). Developmental and structuralist approaches to the classification of adaptive and personality organizations: Infancy and early childhood. *American Journal of Psychiatry, 138*, 725–735.

Griffin, E., & Sparks, G. G. (1990). Friends forever: A longitudinal exploraton of intimacy in same-sex friends and platonic pairs. *Journal of Social and Personal Relationships, 7*, 29–46.

Grigsby, J. P., & Weatherley, D. (1983). Gender and sex-role differences in intimacy of self-disclosure. *Psychological Reports, 53,* 891–897.

Grossmann, K. E., & Grossmann, K. (1991). Attachment quality as an organizer of emotional and behavioral responses in a longitudinal perspective. In C. M. Parkes, J. Stevenson-Hinde, & P. Marris (Eds.), *Attachment Across the Life Cycle* (pp. 93–114). London: Routledge.

Grossmann, K. E., Grossmann, K., & Schwan, A. (1986). Capturing the wider view of attachment: A reanalysis of Ainsworth's Strange Situation. In C.E. Izard & P.B. Read (Eds.), *Measuring Emotions in Infants and Children* (Vol. 2, pp. 124–171). New York: Cambridge University Press.

Grotevant, H. D., & Cooper, C. R. (1985). Patterns of interaction in family relationships and the development of identity exploration in adolescence. *Child Development, 56,* 415–428.

Grotevant, H. D., & Cooper, C. R. (1986). Individuation in family relationships: A perspective on individual differences in the development of identity and role-taking skill in adolescence. *Human Development, 29,* 82–100.

Grotevant, H. D., & Cooper, C. R. (1988). The role of family experience in career exploration: A life-span perspective. In P. B. Baltes, D. L. Featherman, & R. M. Lerner (Eds.), *Life Span Development and Behavior* (pp. 231–258). Hillsdale, NJ: Erlbaum.

Guerrero, L. K., & Andersen, P. A. (1991). The waxing and waning of relational intimacy: Touch as a function of relational stage, gender and touch avoidance. *Journal of Social and Personal Relationships, 8,* 147–165.

Guerrero, L. K., Eloy, S. V., & Wabnik, A. I. (1993). Linking maintenance strategies to relationship development and disengagement: A reconceptualization. *Journal of Social and Personal Relationships, 10,* 273–283.

Guisinger, S., & Blatt, S. J. (1994). Individuality and relatedness: Evolution of a fundamental dialectic. *American Psychologist, 49,* 104–111.

Guldner, G. T., & Swensen, C. H. (1995). Time spent together and relationship quality: Long-distance relationships as a test case. *Journal of Social and Personal Relationships, 12,* 313–320.

Gulley, M. R., Barbee, A. P., & Cunningham, M. R. (1992, August). *Effects of gender in the seeking and giving of social support.* Paper presented at the Annual Meeting, American Psychological Association, Washington, DC.

Guntrip, H. (1968). *Schizoid Phenomena, Object Relations, and the Self.* New York, NY: International Universities Press.

Gurtman, M. B. (1992). Trust, distrust, and interpersonal problems: A circumplex analysis. *Journal of Personality and Social Psychology, 62,* 989–1002.

Gutmann, D. L. (1980). Psychoanalysis and aging: A developmental view. In S.I. Greenspan & G.H. Pollack (Eds.), *The Cause of Life: Psychoanalytic Contributions toward Understanding Personality Development* (Vol. 3). Washington, DC: National Institute of Mental Health.

Hackel, L. A., & Ruble, D. N. (1992). Changes in the marital relationship after the first baby is born: Predicting the impact of expectancy disconfirmation. *Journal of Personality and Social Psychology, 62,* 944–957.

Haft, W. L., & Slade, A. (1989). Affect attunement and maternal attachment: A pilot study. *Infant Mental Health Journal, 10,* 157–172.

Hale, J. L., Lundy, J. C., & Mongeau, P. A. (1989). Perceived relational intimacy and relational message content. *Communication Research Reports, 6,* 94–99.

Handkins, R. E., & Munz, D. C. (1978). Essential hypertension and self-disclosure. *Journal of Clinical Psychology, 34,* 870–875.

Hansen, K. V. (1992). "Our eyes behold each other": Masculinity and intimate friendship in antebellum New England. In P. Nardi (Ed.), *Men's Friendships* (pp. 35–58). Newbury Park, CA: Sage.

Harman, J. I. (1986). Relations among components of the empathic process. *Journal of Counseling Psychology, 33,* 371–376.

Harriman, L. C. (1983). Personal and marital changes accompanying parenthood. *Family Relations, 32,* 387–394.

Harry, J. (1984). *Gay Couples.* New York: Praeger.

Harter, S. (1990). Self and identity development. In S. S. Feldman & G. R. Elliot (Eds.), *At the Threshold: The Developing Adolescent* (pp. 352–387). Cambridge, MA: Harvard University Press.

Harter, S., & Lee, L. (1989, April). *Manifestations of true and false selves in early adolescence.* Paper presented at the Biennial Meeting of the Society for Research on Child Development, Kansas City, MO.

Hartup, W. W. (1986). On relationships and development. In W. W. Hartup & Z. Rubin (Eds.), *Relationships and Development* (pp. 1–26). Erlbaum.

Hartup, W. W. (1989a). Social relationships and their developmental significance. *American Psychologist, 44,* 120–126.

Hartup, W. W. (1989b). Behavioral manifestations of children's friendships. In T. J. Berndt & G. W. Ladd (Eds.), *Peer Relations in Child Development.* New York: Wiley.

Hartup, W. W., & Moore, S. G. (1990). Early peer relations: Developmental significance and prognostic implications. *Early Childhood Research Quarterly, 5,* 1–17.

Hatfield, E. (1988). Passionate and companionate love. In R. J. Sternberg & M. L. Barnes (Eds.), *The Psychology of Love* (pp. 191–217). New Haven, CT: Yale University Press.

Hatfield, E., & Rapson, R. L. (1987). Gender differences in love and intimacy: The fantasy vs. the reality. In W. Ricketts & H. L. Gochros (Eds.), *Intimate Relationships: Social Work Perspectives on Love* (pp. 15–26). New York: Haworth Press.

Hatfield, E., & Sprecher, S. (1986). Measuring passionate love in intimate relationships. *Journal of Adolescence, 9,* 383–410.

Hatfield, E., Sprecher, S., Pillemer, J. T., Greenberger, D., & Wexler, P. (1988). Gender differences in what is desired in the sexual relationship. *Journal of Psychology and Human Sexuality, 1,* 39–52.

Hauser, S. T. (1978). Ego development and interpersonal style. *Journal of Youth and Adolescence, 7,* 333–352.

Havighurst, R. J. (1972). *Developmental Tasks and Education* (3rd ed.). New York: McKay.

Hawkins, A. J., & Belsky, J. (1989). The role of father involvement in personality change in men across the transition to parenthood. *Family Relations, 38,* 378–384.

Hayes, S. C., Jacobson, N. S., Follette, V. M., & Dougher, M. J. (Eds.). (1994). *Acceptance and Change: Content and Context in Psychotherapy.* Reno, NV: Context Press.

Hays, R. B. (1985). A longitudinal study of friendship development. *Journal of Personality and Social Psychology, 48,* 909–924.

Hays, R. B. (1988). Friendship. In S. W. Duck (Ed.), *Handbook of Personal Relationships* (pp. 391–408). New York: Wiley.

Hays, R. B. (1989). The day-to-day functioning of close versus casual friendships. *Journal of Social and Personal Relationships, 6,* 21–37.

Hazan, C., & Shaver, P. (1987). Romantic love conceptualized as an attachment process. *Journal of Personality and Social Psychology, 52,* 511–524.

Hazan, C., & Shaver, P. R. (1990). Love and work: An attachment-theoretical perspective. *Journal of Personality and Social Psychology, 59,* 270–280.

Heavy, C. L., Layne, C., & Christensen, A. (1993). Gender and conflict structure in marital interaction: A replication and extension. *Journal of Consulting and Clinical Psychology, 61,* 16–27.

Helgeson, V. S., Shaver, P., & Dyer, M. (1987). Prototypes of intimacy and distance in same-sex and opposite-sex relationships. *Journal of Social and Personal Relationships, 4,* 195–233.

Henderson-King, D. H., & Veroff, J. (1994). Sexual satisfaction and marital well-being in the first years of marriage. *Journal of Social and Personal Relationships, 11,* 509–534.

Hendrick, C., & Hendrick, S. S. (1989). Research on love: Does it measure up? *Journal of Personality and Social Psychology, 56,* 784–794.

Hendrick, C., & Hendrick, S. (1986). A theory and method of love. *Journal of Personality and Social Psychology, 50,* 392–402.

Hendrick, S. S. (1981). Self-disclosure and marital satisfaction. *Journal of Personality and Social Psychology, 40,* 1150–1159.

Hendrick, S. S., & Hendrick, C. (1987). Love and sexual attitudes, self-disclosure and sensation-seeking. *Journal of Social and Personal Relationships, 4,* 281–297.

Hendrick, S. S., Hendrick, C., & Adler, N. L. (1988). Romantic relationships: Love, satisfaction and staying together. *Journal of Personality and Social Psychology, 54,* 980–988.

Hermans, H. J. M., Kempen, H. J. G., & van Loon, R. J. P. (1992). The dialogical self: Beyond individualism and rationalism. *American Psychologist, 47,* 23–33.

Hershberger, S. L., & D'Augelli, A. R. (1995). The impact of victimization on the mental health and suicidality of lesbian, gay, and bisexual youth. *Developmental Psychology, 31,* 65–74.

Hetherington, S. E., & Soeken, K. L. (1990). Measuring changes in intimacy and sexuality: A self-administered scale. *Journal of Sex Education and Therapy*, *16*, 155–163.

Hicks, M. W., & Platt, M. (1970). Marital happiness and stability: A review of the research in the sixties. *Journal of Marriage and the Family*, *32*, 533–574.

Highlen, P. S., & Gillis, S. F. (1978). Effects of situational factors, sex, and attitude on affective self-disclosure and anxiety. *Journal of Counseling Psychology*, *25*, 270–276.

Hightower, E. (1990). Adolescent interpersonal and familial precursors of positive mental health at midlife. *Journal of Youth and Adolescence*, *19*, 257–275.

Hill, C. E., & Corbett, M. M. (1993). A perspective on the history of process and outcome research in counseling psychology. *Journal of Counseling Psychology*, *40*, 3–24.

Hill, C. T., & Stull, D. E. (1987). Gender and self-disclosure: Strategies for exploring the issues. In V. J. Derlega & J. H. Berg (Eds.), *Self-Disclosure: Theory, Research and Therapy* (pp. 81–100). New York: Plenum.

Hill, J. P., & Holmbeck, G. N. (1986). Attachment and autonomy during adolescence. *Annals of Child Development*, *3*, 145–189.

Hill, J. P., & Lynch, M. E. (1983). The intensification of gender-related role expectations during early adolescence. In J. Brooks-Gunn & A. C. Petersen (Eds.), *Girls at Puberty* (pp. 201–222). New York: Plenum Press.

Hinde, R. A. (1981). The bases of a science of interpersonal relationships. In S. Duck & R. Gilmour (Eds.), *Personal Relationships* (pp. 1–22). London: Academic Press.

Hite, S. (1987). *Women and Love: A Cultural Revolution in Progress*. New York: Knopf.

Hobfoll, S. E., & Leiberman, J. R. (1989). Effects of mastery and intimacy on anxiety following pregnancy: For whom is support supportive and from whom? *Anxiety Research*, *1*, 327–341.

Hobfoll, S. E., & Lerman, M. (1988). Personal relationships, personal attributes, and stress resistance: Mothers' reactions to their child's illness. *American Journal of Community Psychology*, *16*, 565–589.

Hobfoll, S. E., Nadler, A., & Leiberman, J. (1986). Satisfaction with social support during crisis: Intimacy and self-esteem as critical determinants. *Journal of Personaltity and Social Psychology*, *51*, 296–304.

Hodgson, J. W., & Fischer, J. L. (1979). Sex differences in identity and intimacy development in college youth. *Journal of Youth and Adolescence*, *8*, 37–50.

Hoehn-Hyde, D., Schlottmann, R. S., & Rush, A. J. (1982). Perception of social interactions in depressed psychiatric patients. *Journal of Consulting and Clinical Psychology*, *50*, 209–212.

Hoffman, L. W. (1979). Maternal employment: 1979. *American Psychologist*, *34*, 859–865.

Holmes, J. G. (1991). Trust and appraisal process in close relationships. In W. H. Jones & D. Perlman (Eds.), *Advances in Personal Relationships* (pp. 57–104). London: Kingsley.

Holmes, T. S., & Rahe, R. H. (1967). The Social Readjustment Scale. *Journal of Psychosomatic Research, 14*, 121–132.

Holt, M. L. (1977). *Human intimacy in young adults: An experimental developmental scale.* Unpublished doctoral dissertation, University of Georgia.

Hood, J. (1986). The provider role: Its meaning and measurement. *Journal of Marriage and the Family, 48*, 349–359.

Hopper, R., Knapp, M. L., & Scott, L. (1981). Couples' personal idioms: Exploring intimate talk. *Journal of Communication, 31*, 23–33.

Hops, H., Biglan, A., Sherman, L., Arthur, J., Friedman, L., & Osteen, V. (1987). Home observations of family interactions of depressed women. *Journal of Consulting and Clinical Psychology, 55*, 341–346.

Hops, H., Wills, T. A., Patterson, G. R., & Weiss, R. L. (1972). *The Marital Interaction Coding System (MICS).* Unpublished manuscript, University of Oregon.

Horney, K. (1950). *Neuroses and Human Growth.* New York: Norton.

Hornstein, G. A., & Truesdell, S. E. (1988). Development of intimate conversation in close relationships. *Journal of Social and Clinical Psychology, 7*, 49–64.

House, J. S., Landis, K. R., & Umberson, D. (1988). Social relationships and health. *Science, 241*, 540–545.

Howell, A., & Conway, M. (1990). Perceived intimacy of expressed emotion. *Journal of Social Psychology, 130*, 467–476.

Howes, C. (1988). Peer interaction of young children. *Monographs of the Society for Research in Child Development, 53*(1, Serial No. 217).

Huber, J. (1993). Gender role change in families: A macrosociological view. In T. H. Brubaker (Ed.), *Family Relations: Challenges for the Future* (pp. 41–58). Newbury Park, CA: Sage.

Hunter, F. T. (1985). Individual adolescents' perceptions of interactions with friends and parents. *Journal of Early Adolescence, 5*, 295–303.

Hunter, F. T., & Youniss, J. (1982). Changes in function of three relations during adolescence. *Developmental Psychology, 18*, 806–811.

Huston, T. L., & Chorost, A. F. (1994). Behavioral buffers on the effect of negativity on marital satisfaction: A longitudinal study. *Personal Relationships, 1*, 223–240.

Huston, T. L., McHale, S. M., & Crouter, A. C. (1986). When the honeymoon's over: Changes in the marriage relationship over the first year. In R. Gilmour & S. Duck (Eds.), *The Emerging Field of Personal Relationships* (pp. 53–90). New York: Academic Press.

Huston, T. L., Robins, E., Atkinson, J., & McHale, S. M. (1987). Surveying the landscape of marital behavior: A behavioral self-report approach to studying marriage. In S. Oskamp (Ed.), *Family Processes and Problems: Social Psychological Aspects* (pp. 43–72). Newbury Park, CA: Sage.

Huston, T. L., & Vagelisti, A. L. (1991). Socioemotional behavior and satisfaction in marital relationships: A longitudinal study. *Journal of Personality and Social Psychology, 61*, 721–733.

Ickes, W. (1982). A basic paradigm for the study of personality, roles, and social behavior. In W. Ickes & E. S. Knowles (Eds.), *Personality, Roles, and Social Behavior* (pp. 305–341). New York: Springer-Verlag.

Ickes, W., Stinson, L., Bissonnette, V., & Garcia, S. (1990). Naturalistic social cognition: Empathic accuracy in mixed-sex dyads. *Journal of Personality and Social Psychology, 51,* 66–82.

Israelstam, K. (1989). Intimacy and distance regulation: From homeostasis to structural coupling and coherence. *Australian and New Zealand Journal of Family Therapy, 10,* 7–11.

Ivey, A. E. (1971). *Microcounseling: Innovations in Interviewing Training.* Springfield, IL: Thomas.

Izard, C. E. (1990). Facial expressions and the regulation of emotions. *Journal of Personality and Social Psychology, 58,* 487–498.

Izard, C. E., Huebner, R. R., Risser, D., McGinnes, G., & Dougherty, L. (1980). The young infant's ability to reproduce discrete emotion expressions. *Developmental Psychology, 16,* 132–140.

Jack, D. C., & Dill, D. (1992). The silencing the self scale: Schemas of intimacy associated with depression in women. *Psychology of Women Quarterly, 16,* 97–106.

Jacobson, N. S. (1989). The politics of intimacy. *The Behavior Therapist, 12,* 29–32.

Jacobson, N. S., Dobson, K., Fruzzetti, A., Schmaling, K. B., & Salusky, S. (1991). Marital therapy as a treatment for depression. *Journal of Consulting and Clinical Psychology, 59,* 547–557.

Janus, S., & Janus, C. L. (1993). *The Janus Report on Sexual Behavior.* New York: Wiley.

Jaycox, L. H., & Repetti, R. L (1993). Conflict in families and the psychological adjustment of preadolescent children. *Journal of Family Psychology, 7,* 344–355.

Jerrome, D. (1992). *Good Company: An Anthropological Study of Old People in Groups.* Edinburgh: Edinburgh University Press.

Johnson, M. P., Huston, T. L., Gaines, S. O., & Levinger, G. (1992). Patterns of married life among young couples. *Journal of Social and Personal Relationships, 9,* 343–364.

Johnson-George, C., & Swap, W. C. (1982). Measurement of specific interpersonal trust: Construction and validation of a scale to assess trust in a specific other. *Journal of Personality and Social Psychology, 43,* 1306–1317.

Jones, D. C. (1992). Parental divorce, family conflict and friendship networks. *Journal of Social and Personal Relationships, 9,* 219–235.

Jones, D. C., Bloys, N., & Wood, M. (1990). Sex roles and friendship patterns. *Sex Roles, 23,* 159–168.

Jones, G. P., & Dembo, M. H. (1989). Age and sex-role differences in intimate friendships during childhood and adolescence. *Merrill-Palmer Quarterly, 35,* 445–462.

Jones, S. E., & Yarbrough, E. (1985). A naturalistic study of the meanings of touch. *Communication Monographs, 52,* 19–56.

Jordan, J. V., Kaplan, A. G., Miller, J. B., Stiver, I. P., & Surrey, J. L. (1991). *Women's Growth in Connection: Writings from the Stone Center.* New York: Guilford Press.

Jorgensen, S. R., King, S. L., & Torrey, B. A. (1980). Dyadic and social network influences on adolescent exposure to pregnancy risk. *Journal of Marriage and the Family, 42,* 141–155.

Josselson, R. (1987). *Finding Herself: Pathways to Identity Development in Women.* San Francisco: Jossey-Bass.

Jourard, S. M. (1959). Self-disclosure and other cathexis. *Journal of Abnormal and Social Psychology, 59,* 428–431.

Jourard, S. M. (1968). *Disclosing Man to Himself.* New York: Van Nostrand.

Jourard, S. M. (1971). *The Transparent Self.* New York: Van Nostrand.

Jourard, S. M., & Lasakow, P. (1958). Some factors in self-disclosure. *Journal of Abnormal and Social Psychology, 56,* 91–98.

Julien, D., Markman, H. J., Leveille, S., Chartrand, E., & Begin, J. (1994). Networks' support and interference with regard to marriage: Disclosures of marital problems to confidants. *Journal of Family Psychology, 8,* 16–31.

Kaplan, A. G., & Sedney, M. A. (1980). *Psychology and Sex-Roles: An Androgynous Perspective.* Boston: Little, Brown.

Kaplan, H. S. (1974). *The New Sex Therapy: Active Treatment of Sexual Dysfunctions.* New York: Brunner/Mazel.

Kaplan, H. S. (1990). Sex, intimacy, and the aging process. *Journal of the American Academy of Psychoanalysis, 18,* 185–205.

Kaplan, K. J., Firestone, I. J., Klein, K. W., & Sodikoff, C. (1983). Distancing in dyads: A comparison of four models. *Social Psychology Quarterly, 46,* 108–115.

Karpel, M. (1976). Individuation: From fusion to dialogue. *Family Process, 15,* 65–82.

Katz, P. A., & Ksansnak, K. R. (1994). Developmental aspects of gender role flexibility and traditionality in middle childhood and adolescence. *Developmental Psychology, 30,* 272–282.

Keating, N. C., & Cole, P. (1980). What do I do with him 24 hours a day? Changes in the housewife role after retirement. *The Gerontologist, 20,* 84–89.

Keeley, M. P., & Hart, A. J. (1994). Nonverbal behavior in dyadic interactions. In S. W. Duck (Ed.), *Dynamics of Relationships* (pp. 135–162). Thousand Oaks, CA: Sage.

Keitner, G. I., & Miller, I. W. (1990). Family functioning and major depression: An overview. *American Journal of Psychiatry, 147,* 1128–1137.

Kelley, D. L., & Burgoon, J. K. (1991). Understanding marital satisfaction and couple type as functions of relational expectations. *Human Communication Research, 18,* 40–69.

Kelley, H. H., Berscheid, E., Christensen, A., Harvey, J. H., Huston, T. L., Levinger, G., McClintock, E., Peplau, L. A., & Peterson, D. (1983). Analyzing close relationships. In H. H. Kelley, E. Berscheid, A. Christensen, J. H. Harvey, T. L. Huston, G. Levinger, E. McClintock, L. A. Peplau, & D. R. Peterson (Eds.), *Close Relationships: Development and Change*. New York: Freeman.

Kelvin, P. (1977). Predictability, power and vulnerability in interpersonal attraction. In S. Duck (Ed.), *Theory and Practice in Interpersonal Attraction* (pp. 355–378). New York: Academic Press.

Keniston, K. (1982). Youth: A "new" stage of life. In L. R. Allman & D. T. Jaffe (Eds.), *Readings in Adult Psychology: Contemporary Perspectives* (pp. 80–99). Cambridge, MA: Harper & Row.

Kent, J. H. K. (1975). Relation of personality, expectancy, and situational variables to self-disclosing behavior. *Journal of Consulting and Clinical Psychology, 43*, 120–121.

Kerckhoff, R. K. (1976). Marriage and middle age. *The Family Coordinator, 25*, 5–11.

Kerckhoff, R. K., & Bean, F. (1970). Social status and interpersonal patterns among married couples. *Social Forces, 49*, 264–271.

Kerns, D. A., & Barth, J. M. (1995). Attachment and play: Convergence across components of parent–child relationships and their relations to peer competence. *Journal of Social and Personal Relationships, 12*, 243–260.

Kerr, M. E., & Bowen, M. (1988). *Family Evaluation: An Approach Based on Bowen Theory*. New York: Norton.

Kestenbaum, R., Farber, E. A., & Sroufe, L. A. (1989). Individual differences in empathy among preschoolers: Relation to attachment history. In N. Eisenberg (Ed.), *Empathy and Related Emotional Responses* (pp. 51–64). San Francisco: Jossey-Bass.

Kiecolt-Glaser, J. K., Fisher, B. S., Ogrocki, P., Stout, J. C., Speicher, C. E., & Glaser, R. (1988). Marital discord and immunity in males. *Psychosomatic Medicine, 50*, 213–229.

King, C. E., & Christensen, A. (1983). The Relationship Events Scale: A Guttman scaling of progress in courtship. *Journal of Marriage and the Family, 45*, 671–678.

Kinsey, A. C., Pomeroy, W. B., & Martin, C. E. (1948). *Sexual Behavior in the Human Male*. Philadelphia: Saunders.

Kinsey, A. C., Pomeroy, W. B., Martin, C. E., & Gebhard, P. H. (1953). *Sexual Behavior in the Human Female*. Philadelphia: Saunders.

Kirkpatrick, L. A., & Davis, K. E. (1994). Attachment style, gender, and relationship stability: A longitudinal analysis. *Journal of Personality and Social Psychology, 66*, 502–512.

Klein, M. (1935). A contribution to the psychogenesis of manic–depressive states. *International Journal of Psycho-Analysis, 16*, 145–174. (Reprinted in Buckley, P. (Ed.). (1986). *Essential Papers on Object Relations* (pp. 40–70). New York: New York University Press.)

Kleinke, C. L. (1986). Gaze and eye contact: A research review. *Psychological Bulletin, 100,* 78–100.

Kleinke, C. L., Bustos, A. A., Meeker, F. B., & Standeski, R. A. (1973). Effects of self-attributed and other-attributed gaze on interpersonal evaluations between males and females. *Journal of Experimental Social Psychology, 9,* 154–163.

Kleinke, C. L., Meeker, F. B., & La Fong, C. (1974). Effects of gaze, touch and use of name on evaluation of "engaged" couples. *Journal of Research in Personality, 7,* 368–373.

Klos, D. S., & Loomis, D. F. (1978). A rating scale of intimate disclosure between late adolescents and their friends. *Psychological Reports, 42,* 815–820.

Knapp, C. W., & Harwood, B. T. (1977). Factors in the determination of same-sex friendship. *Journal of Genetic Psychology, 131,* 83–90.

Kobak, R. R., & Hazan, C. (1991). Attachment in marriage: Effects of security and accuracy of working models. *Journal of Personality and Social Psychology, 60,* 861–869.

Kohlberg, L. (1966). A cognitive-developmental analysis of children's sex-role concepts and attitudes. In E. Maccoby (Ed.), *The Development of Sex Differences* (pp. 82–173). Stanford, CA: Stanford University Press.

Kohut, H. (1980). *Advances in Self Psychology.* New York: International Universities Press.

Komarovsky, M. (1967). *Blue Collar Marriage.* New York: Vintage.

Kon, I. S., Losenkov, V. A., de Lissovoy, C., & de Lissovoy, V. (1978). Friendship in adolescence: Values & behavior. *Journal of Marriage and the Family, 40,* 143–155.

Kowalik, D. L., & Gotlib, I. H. (1987). Depression and marital interaction: Concordance between intent and perception of communication. *Journal of Abnormal Psychology, 96,* 127–134.

Kurash, C., & Schaul, J. (1980, September). *The transition into early adulthood: An empirical study.* Paper presented at the Annual Meeting, American Psychological Association, Montreal.

Kurdek, L. (1990). Spouse attributes and spousal interactions as dimensions of relationship quality in first-married and remarried newlywed men and women. *Journal of Family Issues, 11,* 91–100.

Kurdek, L. A. (1991a). Predictors of increases in marital distress in newlywed couples. *Developmental Psychology, 27,* 627–636.

Kurdek, L. A. (1991b). Correlates of relationship satisfaction in cohabiting gay and lesbian couples: Integration of contextual, investment, and problem-solving models. *Journal of Personality and Social Psychology, 61,* 910–922.

Kurdek, L. A. (1994). The nature and correlates of relationship quality in gay, lesbian, and heterosexual cohabiting couples: A test of the individual difference, interdependence, and discrepancy models. In B. Greene & G.M. Herek (Eds.), *Lesbian and Gay Psychology* (pp. 133–155). Thousand Oaks, CA: Sage.

Kurdek, L. A., & Schmitt, J. P. (1986a). Early development of relationship quality in heterosexual married, heterosexual cohabiting, gay and lesbian couples. *Developmental Psychology, 22*, 305–309.

Kurdek, L. A., & Schmitt, J. P. (1986b). Interaction of sex-role self-concept with relationship quality and relationship beliefs in married, heterosexual cohabiting, gay and lesbian couples. *Journal of Personality and Social Psychology, 51*, 365–370.

L'Abate, L., & L'Abate, B. L. (1979). The paradoxes of intimacy. *Family Therapy, 3*, 175–184.

L'Abate, L., & Sloan, S. (1984). A workshop format to facilitate intimacy in married couples. *Family Relations, 33*, 245–250.

Ladd, G. W., Profilet, S. M., & Hart, C. H. (1992). Parents' management of children's peer relations: Facilitating and supervising children's activities in the peer culture. In R. D. Parke & G. W. Ladd (Eds.), *Family–Peer Relationships: Modes of Linkage* (pp. 215–254). Hillsdale, NJ: Erlbaum.

LaFollette, H., & Graham, G. (1986). Honesty and intimacy. *Journal of Social and Personal Relationships, 3*, 3–18.

LaFreniere, P. J., & Sroufe, L. A. (1985). Profiles of peer competence in the preschool: Interrelations between measures, influence of social ecology, and relation to attachment history. *Developmental Psychology, 21*, 56–69.

Lamb, M. E., & Gilbride, K. E. (1985). Compatibility in parent–infant relationships: Origins and processes. In W. Ickes (Ed.), *Compatible and Incompatible Relationships* (pp. 33–60). New York: Springer-Verlag.

Lamb, M. E., & Nash, A. (1989). Infant–mother attachment, sociability, and peer competence. In T. J. Berndt & G. W. Ladd (Eds.), *Peer Relations in Child Development* (pp. 219–245). New York: Wiley.

LaRossa, R., & LaRossa, M. M. (1989). Baby care: Fathers vs. mothers. In B. J. Risman & P. Schwartz (Eds.), *Gender in Intimate Relationships* (pp. 138-154). Belmont, CA: Wadsworth.

Larson, D. G., & Chastain, R. L. (1990). Self-concealment: Conceptualization, measurement and health implications. *Journal of Social and Clinical Psychology, 9*, 439–455.

Larson, R. W. (1990). The solitary side of life: An examination of the time people spend alone from childhood to old age. *Developmental Review, 10*, 155–183.

Larson, R. W., Csikszentmihalyi, M., & Graef, R. (1982). Time alone in daily experience: Loneliness or renewal? In L.A. Peplau & D. Perlman (Eds.), *Loneliness: A Sourcebook of Current Theory, Research, and Therapy*. New York: Wiley-Interscience.

Larson, R. W., Richards, M. H., & Perry-Jenkins, M. (1994). Divergent worlds: The daily emotional experience of mothers and fathers in the domestic and public spheres. *Journal of Personality and Social Psychology, 67*, 1034–1046.

Lazowski, L. E., & Anderson, S. M. (1990). Self-disclosure and social perceptions: Impact of private, negative, and extreme communications. *Journal of Social Behavior and Personality, 5*, 131–154.

Leaper, C., Hauser, S. T., Kremen, A., Powers, S. I., Jacobson, A. M., Noam, G. G., Weiss-Perry, B., & Follansbee, D. (1989). Adolescent–parent interactions in relation to adolescents' gender and ego development pathway: A longitudinal study. *Journal of Early Adolescence, 9,* 335–361.

Leatham, G. B., & Duck, S. W. (1990). Conversations with friends and the dynamics of social support. In S. W. Duck (Ed.), *Personal Relationships and Social Support* (pp. 1–29). London: Sage.

Lee, J. A. (1973). *Colors of Love.* Toronto: New Press.

Lee, J. A. (1988). Love-styles. In R. J. Sternberg & M. L. Barnes (Eds.), *The Psychology of Love* (pp. 38-67). New Haven, CT: Yale University Press.

Leigh, B. C. (1989). Reasons for having and avoiding sex: Gender, sexual orientation, and relationship to sexual behavior. *Journal of Sex Research, 26,* 199–209.

Lemmer, C. (1987). Becoming a father: A review of nursing research on expectant fatherhood. *Maternal Child Nursing Journal, 16,* 261–275.

Lerner, H. G. (1989). *The Dance of Intimacy: A Woman's Guide to Courageous Acts of Change in Key Relationships.* New York: Harper & Row.

Lerner, H. G. (1993). *The Dance of Deception: Pretending and Truth-Telling in Women's Lives.* New York: HarperCollins.

Lerner, R. M. (1989). Individual development and the family system: A life-span perspective. In K. Kreppner & R. M. Lerner (Eds.), *Family Systems and Life-Span Development* (pp. 15–32). Hillsdale, NJ: Erlbaum.

Levenson, R. W., Carstensen, L. L., & Gottman, J. M. (1994). The influence of age and gender on affect, physiology, and their interrelations: A study of long-term marriages. *Journal of Personality and Social Psychology, 67,* 56–68.

Levensen, R. W., & Gottman, J. M. (1983). Physiological and affective predictors of change in relationship satisfaction. *Journal of Personality and Social Psychology, 49,* 85–94.

Levinger, G. (1965). Marital cohesiveness and dissolution: An integrative review. *Journal of Marriage and the Family, 27,* 19–28.

Levinger, G. (1977). Re-viewing the close relationships. In G. Levinger & H. L. Raush (Eds.), *Close Relationships: Perspectives on the Meaning of Intimacy* (pp. 137–162). Amherst, MA: University of Massachusetts Press.

Levinger, G. (1983). Development and change. In H. Kelly (Ed.), *Close Relationships: Development and Change.* New York: Freeman.

Levinger, G., & Huston, T. L. (1990). The social psychology of marriage. In F. D. Fincham & T. N. Bradbury (Eds.), *The Psychology of Marriage: Basic Issues and Applications* (pp. 19–58). New York: Guilford Press.

Levinger, G., & Levinger, A. C. (1986). The temporal course of close relationships: Some thoughts about the development of children's ties. In W. W. Hartup & Z. Rubin (Eds.), *Relationships and Development* (pp. 111–133). Hillsdale, NJ: Erlbaum.

Levinger, G., & Senn, D. J. (1967). Disclosure of feelings in marriage. *Merril-Palmer Quarterly, 13,* 237–249.

Levinson, D. J., Darrow, C. N., Klein, E. B., Levinson, M. H., & McKee, B. (1978). *The Seasons of a Man's Life.* New York: Ballantine.

Levi-Shiff, R., & Israelashvili, R. (1988). Antecedents of fathering: Some further exploration. *Developmental Psychology, 24,* 434–440.

Lewis, M., & Feiring, C. (1989). Early predictors of children's friendships. In T.J. Berndt & G.W. Ladd (Eds.), *Peer Relationships in Child Development* (pp. 246–273). New York: Wiley.

Lewis, R. A. (1978). Emotional intimacy among men. *Journal of Social Issues, 34,* 108–121.

Lewittes, H. J. (1989). Just being friendly means a lot: Women, friendship, and aging. *Women and Health, 14,* 139–159.

Liben, L. S., & Signorella, M. L. (1993). Gender-schematic processing in children: The role of initial interpretations of stimuli. *Developmental Psychology, 29,* 141–149.

Lieberman, A. F. (1977). Preschoolers' competence with a peer: Relations with attachment and peer experience. *Child Development, 48,* 1277–1287.

Lindahl, K. M., & Markman, H. J. (1990). Communication and negative affect regulation in the family. In E. A. Blechman (Ed.), *Emotions and the Family* (pp. 99–115). Hillsdale, NJ: Erlbaum.

Lipman, A. (1960). Marital roles of the retired aged. *Merrill-Palmer Quarterly, 6,* 192–195.

Lipman, A. (1961). Role conceptions and morale of couples in retirement. *Journal of Gerontology, 16,* 267–271.

Lipman, A. (1986). Homosexual relationships. *Generations, 11,* 51–54.

Loevinger, J. (1976). *Ego Development.* San Francisco: Jossey-Bass.

Long, E. C. J., & Andrews, D. W. (1990). Perspective taking as a predictor of marital adjustment. *Journal of Personality and Social Psychology, 59,* 126–131.

Lopata, H. Z. (1971). *Occupation: Housewife.* New York: Oxford University Press.

Lopata, H. Z. (1979). *Women as Widows: Support Systems.* New York: Elsevier.

Lopez, F. G., Campbell, V. L., & Watkins, C. E., Jr. (1988). Family structure, psychological separation, and college adjustment: A canonical analysis and cross-validation. *Journal of Counseling Psychology, 35,* 402–409.

Lopez, F. G., Campbell, V. L., & Watkins, C. E., Jr. (1989a). Constructions of current family functioning among depressed and nondepressed college students. *Journal of College Student Development, 30,* 221–228.

Lopez, F. G., Campbell, V. L., & Watkins, C. E., Jr. (1989b). Effects of marital conflict and family coalition patterns on college student adjustment. *Journal of College Student Development, 30,* 46–52.

Lott, B., & Maluso, D. (1993). The social learning of gender. In A. E. Beall & R. J. Sternberg (Eds.), *The Psychology of Gender* (pp. 99–123). New York: Guilford Press.

Lowenthal, M. F., & Haven, C. (1968). Interaction and adaptation: Intimacy as a critical variable. *American Sociological Review, 33,* 20–30.

Lowenthal, M. F., Thurnher, M., & Chiriboga, D. (1977). *Four Stages of Life.* San Francisco: Jossey-Bass.

Lutgendorf, S. K., Antoni, M. H., Kumar, M., & Scheiderman, N. (1994). Changes in cognitive coping strategies predict EBV-antibody titre change following a stressor disclosure induction. *Journal of Psychosomatic Research*, 38, 63–78.

Lytton, H., & Romney, D. M. (1991). Parents' differential socialization of boys and girls: A meta-analysis. *Psychological Bulletin, 109*, 267–296.

Maccoby, E. E. (1990a). Gender and relationships. *American Psychologist, 45*, 513–520.

Maccoby, E. E. (1990b). The role of gender identity and gender constancy in sex-differentiated development. *New Directions for Child Development, 47*, 5–20.

Maccoby, E. E., & Martin, J. A. (1983). Socialization in the context of the family: Parent–child interaction. In P. Mussen (Series Ed.) & E. M. Hetherington (Vol. Ed.), *Handbook of Child Psychology: Vol. 4. Socialization, Personality, and Social Development* (4th ed., pp. 1–102). New York: Wiley.

MacDermid, S. M., Huston, T. L., & McHale, S. M. (1990). Changes in marriage associated with the transition to parenthood: Individual differences as a function of sex-role attitudes and changes in the division of household labor. *Journal of Marriage and the Family, 52*, 475–486.

MacDonald, K. (1987). Parent–child physical play with rejected, neglected, and popular boys. *Developmental Psychology, 23*, 705–711.

MacKinnon-Lewis, C., Volling, B. L., Lamb, M. E., Dechman, K., Rabiner, D., & Curtner, M. E. (1994). A cross-contextual analysis of boys' social competence: From family to school. *Developmental Psychology, 30*, 325–333.

Magnussen, D. (1990). Personality development from an interactional perspective. In L. A. Pervin (Ed.), *Handbook of Personality: Theory and Research* (pp. 193–224). New York: Guilford Press.

Mahler, M. S. (1975). On the current status of the infantile neurosis. *Journal of the American Psychoanalytic Association, 23*, 327–333.

Mahler, M. S. (1986). On human symbiosis and the vicissitudes of individuation. In P. Buckley (Ed.), *Essential Papers on Object Relations* (pp. 200–221). New York: New York University Press.

Mahler, M. S., & McDevitt, J. B. (1980). The separation-individuation process and identity formation. In S. I. Greenspan & G. H. Pollock (Eds.), *The Course of Life: Psychoanalytic Contributions toward Understanding Personality Development* (pp. 395–423). Adelphi, MD: Mental Health Study Center.

Main, M. (1991). Metacognitive knowledge, metacognitive monitoring, and singular (coherent) vs. multiple (incoherent) model of attachment. In C. M. Parkes, J. Stevenson-Hinde, & P. Marris (Eds.), *Attachment Across the Life Cycle* (pp. 127–159). London: Routledge.

Main, M., & Goldwyn, R. (1984). Predicting rejection of her own infant from mother's representation of her own experience: Implication for the abused-abusing intergenerational cycle. *Child Abuse and Neglect, 8*, 203–217.

Main, M., Kaplan, N., & Cassidy, J. (1985). Security in infancy, childhood, and adulthood: A move to the level of representation. In I. Bretherton & E. Waters (Eds.), Growing points of attachment theory and research. *Mono-*

graphs of the Society for Research in Child Development, 50 (Serial No. 209), 66–104.

Main, M., & Weston, D. R. (1981). The quality of toddler's relationship to mother and to father: Related to conflict behavior and the readiness to establish new relationships. *Child Development, 52,* 932–940.

Mandler, G. (1980). The generation of emotion: A psychological theory. In R. Plutchik & H. Kellerman (Eds.), *Emotion: Theory, Research and Experience: Vol. 1. Theories of Emotion.* New York: Academic Press.

Mannarino, A. P. (1976). Friendship patterns and altruistic behavior. *Developmental Psychology, 12,* 555–556.

Marcia, J. (1966). Development and validation of ego identity status. *Journal of Personality, 36,* 118–133.

Marcia, J. E. (1980). Identity in adolescence. In J. Adelson (Ed.), *Handbook of Adolescent Psychology* (pp. 159–187). New York: Wiley.

Marcia, J., & Friedman, M. L. (1970). Ego identity status in college women. *Journal of Personality, 38,* 249–263.

Marcoen, A., & Brumagne, M. (1985). Loneliness among children and young adolescents. *Developmental Psychology, 6,* 1025–1031.

Maret, E., & Finlay, B. (1984). The distribution of household labor among women in dual-earner families. *Journal of Marriage and the Family, 46,* 357–364.

Margolin, G. (1982). A social learning approach to intimacy. In M. Fisher & G. Stricker (Eds.), *Intimacy* (pp. 175–201). New York: Plenum.

Margolin, G., & Wampold, B. E. (1981). Sequential analysis of conflict and accord in distressed and nondistressed marital partners. *Journal of Consulting and Clinical Psychology, 49,* 554–567.

Margulis, S. (1977). Conceptions of privacy: Current status and next steps. *Journal of Social Issues, 33,* 5–21.

Mark, E. W., & Alper, T. G. (1980). Sex differences in intimacy motivation. *Psychology of Women Quarterly, 5,* 164–169.

Markman, H. J. (1981). Prediction of marital distress: A 5-year follow-up. *Journal of Consulting and Clinical Psychology, 49,* 760–762.

Markman, H. J., & Kraft, S. A. (1989). Men and women in marriage: Dealing with gender differences in marital therapy. *Behavior Therapist, 12,* 51–56.

Markman, H. J., & Notarius, C. I. (1987). Coding marital and family interaction: Current status. In T. Jacob (Ed.), *Family Interaction and Psychopathology* (pp. 329–390). New York: Plenum.

Markus, H. R., & Kitayama, S. (1991). Culture and the self: Implications for cognition, emotion, and motivation. *Psychological Review, 98,* 224–253.

Markus, H., & Zajonc, R. B. (1985). The cognitive perspective in social psychology. In G. Lindzey & E. Aronson (Eds.), *Handbook of Social Psychology* (3rd ed.; Vol. 1, pp. 137–230). New York: Random House.

Marston, P. J., Hecht, M. L., & Robers, T. (1987). "True love ways": The subjective experience and communication of romantic love. *Journal of Social and Personal Relationships, 4,* 387–407.

Maslin, C. A., Bretherton, I., & Morgan, G. A. (1986, April). *The influence of attachment security and maternal scaffolding on toddler mastery motivation*. Paper presented at the International Conference on Infant Studies, Beverly Hills, CA.

Maslow, A. H. (1968). *Toward a Psychology of Being* (2nd ed.). New York: Van Nostrand.

Matas, L., Arend, R. A., & Sroufe, L. A. (1978). Continuity of adaptation in the second year: The relationship between quality of attachment and later competence. *Child Development, 49*, 547–556.

Matthews, S. H. (1986). *Friendships Through the Life Course: Oral Biographies in Old Age*. Beverly Hills, CA: Sage.

Maxwell, G. M. (1985). Behaviour of lovers: Measuring the closeness of relationships. *Journal of Social and Personal Relationships, 2*, 215–238.

McAdams, D. P. (1980). A thematic coding system for the intimacy motive. *Journal of Research in Personality, 14*, 413–432.

McAdams, D. P. (1982a). Experience of intimacy and power: Relationships between social motives and autobiographical memory. *Journal of Personality and Social Psychology, 42*, 292–302.

McAdams, D. P. (1984). Human motives and personal relationships. In V. J. Derlega (Ed.), *Communication, Intimacy and Close Relationships* (pp. 41–70). Orlando, FL: Academic Press.

McAdams, D. P. (1988a). Personal needs and personal relationships. In S. W. Duck (Ed.), *Handbook of Personal Relationships* (pp. 7–22). New York: Wiley.

McAdams, D. P. (1988b). *Power, Intimacy and the Life Story*. New York: Guilford Press.

McAdams, D. P., & Bryant, F. B. (1987). Intimacy motivation and subjective mental health in a nationwide sample. *Journal of Personality, 55*, 395–413.

McAdams, D. P., & Constantian, C. A. (1983). Intimacy and affiliation motives in daily living: An experience-sampling analysis. *Journal of Personality and Social Psychology, 45*, 851–861.

McAdams, D. P., Healy, S., & Krause, S. (1984). Social motives and patterns of friendship. *Journal of Personality and Social Psychology, 47*, 828–838.

McAdams, D. P., Jackson, R. J., & Kirshnit, C. (1984). Looking, laughing, and smiling in dyads as a function of intimacy motivation and reciprocity. *Journal of Personality, 52*, 261–273.

McAdams, D. P., Lester, R. M., Brand, P. A., McNamara, W. J., & Lensky, D. B. (1988). Sex and the TAT: Are women more intimate than men? Do men fear intimacy? *Journal of Personality Assessment, 52*, 397–409.

McAdams, D. P., & Powers, J. (1981). Themes of intimacy in behavior and thought. *Journal of Personality and Social Psychology, 40*, 573–587.

McCallum, J. (1986). Retirement and widowhood transitions. In H. L. Kendig (Ed.), *Aging and Families: A Support Networks Perspective* (pp. 129–148). Sydney, Australia: Allen & Unwin.

McCarthy, B. W. (1987). Developing positive intimacy cognitions in males with a history of nonintimate sexual experiences. *Journal of Sex and Marital Therapy, 13*, 253–259.

McClelland, D. C. (1985). *Human Motivation*. Glenview, IL: Scott, Foresman.

McGiboney, K. E. (1993). *An examination of loneliness among aggressive and withdrawn children*. Unpublished doctoral dissertation, University of Texas at Dallas.

McGuire, K. D., & Weisz, J. R. (1982). Social cognition and behavior correlates of preadolescent chumship. *Child Development, 53*, 1478–1484.

McHale, S. M., & Huston, T. L. (1985). The effect of the transition to parenthood on the marriage relationship: A longitudinal study. *Journal of Family Issues, 6*, 409–433.

McNulty, S. E., & Swann, W. B. (1994). Identity negotiation in roommate relationships: The self as architect and consequence of social reality. *Journal of Personality and Social Psychology, 6*, 1012–1023.

McWhirter, D. P., & Mattison, A. M. (1984). *The Male Couple: How Relationships Develop*. Englewood Cliffs, NJ: Prentice-Hall.

Medin, D. L. (1989). Concepts and conceptual structure. *American Psychologist, 44*, 1469–1481.

Mehrabian, A. (1969). Some referents and measures of nonverbal behavior. *Behavior Research Methods and Instrumentation, 1*, 203–207.

Mehrabian, A. (1970). A semantic space for nonverbal behavior. *Journal of Consulting and Clinical Psychology, 35*, 248–257.

Mehrabian, A. (1971). *Silent Messages*. Belmont, CA: Wadsworth.

Merves-Okin, L., Amidon, E., & Bernt, F. (1991). Perceptions of intimacy in marriage: A study of married couples. *American Journal of Family Therapy, 19*, 110–118.

Messer, M. (1968). Age grouping and the family status of the elderly. *Sociology and Social Research, 53*, 271–279.

Mettetal, G. (1983). Fantasy, gossip, and self-disclosure: Children's conversations with friends. In R. N. Bostrom (Ed.), *Communication Yearbook 7* (pp. 717–736). Beverly Hills, CA: Sage.

Miell, D., & Duck, S. (1986). Strategies in developing friendships. In V. J. Derlega & B. Winstead (Eds.), *Friendship and Social Interaction* (pp. 129–143). New York: Springer-Verlag.

Mikulincer, M., & Nachshon, O. (1991). Attachment styles and patterns of self-disclosure. *Journal of Personality and Social Psychology, 61*, 321–331.

Milardo, R. M., Johnson, M. P., & Huston, T. L. (1983). Developing close relationships: Changing patterns of interaction between pair members and social networks. *Journal of Personality and Social Psychology, 44*, 964–976.

Milardo, R. M., & Wellman, B. (1992). The personal is social. *Journal of Social and Personal Relationships, 9*, 339–342.

Milgram, S. (1974). *Obedience to Authority: An Experimental View*. New York: Harper & Row.

Miller, B. C. (1976). A multivariate developmental model of marital satisfaction. *Journal of Marriage and the Family, 38,* 643–657.

Miller, J. B. (1991). The development of women's sense of self. In J. V. Jordan, A. G. Kaplan, J. B. Miller, I. P. Stiver, & J. L. Surrey, *Women's Growth in Connection: Writings from the Stone Center* (pp. 11–26). New York: Guilford Press.

Miller, K. E. (1990). Adolescents' same-sex and opposite-sex peer relations: Sex differences in popularity, perceived social competence and social cognitive skills. *Journal of Adolescent Research, 5,* 222–241.

Miller, L. C. (1990). Intimacy and liking: Mutual influence and the role of unique relationships. *Journal of Personality and Social Psychology, 59,* 50–60.

Miller, L. C., & Berg, J. (1984). Selectivity and urgency in interpersonal exchange. In V. J. Derlega (Ed.), *Communication, Intimacy, and Close Relationships* (pp. 161–206). Orlando, FL: Academic Press.

Miller, L. C., Berg, J. H., & Archer, R. L. (1983). Openers: Individuals who elicit intimate self-disclosure. *Journal of Personality and Social Psychology, 44,* 1234–1244.

Miller, L. C., & Kenny, D. A. (1986). Reciprocity of self-disclosure at the individual and dyadic levels: A social relations analysis. *Journal of Personality and Social Psychology, 50,* 713–719.

Miller, L. C., & Read, S. J. (1987). Why am I telling you this? Self-disclosure in a goal-based model of personality. In V. J. Derlega & J. H. Berg (Eds.), *Self-disclosure: Theory, research & therapy* (pp. 35–58). New York: Plenum.

Miller, L. C., & Read, S. J. (1991). On the coherence of mental models of persons and relationships: A knowledge structure approach. In G. J. O. Fletcher & F. D. Fincham (Eds.), *Cognition in Close Relationships* (pp. 69–100). Hillsdale, NJ: Erlbaum.

Miller, P. C., Lefcourt, H. M., Holmes, J. G., Ware, E. E., & Saleh, W. E. (1986). Marital locus of control and marital problem-solving. *Journal of Personality and Social Psychology, 51,* 161–169.

Miller, R. S., & Lefcourt, H. M. (1982). The assessment of social intimacy. *Journal of Personality Assessment, 46,* 514–518.

Miller, R. S., & Lefcourt, H. M. (1983). Social intimacy: An important moderator of stressful life events. *American Journal of Community Psychology, 11,* 127–139.

Mischel, W. (1973). Toward a cognitive social learning reconceptualization of personality. *Psychological Review, 80,* 252–283.

Mischel, W. (1981). *Introduction to Personality* (3rd ed.). New York: Holt, Rinehart & Winston.

Mischel, W. (1993). *Introduction to Personality* (5th ed.). New York: Harcourt Brace.

Moen, P. (1985). Continuities and discontinuities in women's labor force activity. In G.H. Elder, Jr. (Ed.), *Life Course Dynamics* (pp. 113–155). Ithaca, NY: Cornell University Press.

Monsour, M. (1992). Meanings of intimacy in cross and same-sex friendships. *Journal of Social and Personal Relationships*, 9, 277–296.

Montgomery, B. M. (1984a). Behavioral characteristics predicting self and peer perceptions of open communication. *Communication Quarterly*, 32, 233–242.

Montgomery, B. M. (1984b). Communication in intimate relationships: A research challenge. *Communication Quarterly*, 32, 318–323.

Montgomery, B. M., & Duck, S. (Eds.). (1991). *Studying Interpersonal Interaction*. New York: Guilford Press.

Moos, R. H., & Moos, B. S. (1983). Clinical applications of the family environment scale. In E. E. Filsinger (Ed.), *Marriage and Family Assessment* (pp. 253–273). Beverly Hills, CA: Sage.

Morgan, B. S. (1976). Intimacy of disclosure topics and sex differences in self-disclosure. *Sex Roles*, 2, 161–166.

Morgan, D. L. (1990). Combining the strengths of social networks, social support, and personal relationships. In S. W. Duck (Ed.), *Personal Relationships and Social Support* (pp. 190–244). London: Sage.

Morgan, W. R., Parnes, H. S., & Less, L. J. (1985). Leisure activities and social networks. In H. S. Parnes (Eds), *Retirement among American Men* (pp. 119–146). Lexington, MA: Lexington Books.

Morris, D. (1982). Attachment and intimacy. In M. Fisher & G. Stricker (Eds.), *Intimacy*. New York: Plenum.

Mortimer, J., & Lorence, J. T. (1979). Work experience and occupational value socializaton: A longitudinal study. *American Journal of Sociology*, 84, 1361–1385.

Morton, T. L. (1978). Intimacy and reciprocity of exchange: A comparison of spouses and strangers. *Journal of Personality and Social Psychology*, 36, 72–81.

Moss, B. F., & Schwebel, A. I. (1993). Intimacy in enduring romantic relationships. *Family Relations*, 42, 31–37.

Moustakas, C. E. (1975). *The Touch of Loneliness*. Englewood Cliffs, NJ: Prentice-Hall.

Mueller, I., & Brenner, J. (1977). The origins of social skills and interaction among playgroup toddlers. *Child Development*, 48, 854–861.

Munro, G., & Adams, G. R. (1977). Ego-identity formation in college students and working youth. *Developmental Psychology*, 13, 523–524.

Murphy, D. J., & Messer, D. J. (1977). Mothers and infants pointing: A study of gesture. In R. H. Schaffer (Ed.), *Studies in Mother–Infant Interaction* (pp. 323–354). New York: Academic Press.

Murray, H. A. (1938). *Explorations in Personality*. New York: Oxford University Press.

Murray, H. A. (1943). *Thematic Apperception Test Manual*. Cambridge, MA: Harvard University Press.

Murray, S. L., & Holmes, J. G. (1993). Seeing virtues in faults: Negativity and the transformation of interpersonal narratives in close relationships. *Journal of Personality and Social Psychology*, 65, 707–722.

Nardi, P. M. (1992a). That's what friends are for: Friends as family in the gay and lesbian community. In K. Plummer (Ed.), *Modern Homosexualities* (pp. 108–120). London: Routledge.

Nardi, P. M. (1992b). "Seamless souls": An introduction to men's friendships. In P. M. Nardi (Ed.), *Men's Friendships* (pp. 1–14). Newbury Park, CA: Sage.

Nardi, P. M., & Sherrod, D. (1994). Friendship in the lives of gay men and lesbians. *Journal of Social and Personal Relationships, 11*, 185–200.

Nash, A. (1988). Ontogeny, phylogeny, & relationships. In S. W. Duck (Ed.), *Handbook of Personal Relationships* (pp. 121–141). New York: Wiley.

Nash, A., & Lamb, M. E. (1987, April). *Becoming acquainted with unfamiliar adults and peers in infancy*. Paper presented to the Society for Research in Child Development, Baltimore.

Narus, L. R., & Fischer, J. L. (1982). Strong but not silent: A reexamination of expressivity in the relationships of men. *Sex Roles, 8*, 159–168.

Neugarten, B. L. (1976). Adaptation and the life cycle. *Counseling Psychologist, 6*, 6–20.

Newcomb, A. F., & Brady, J. E. (1982). Mutuality in boys' friendship relations. *Child Development, 50*, 878–881.

Nezlek, J. B., Wheeler, L., & Reis, H. T. (1983). Studies of social participation. *New Directions for Methodology of Social and Behavioral Science, 15*, 57–73.

O'Conner, E. M., & Simms, C. M. (1990). Self-revelation as manipulation: The effects of sex and Machiavellianism on self-disclosure. *Social Behavior and Personality, 18*, 95–100.

O'Connor, P. (1992). *Friendships Between Women: A Critical Review*. New York: Guilford Press.

O'Leary, K. D. (Ed.). (1987). *Assessment of Marital Discord: An Integration for Research and Clinical Practice*. Hillsdale, NJ: Erlbaum.

Oliker, S. J. (1989). *Best Friends and Marriage*. Berkeley: University of California Press.

Olsen, D., & Zubek, J. (1970). Effect of one-day sensory deprivation on a battery of open-ended cognitive tests. *Percpetual and Motor Skills, 31*, 919–923.

Olson, D. H. (1993). Family continuity and change: A family life-cycle perspective. In T. H. Brubaker (Ed.), *Family Relations: Challenges for the Future*, (pp. 17–40). Newbury Park, CA: Sage.

Olson, D. H., & Portner, J. (1983). Family adaptability and cohesion evaluation scales. In E. E. Filsinger (Ed.), *Marriage and Family Assessment* (pp. 299–315). Beverly Hills, CA: Sage.

Olson, D. H., Portner, J., & Bell, R. (1982). *The Family Adaptability and Cohesion Evaluation Scales (FACES)*. St Paul: Family Social Science, University of Minnesota.

O'Meara, J. D. (1994). Cross-sex friendship's opportunity challenge: Uncharted terrain for exploration. *Personal Relationship Issues, 2*, 4–7.

O'Meara, J. D. (1989). Cross-sex friendship: Four basic challenges of an ignored relationship. *Sex Roles, 21*, 523–543.

Orlofsky, J. L. (1976). Intimacy status: Relationship to interpersonal perception. *Journal of Youth and Adolescence, 5*, 73–88.

Orlofsky, J. L. (1978). The relationship between intimacy status and antecedent personality components. *Adolescence, 13*, 419–441.

Orlofsky, J. L. (1988). Intimacy status: Theory and research. In J. E. Marcia (Ed.), *Identity in Adolescence*. Hillsdale, NJ: Erlbaum.

Orlofsky, J. L., & Ginsburg, S. D. (1981). Intimacy status: Relation to affect cognition. *Adolescence, 16*, 91–100.

Orlofsky, J. L., Marcia, J. E., & Lesser, I. M. (1973). Ego identity status and the intimacy vs. isolation crisis of young adulthood. *Journal of Personality and Social Psychology, 27*, 211–219.

Osgood, C. E., Suci, G. J., & Tannenbaum, P. H. (1957). *The Measurement of Meaning*. Urbana: University of Illinois Press.

Oyserman, D. (1993). The lens of personhood: Viewing the self and others in a multicultural society. *Journal of Personality and Social Psychology, 65*, 993–1009.

Paikoff, R. L., & Brooks-Gunn, J. (1991). Do parent–child relationships change during puberty? *Psychological Bulletin, 110*, 47–66.

Palys, T. S., & Little, B. R. (1983). Perceived life satisfaction and the organizaton of personal project systems. *Journal of Personality and Social Psychology, 44*, 1121–1230.

Papini, D. R., Farmer, F. L., Clark, S. M., & Snell, W. E. (1988). An evaluation of adolescent patterns of sexual self-disclosure to parents and friends. *Journal of Adolescent Research, 3*, 387–401.

Park, B. (1986). A method for studying the development of impressions of real people. *Journal of Personality and Social Psychology, 51*, 907–917.

Park, K. A., & Waters, E. (1989). Security of attachment and preschool friendships. *Child Development, 60*, 1076–1081.

Parke, R. D., & Ladd, G. W. (1992). *Family–Peer Relationships: Modes of Linkage*. Hillsdale, NJ: Erlbaum.

Parke, R. D., MacDonald, K. B., Beitel, A., & Bhavnagri, N. (1988). The role of the family in the development of peer relationships. In R. Peters & J. McMahon (Eds.), *Social Learning Systems Approaches to Marriage and the Family* (pp. 17–44). New York: Brunner/Mazel.

Parker, J. G., & Asher, S. R. (1987). Peer relations and later personal adjustment: Are low-accepted children at risk? *Psychological Bulletin, 102*, 357–389.

Parker, J. G., & Gottman, J. M. (1989). Social and emotional development in a relational context. In T. J. Berndt & G. W. Ladd (Eds.), *Peer Relationships in Child Development* (pp. 95–131). New York: Wiley.

Parks, M. R., & Eggert, L. L. (1991). Social context in the dynamics of relationships. In W. H. Jones & D. Perlman (Eds.), *Advances in Personal Relationships* (Vol. 2, pp. 1–34). London: Kingsley.

Parmelee, P. A. (1987). Sex role identity, role performance, and marital satisfaction of newly-wed couples. *Journal of Social and Personal Relationships, 4*, 429–444.

Patterson, C. J. (1995). Sexual orientation and human development: An overview. *Developmental Psychology, 31*, 3–11.

Patterson, C. J., Kupersmidt, J. B., & Griesler, P. C. (1990). Children's perceptions of self and of relationships with others as a function of sociometric status. *Child Development, 61,* 1335–1349.

Patterson, C. J., Kupersmidt, J. B., & Vaden, N. A. (1990). Income level, gender, ethnicity, and household composition as predictors of children's school-based competence. *Child Development, 61,* 485–494.

Patterson, M. L. (1976). An arousal model of interpersonal intimacy. *Psychological Review, 83,* 235–245.

Patterson, M. L. (1982). A sequential functional model of nonverbal exchange. *Psychological Review, 89,* 231–249.

Patterson, M. L. (1984). Intimacy, social control, and nonverbal involvement: A functional approach. In V. J. Derlega (Ed.), *Communication, Intimacy and Close Relationships* (pp. 13–42). Beverly Hills, CA: Sage.

Patterson, M. L. (1987). Presentation and affect-management functions of nonverbal involvement. *Journal of Nonverbal Behavior, 11,* 110–122.

Patterson, M. L. (1988). Functions of nonverbal behavior in close relationships. In S. W. Duck (Ed.), *Handbook of Personal Relationships* (pp. 41–56). New York: Wiley.

Patton, D., & Waring, E. M. (1984). The quality and quantity of marital intimacy in the marriages of psychiatric patients. *Journal of Sex and Marital Therapy, 10,* 201–206.

Patton, D., & Waring, E. M. (1985). Sex and marital intimacy. *Journal of Sex and Marital Therapy, 11,* 176–184.

Paul, E. L., & White, K. M. (1990). The development of intimate relationships in late adolescence. *Adolescence, 25,* 375–400.

Pedersen, D. M. (1988). Correlates of privacy regulation. *Perceptual and Motor Skills, 66,* 595–601.

Pederson, D. M., & Breglio, V. J. (1968). Personality correlates of self-disclosure. *Psychological Reports, 22,* 495–501.

Pellman, J. (1992). Widowhood in elderly women: Exploring its relationship to community integration, hassles, stress, social support and social support seeking. *International Journal of Aging and Human Development, 35,* 253–264.

Pennebaker, J. W., Barger, S. D., & Tiebout, J. (1989). Disclosure of traumas and health among holocaust survivors. *Psychosomatic Medicine, 51,* 577–589.

Pennebaker, J. W., & Beall, S. K. (1986). Confronting a traumatic event: Toward an understanding of inhibition and disease. *Journal of Abnormal Psychology, 95,* 274–281.

Pennebaker, J. W., Colder, M., & Sharp, L. K. (1990). Accelerating the coping process. *Journal of Personality and Social Psychology, 58,* 528–537.

Pennebaker, J. W., Dyer, M. A., Caulkins, R. S., Litowitz, D. L., Ackerman, P. L., Anderson, D. B., & McGraw, K. M. (1979). Don't the girls get prettier at closing time: A country and western application to psychology. *Personality and Social Psychology Bulletin, 5,* 122–125.

Peplau, L. A., Bikson, T. K., Rook, K. S., & Goodchilds, J. D. (1982). Being old and living alone. In L. A. Peplau & D. Perlman (Eds.), *Loneliness: A Source-*

book of Current Theory, Research and Therapy (pp. 327–347). New York: Wiley.

Peplau, L. A., & Cochran, S. (1990). A relationship perspective on homosexuality. In D. P. McWhirter, S. A. Sanders, & J. M. Reinisch (Eds.), *Homosexuality/Heterosexuality: Concepts of Sexual Orientation* (pp. 321–349). New York: Oxford University Press.

Peplau, L. A., Cochran, S., Rook, K., & Padesky, C. (1978). Loving women: Attachment and autonomy in lesbian relationships. *Journal of Social Issues, 34*, 7–27.

Peretti, P. O., & Lowrey, B. (1984–1986). Intimacy in the confidant role in closest friendships of nonconfined aged males. *Psychology and Human Development, 1*, 75–79.

Perlman, D., & Fehr, B. (1987). The development of intimate relationships. In D. Perlman & S. Duck (Eds.), *Intimate Relationships: Development, Dynamics, and Deterioration* (pp. 13–42). Newbury Park, CA: Sage.

Pervin, L. A. (1989). Goal concepts in personality and social psychology: A historical perspective. In L. A. Pervin (Ed.), *Goal Concepts in Personality and Social Psychology* (pp. 1–17). Hillsdale, NJ: Erlbaum.

Peterson, A. C. (1983). The nature of biological–psychosocial interactions: The sample case of early adolescence. In R. M. Lerner & T. T. Fock (Eds.), *Biological–Psychosocial Interactions in Early Adolescence* (pp. 35–61). Hillsdale, NJ: Erlbaum.

Peterson, A. C., Compas, B. E., Brooks-Gunn, J., Stemmler, M., Ey, S., & Grant, K. E. (1993). Depression in adolescence. *American Psychologist, 48*, 155–168.

Peterson, B. E., & Stewart, A. J. (1993). Generativity and social motives in young adults. *Journal of Personality and Social Psychology, 65*, 186–198.

Peterson, D. R. (1983). Conflict. In H. H. Kelley, E. Bersheid, A. Christensen, J. H. Harvey, T. L. Huston, G. Levinger, E. McClintock, L. A. Peplau, & D. R. Peterson (Eds.), *Close Relationships: Development and Change*. New York: Freeman.

Peterson, E. T. (1989). Elderly parents and their offspring. In S. J. Bahr & E. T. Peterson (Eds.), *Aging and the Family* (pp. 175–192). Lexington, MA: Lexington.

Pettit, G. S., Dodge, K. A., & Brown, M. M. (1988). Early family experience, social problem-solving patterns, and children's social competence. *Child Development, 59*, 107–120.

Piaget, J. (1954). *The Construction of Reality in the Child*. New York: Basic Books.

Piaget, J. (1965). *The Moral Judgment of the Child*. Glencoe, IL: Free Press. (Original work published 1932)

Pilkington, C. J., & Richardson, D. R. (1988). Perceptions of risk in intimacy. *Journal of Social and Personal Relationships, 5*, 503–508.

Pilkington, C. J., & Tesser, A. (1991). On the uniqueness of self-definition: A self-evaluation maintenance perspective. *Cahiers de Psychologie Cognitive, 11*, 645–668.

Pilkington, C. J., Tesser, A., & Stephens, D. (1991). Complementarity in romantic relationships: A self-evaluation maintenance perspective. *Journal of Social and Personal Relationships, 8*, 481–504.

Pitcher, B. L., & Larson, D. C. (1989). Elderly widowhood. In S. J. Bahr & E. T. Peterson (Eds.), *Aging and the Family* (pp. 59–81). Lexington, MA: Lexington Books.

Pittman, J. F., Price-Bonham, S., & McKenry, P. C. (1983). Marital cohesion: A path model. *Journal of Marriage and the Family, 45*, 521–531.

Pleck, J. H. (1981). *The Myth of Masculinity*. Cambridge, MA: MIT Press.

Pleck, J. H. (1985). *Working Wives/Working Husbands*. Newbury Park, CA: Sage.

Pogrebrin, L. C. (1987). *Among Friends: Who We Like, Why We Like Them, and What We Do With Them*. New York: McGraw-Hill.

Post, A. L., Wittmaier, B. C., & Radin, M. E. (1978). Self-disclosure as a function of state and trait anxiety. *Journal of Consulting and Clinical Psychology, 46*, 12–19.

Prager, K. J. (1983a). Intimacy development in young adults: A multidimensional view. *Psychological Reports, 52*, 751–756.

Prager, K. J. (1983b). Identity status, sex-role orientation, and self-esteem in late adolescent females. *Journal of Genetic Psychology, 143*, 159–167.

Prager, K. J. (1986). Intimacy status: Its relationship to locus of control, self-disclosure and anxiety. *Personality and Social Psychology Bulletin, 12*, 91–109.

Prager, K. J. (1989). Intimacy status and couple communication. *Journal of Social and Personal Relationships, 6*, 435–449.

Prager, K. J. (1991). Intimacy status and couple conflict resolution. *Journal of Social and Personal Relationships*, 505–526.

Prager, K. J., & Buhrmester, D. (1992, August). *Assessing agentic and communal need fulfillment and life satisfaction*. Paper presented at the Annual Meeting, American Psychological Association, Washington, DC.

Prager, K. J., Fuller, D. O., & Gonzalez, A. S. (1989). The function of self-disclosure in social interaction. *Journal of Social Behavior and Personality, 4*, 563–580.

Pretzer, J., Epstein, N., & Fleming, B. (1991). Marital Attitude Survey: A measure of dysfunctional attributions and expectancies. *Journal of Cognitive Psychotherapy: An International Quarterly, 5*, 131–148.

Putallaz, M., & Heflin, A. H. (1990). Parent–child interaction. In S. R. Asher & J. C. Coie (Eds.), *Children's Status in the Peer Group* (pp. 189–216). New York: Cambridge University Press.

Raffaelli, M., & Duckett, E. (1989). "We were just talking . . . ": Conversations in early adolescence. *Journal of Youth and Adolescence, 18*, 567–582.

Raphael, S. M., & Robinson, M. K. (1980). The older lesbian. *Alternative Lifestyles, 3*, 207–229.

Raush, H. L., Barry, W. A., Hertel, R. K., & Swain, M. A. (1974). *Communication, Conflict and Marriage*. San Francisco: Jossey-Bass.

Rawlins, W. K. (1992). *Friendship Matters*. New York: Aldine de Gruyter.

Rawlins, W. K. (1994). Reflecting on (cross-sex) friendship: De-scripting the drama. *Personal Relationship Issues, 2*, 1–3.

Rawlins, W. K., & Holl, M. (1987). The communicative achievement of friendship during adolescence: Predicaments of trust and violation. *Western Journal of Speech Communication, 51*, 345–363.

Read, S. J., & Miller, L. C. (1989). Inter-personalism: Toward a goal-based theory of persons in relationships. In L. A. Pervin (Ed.), *Goal Concepts in Personality and Social Psychology* (pp. 413–472). Hillsdale, NJ: Erlbaum.

Reddon, J. R., Patton, D., & Waring, E. M. (1985). The item-factor structure of the Waring Intimacy Questionnaire. *Educational and Psychological Measurement, 45*, 233–244.

Register, L. M., & Henley, T. B. (1992). The phenomenology of intimacy. *Journal of Social and Personal Relationships, 9*, 467–481.

Reid, H. M., & Fine, G. A. (1992). Self-disclosure in men's friendships. In P. M. Nardi (Ed.), *Men's Friendships* (pp. 132–152). Newbury Park, CA: Sage.

Reis, H. T. (1984a). Social interaction and well-being. In S. Duck (Ed.), *Personal Relationships: Repairing Personal Relationships* (pp. 21–45). London: Academic Press.

Reis, H. T. (1984b). The role of the self in the initiation and course of social interaction. In W. Ickes (Ed.), *Compatible and Incompatible Relationships* (pp. 209–231). New York: Springer-Verlag.

Reis, H. T. (1990). The role of intimacy in interpersonal relations. *Journal of Social and Clinical Psychology, 9*, 15–30.

Reis, H. T., & Franks, P. (1994). The role of intimacy and social support in health outcomes: Two processes or one? *Personal Relationships, 1*, 185–197.

Reis, H. T., Senchak, M., & Solomon, B. (1985). Sex differences in intimacy of social interaction: Further examination of potential explanations. *Journal of Personality and Social Psychology, 48*, 1204–1217.

Reis, H. T., & Shaver, P. (1988). Intimacy as interpersonal process. In S. Duck (Ed.), *Handbook of Personal Relationships: Theory, Relationships, and Interventions* (pp. 367–389). Chichester, UK: Wiley.

Reis, H. T., Wheeler, L., Kernis, M. H., Spiegel, N., & Nezlek, J. (1985). On specificity in the impact of social participation on physical and psychological health. *Journal of Personality and Social Psychology, 48*, 456–471.

Reisman, J. M. (1985). Friendship and its implications for mental health or social competence. *Journal of Early Adolescence, 5*, 383–394.

Reisman, J. M. (1990). Intimacy in same-sex friendships. *Sex Roles, 23*, 65–82.

Reissman, C., Aron, A., & Bergen, M. R. (1993). Shared activities and marital satisfaction: Causal direction and self-expansion versus boredom. *Journal of Social and Personal Relationships, 10*, 243–254.

Rempel, J. K., Holmes, J. G., & Zanna, M. P. (1985). Trust in close relationships. *Journal of Personality and Social Psychology, 49*, 95–112.

Rhodes, J. E., Ebert, L., & Meyers, A. B. (1994). Social support, relationship problems and the psychological functioning of young African-American mothers. *Journal of Social and Personal Relationships, 11*, 587–599.

Richardson, R. A., Galambos, N. L., & Petersen, A. C. (1984). Young adolescents' perceptions of the family environment. *Journal of Early Adolescence, 4*, 131–153.

Risman, B. J., & Schwartz, P. (1989). Being gendered: A microstructural view of intimate relationships. In B. J. Risman & P. Schwartz (Eds.), *Gender in Intimate Relationships: A Microstructural Approach* (pp. 1–9). Belmont, CA: Wadsworth.

Robbins, E. S., & Haase, R. F. (1985). Power of nonverbal cues in counseling interactions: Availability, vividness, or salience? *Journal of Counseling Psychology, 32,* 502–513.

Roberts, P., & Newton, P. M. (1987). Levinsonian studies of women's adult development. *Psychology and Aging, 2,* 154–163.

Robins, E. (1990). The study of interdependence in marriage. In F. D. Fincham & T. N. Bradbury (Eds.), *The Psychology of Marriage: Basic Issues and Applications* (pp. 59–86). New York: Guilford Press.

Robinson, B. E., & Barret, R. L. (1986). *The Developing Father: Emerging Roles in Contemporary Society.* New York: Guilford Press.

Robinson, G. E., Olmsted, M. P., & Garner, D. M. (1989). Predictors of postpartum adjustment. *Acta Psychiatrica Scandinavica, 80,* 561–565.

Rogers, C. R. (1951). *Client-Centered Therapy.* Boston: Houghton Mifflin.

Rogers, C. R. (1959). A theory of therapy, personality and interpersonal relationships, as developed in the client-centered framework. In S. Koch (Ed.), *Psychology: A Study of a Science* (Vol. 3, pp. 184–526). New York: McGraw-Hill.

Rogers, C. R. (1974). Remarks on the future of client-centered therapy. In D. A. Wexler & L. N. Rice (Eds.), *Innovations in Client-Centered Therapy* (pp. 7–13). New York: Wiley.

Rogers, C. R. (1980). *A Way of Being.* Boston: Houghton Mifflin.

Rogers-Doll, E., Bateman, M., Van Egeren, L, Wilner, B., Yurk, H., & Mitchell, M. E. (1992, November). *Predicting intimacy in engaged and married couples: Some preliminary findings.* Paper presented at the Annual Meeting, Association for the Advancement of Behavior Therapy, New York.

Rosch, E., & Mervis, C. B. (1975). Family resemblances: Studies in the internal structure of categories. *Cognitive Psychology, 7,* 573–605.

Rosch, E., Mervis, C. B., Gray, W. D., Johnson, D. M., & Boyes-Braem, P. (1976). Basic objects in natural categories. *Cognitive Psychology, 8,* 382–439.

Roscoe, B., Kennedy, D., & Pope, T. (1987). Adolescents' views of intimacy: Distinguishing intimate from nonintimate relationships. *Adolescence, 22,* 511–516.

Rose, S. M. (1985). Same- and cross-sex friendships and the psychology of homosociality. *Sex Roles, 12,* 63–74.

Rosenbaum, J. E. (1984). *Career Mobility in a Corporate Hierarchy.* New York: Academic Press.

Rosenberg, S. D., & Farrell, M. P. (1977–1978). Identity and crisis in middle-aged men. *International Journal of Aging and Human Development, 7,* 153–170.

Rosenbluth, S. C., & Steil, J. M. (1995). Predictors of intimacy for women in heterosexual and homosexual couples. *Journal of Social and Personal Rela-*

tionships, 12, 163–175.

Rosenfeld, H. M., Breck, B. E., Smith, S. H., & Kehoe, S. (1984). Intimacy-mediators of the proximity-gaze compensation effect: Movement, conversational role, acquaintance and gender. *Journal of Nonverbal Behavior, 8,* 235–249.

Rosenkrantz, P. S., Vogel, S. R., Bee, H., Broverman, I. K., & Broverman, D. M. (1968). Sex role stereotypes and self concepts in college students. *Journal of Consulting and Clinical Psychology, 32,* 287–295.

Rosenthal, D. A., Gurney, R. M., & Moore, S. M. (1981). From trust to intimacy: A new inventory for examining Erikson's stages of psychosocial development. *Journal of Youth and Adolescence, 10,* 525–537.

Rotenberg, K. J., & Hamel, J. (1988). Social interaction and depression in elderly individuals. *International Journal of Aging and Human Development, 27,* 305–318.

Rotenberg, K. J., & Sliz, D. (1988). Children's restrictive disclosure to friends. *Merrill-Palmer Quarterly, 34,* 203–215.

Rotter, J. B. (1982). Social learning theory. In N. T. Feather (Ed.), *Expectations and Actions: Expectancy-Value Models in Psychology* (pp. 241–260). Hillsdale, NJ: Erlbaum.

Rubin, L. (1983). *Intimate Strangers: Men and Women Together.* New York: Harper & Row.

Rubin, L. (1985). *Just Friends: The Role of Friendship in Our Lives.* New York: Harper & Row.

Rubin, L. (1990). *Erotic Wars: What Happened to the Sexual Revolution?* New York: Farrar, Straus & Giroux.

Rubin, Z. (1970). Measurement of romantic love. *Journal of Personality and Social Psychology, 16,* 265–273.

Rubin, Z., Hill, C. T., Peplau, L. A., & Dunkel-Schetter, C. (1980). Self-disclosure in dating couples: Sex roles and the ethic of openness. *Journal of Marriage and the Family, 42,* 305–317.

Rubin, Z., & Shenker, S. (1978). Friendship, proximity, and self-disclosure. *Journal of Personality, 46,* 1–22.

Ruble, D. N., & Brooks-Gunn, J. (1982). The experience of menarche. *Child Development, 53,* 1557–1566.

Ruble, D. N., Fleming, A. S., Hackel, L., & Stangor, C. (1988). Changes in the marital relationship during the transition to first-time motherhood: Effects of violated expectations concerning division of household labor. *Journal of Personality and Social Psychology, 55,* 78–87.

Rusbult, C. E., Johnson, D. J., & Morrow, G. D. (1986). Impact of couple patterns of problem-solving on distress and nondistress in dating relationships. *Journal of Personality and Social Psychology, 50,* 744–753.

Rusbult, C. E., Zembrodt, I. M., & Gunn, L. K. (1982). Exit, voice, loyalty, neglect: Responses to dissatisfaction in romantic involvements. *Journal of Personality and Social Psychology, 43,* 1230–1242.

Russell, L. (1990). Sex and couples therapy: A method of treatment to enhance physical and emotional intimacy. *Journal of Sex and Marital Therapy, 16,* 111–120.

Ryckman, R. M., Sherman, M. F., & Burgess, G. D. (1973). Locus of control and self-disclosure of public and private information by college men and women: Brief note. *Journal of Psychology, 84,* 317–318.

Ryder, R. G. (1973). Longitudinal data relating marriage satisfaction and having a child. *Journal of Marriage and the Family, 35,* 604–606.

Ryff, C. D., & Migdal, S. (1984). Intimacy and generativity: Self-perceived transitions. *Signs: Journal of Women in Culture and Society, 9,* 470–481.

Saarni, C. (1988). Emotional competence: How emotions and relationships become integrated. *Nebraska Symposium on Motivation, 36,* 115–182.

Salokangas, P. K. R., Matilla, V., & Joukamaa, M. (1988). Intimacy and mental disorder in late middle age. *Acta Psychiatrica Scandinavica, 78,* 555–560.

Sanders, R. E. (1991). The two-way relationship between talk in social interactions and actors' goals and plans. In K. Tracy (Ed.), *Understanding Face-to-Face Interaction: Issues Linking Goals and Discourse* (pp. 167–188). Hillsdale, NJ: Erlbaum.

Savin-Williams, R. C. (1995). An exploratory study of pubertal maturation timing and self-esteem among gay and bisexual male youths. *Developmental Psychology, 31,* 56–64.

Savin-Williams, R. C., & Berndt, T. J. (1990). Friendship and peer relations. In S. S. Feldman & G. R. Elliot (Eds.), *At the Threshold: The Developing Adolescent.* Cambridge, MA: Harvard University Press.

Sayers, S. L., & Baucom, D. H. (1991). The role of femininity and masculinity in distressed couples' communication. *Journal of Personality and Social Psychology, 61,* 641–647.

Scaife, M., & Bruner, J. S. (1975). The capacity for joint visual attention in the infant. *Nature, 253,* 265–266.

Schaefer, M. T., & Olson, D. H. (1981). Assessing intimacy: The PAIR Inventory. *Journal of Marital and Family Therapy, 7,* 47–60.

Schenkel, S., & Marcia, J. E. (1972). Attitudes toward premarital intercourse in determining ego identity status in college women. *Journal of Personality, 3,* 472–482.

Schiedel, D. G., & Marcia, J. E. (1985). Ego identity, intimacy, sex role orientation, and gender. *Developmental Psychology, 21,* 149–160.

Sedikides, C., Olsen, N., & Reis, H. T. (1993). Relationships as natural categories. *Journal of Personality and Social Psychology, 64,* 71–82.

Seidler, V. J. (1992). Rejection, vulnerability and friendship. In P. M. Nardi (Ed.), *Men's Friendships* (pp. 15–34). Newbury Park, CA: Sage.

Selman, R. (1980). *The Growth of Interpersonal Understanding: Developmental and Clinical Analyses.* New York: Academic Press.

Selman, R. L., & Byrne, D. F. (1974). A structural-developmental analysis of levels of role taking in middle childhood. *Child Development, 45,* 803–806.

Selman, R. L., & Schultz, L. H. (1990). *Making a Friend in Youth.* Chicago: University of Chicago Press.

Senchak, M., & Leonard, K. E. (1992). Attachment styles and marital adjustment among newlywed couples. *Journal of Social and Personal Relationships, 9*, 51–64.

Sexton, R. E., & Sexton, V. S. (1982). Intimacy: A historical perspective. In M. Fisher & G. Stricker (Eds.), *Intimacy* (pp. 1–20). New York: Plenum.

Shadish, W. R. (1984). Intimate behavior and the assessment of benefits in clinical groups. *Small Group Behavior, 15*, 204–221.

Shadish, W. R. (1986). The validity of a measure of intimate behavior. *Small Group Behavior, 17*, 113–120.

Shaffer, D. R. (1988). *Social and Personality Development* (2nd ed.) Pacific Grove, CA: Brooks/Cole.

Shaffer, D. R., & Ogden, J. K. (1986). On sex differences in self-disclosure during the acquaintance process: The role of anticipated future interaction. *Journal of Personality and Social Psychology, 51*, 92–101.

Shaffer, D. R., Pegalis, L., & Cornell, D. P. (1991). Interactive effects of social context and sex-role identity on female self-disclosure during the acquaintance process. *Sex Roles, 24*, 1–19.

Shaffer, D. R., Smith, J. E., & Tomarelli, M. (1982). Self-monitoring as a determinant of self-disclosure recriprocity during the acquaintance process. *Journal of Personality and Social Psychology, 43*, 163–175.

Shaffer, D. R., & Tomarelli, M. M. (1989). When public and private self-foci clash: Self-consciousness and self-disclosure reciprocity during the acquaintance process. *Journal of Personality and Social Psychology, 56*, 765–776.

Shapiro, A., & Swensen, C. (1969). Patterns of self-disclosure among married couples. *Journal of Counseling Psychology, 16*, 179–180.

Sharabany, R. (1974). The development of capacity for altruism as a function of object relations development and vicissitudes. In E. Staub, D. Bart-Tal, J. Karylowski, & J. Reykowski (Eds.), *Development and Maintenance of Prosocial Behavior* (pp. 201–224). New York: Plenum.

Sharabany, R., Gershoni, R., & Hofman, J. (1981). Girlfriend, boyfriend: Age and sex differences in intimate friendships. *Developmental Psychology, 17*, 800–808.

Sharabany, R., & Wiseman, H. (1993). Close relationships in adolescence: The case of the kibbutz. *Journal of Youth and Adolescence, 22*, 671–695.

Shaver, P. R., & Brennan, K. A. (1992). Attachment styles and the "Big Five" personality traits: Their connections with each other and with romantic relationship outcomes. *Personality and Social Psychology Bulletin, 18*, 536–545.

Shaver, P., Furman, W., & Buhrmester, D. (1985). Transition to college: Network changes, social skills and loneliness. In S. Duck & D. Perlman (Eds.), *Understanding Personal Relationships: An Interdisciplinary Approach* (pp. 193–219). London: Sage.

Shaver, P. R., & Hazan, C. (1985). Incompatibility, loneliness and "limerence." In W. Ickes (Ed.), *Compatible and Incompatible Relationships* (pp. 163–184). New York: Springer-Verlag.

Shaver, P. R., & Hazan, C. (1988). A biased overview of the study of love. *Journal of Social and Personal Relationships, 5*, 473–501.

Shaver, P., Schwartz, J., Kirson, D., & O'Connor, C. (1987). Emotion knowledge: Further exploration of a prototype approach. *Journal of Personality and Social Psychology, 52*, 1061–1086.

Shea, L., Thompson, L., & Blieszner, R. (1988). Resources in older adults' old and new friendships. *Journal of Social and Personal Relationships, 5*, 83–96.

Sheehy, G. (1976). *Passages*. New York: Dutton.

Shildo, A. (1994). Internalized homophobia. In B. Greene & G. M. Herek (Eds.), *Lesbian and Gay Psychology* (pp. 176–205). Thousand Oaks, CA: Sage.

Shulman, N. (1975). Life-cycle variations in patterns of close relationships. *Journal of Marriage and the Family, 37*, 813–821.

Siavelia, R. L., & Lamke, L. K. (1992). Instrumentalness and expressiveness: Predictors of heterosexual relationship satisfaction. *Sex Roles, 26*, 149–159.

Sillars, A. L., Weisberg, J., Burgraf, C. S., & Zietlow, P. H. (1990). Communication and understanding revisited: Married couples' understanding and recall of conversations. *Communication Research, 17*, 500–522.

Simpson, J. A. (1990). Influence of attachment styles on romantic relationships. *Journal of Personality and Social Psychology, 59*, 971–980.

Simpson, J. A., Rholes, W. S., & Nelligan, J. S. (1992). Support seeking and support giving within couples in an anxiety-provoking situation: The role of attachment styles. *Journal of Personality and Social Psychology, 62*, 434–446.

Sinnott, J. D. (1984). Older men, older women: Are their perceived sex roles similar? *Sex Roles, 10*, 847–856.

Skolnick, A. (1986). Early attachment and personal relationships across the life course. In P. B. Baltes, D. L. Featherman, & R. M. Lerner (Eds.), *Life-Span Development and Behavior*, (Vol. 7, pp. 173–206). Hillsdale, NJ: Erlbaum.

Slaby, R. G., & Frey, K. S. (1975). Development of gender constancy and selective attention to same-sex models. *Child Development, 46*, 849–856.

Smith, D. A., Vivian, D., & O'Leary, K. D. (1990). Longitudinal prediction of marital discord from premarital expressions of affect. *Journal of Consulting and Clinical Psychology, 58*, 790–798.

Smith, P. K. (1987). Exploration, play and social development in boys and girls. In D. J. Hargreaves & A. M. Colley (Eds.), *The Psychology of Sex Roles* (pp. 118–141). New York: Hemisphere.

Smith-Rosenberg, C. (1986). *Disorderly Conduct*. New York: Oxford University Press.

Smollar, J., & Youniss, J. (1982). Social development through friendship. In K. H. Rubin & H. S. Ross (Eds.), *Peer Relations and Social Skills in Childhood* (pp. 279–298). New York: Springer Verlag.

Snarey, J. (1993). *How fathers care for the next generation: A four-decade study*. Cambridge, MA: Harvard University Press.

Snarey, J., Son, L., Kuehne, V. S., Hauser, S., & Vaillant, G. (1987). The role of parenting in men's psychosocial development: A longitudinal study of early adulthood infertility and midlife generativity. *Developmental Psychology, 23,* 593–603.

Snell, W. E. (1989). Willingness to self-disclose to female and male friends as a function of social anxiety and gender. *Personality and Social Psychology Bulletin, 15,* 113–125.

Snell, W. E., Belk, S. S., Flowers, A., & Warren, J. (1988). Women's and men's willingness to self-disclose to therapists and friends: The moderating influence of instrumental, expressive, masculine, and feminine topics. *Sex Roles, 18,* 769–776.

Snell, W. E., Belk, S. S., & Hawkins, R. C. (1986). The masculine and feminine self-disclosure scale: The politics of masculine and feminine self-presentation. *Sex Roles, 15,* 249–267.

Snell, W. E., Miller, R. S., & Belk, S. S. (1988). Development of the Emotional Self-disclosure Scale. *Sex Roles, 18,* 59–73.

Snell, W. E., Miller, R. S., Belk, S. S., Garcia-Falconi, R., & Hernandez-Sanchez, J. E. (1989). Men's and women's emotional disclosures: The impact of disclosure recipient, culture and the masculine role. *Sex Roles, 21,* 467–486.

Snyder, D. K., Wills, R. M., & Keiser, T. W. (1981). Empirical validation of the Marital Satisfaction Inventory: An actuarial approach. *Journal of Consulting & Clinical Psychology, 49,* 262–268.

Snyder, M., & Simpson, J. A. (1984). Self-monitoring and dating relationships. *Journal of Personality and Social Psychology, 47,* 1281–1291.

Solano, C. H. (1986). People without friends: Loneliness and its alternatives. In V. J. Derlega & B. Winstead (Eds.), *Friendship and Social Interaction* (pp. 225–246). New York: Springer-Verlag.

Solomon, R. C. (1981). *Love: Emotion, Myth and Metaphor.* Garden City, NY: Anchor Press.

Solomon, R. C. (1988). *About Love: Reinventing Romance for Our Times.* New York: Simon & Schuster.

Sontag, S. (1972). The double standard of aging. (Reprinted in Allman, L. R., & Jaffe, D. T. (Eds.). (1982). *Readings in Adult Psychology: Contemporary Perspectives* (2nd ed., pp. 324–333). New York: Harper & Row.)

Sorce, J. F., & Emde, R. N. (1981). Mother's presence is not enough: Effect of emotional availability on infant exploration. *Developmental Psychology, 17,* 737–745.

Sorce, J. F., Emde, R. N., Campos, J., & Klinnert, M. D. (1985). Maternal emotional signaling: Its effect on the visual cliff behavior of 1-year-olds. *Developmental Psychology, 21,* 195–200.

Spanier, G. B. (1976). Measuring dyadic adjustment: New scales for assessing the quality of marriage and similar dyads. *Journal of Marriage and the Family, 38,* 15–28.

Spanier, G. B., Lewis, R. A., & Cole, C. L. (1975). Marital adjustment over the family life cycle: The issue of curvilinearity. *Journal of Mariage and the Family, 37,* 264–275.

Spence, J. T., & Helmreich, R. L. (1978). *Masculinity and Femininity: Their Psychological Dimensions, Correlates, and Antecedents*. Austin, TX: University of Texas Press.

Spence, J. T. (1985). Achievement American style: The rewards and costs of individualism. *American Psychologist, 40*, 1285–1295.

Spencer, T. (1994). Transforming relationships through ordinary talk. In S. W. Duck (Ed.), *Dynamics of Relationships* (pp. 58–85). Thousand Oaks, CA: Sage.

Spitz, R. A. (1949). The role of ecological factors in emotional development in infancy. *Child Development, 20*, 145–155.

Sprague, J., & Quadagno, D. (1989). Gender and sexual motivation: An exploration of two assumptions. *Journal of Psychology and Human Sexuality, 2*, 57–76.

Sprecher, S. (1987). The effects of self-disclosure given and received on affection for an intimate partner and stability of the relationship. *Journal of Social and Personal Relationships, 4*, 115–128.

Sprecher, S., & McKinney, K. (1993). *Sexuality*. Newbury Park, CA: Sage.

Sroufe, J. W. (1991). Assessment of parent–adolescent relationships: Implications for adolescent development. *Journal of Family Psychology, 5*, 21–45.

Sroufe, L. A. (1983). Infant–caregiver attachment and patterns of adaptation in preschool: The roots of maladaptation and competence. *Minnesota Symposia on Child Psychology, 16*, 41–81.

Sroufe, L. A. (1989). Relationships, self and individual adaptation. In A. S. Roffen & R. N. Emde (Eds.), *Relationship Disturbances in Early Childhood* (pp. 70–94). New York: Basic Books.

Sroufe, L. A., & Cooper, R. G. (1988). *Child Development: Its Nature and Course*. New York: Knopf.

Sroufe, L. A., Egeland, B., & Kreutzer, T. (1990). The fate of early experience following developmental change: Longitudinal approaches to individual adaptation in childhood. *Child Development, 61*, 1363–1373.

Sroufe, L. A., & Fleeson, J. (1986). Attachment and the construction of relationships. In W. W. Hartup & Z. Rubin (Eds.), *Relationships and Development* (pp. 51–72). Hillsdale, NJ: Erlbaum.

Stafford, L., & Bayer, C. L. (1993). *Interaction between Parents and Children*. Newbury Park, Ca: Sage.

Steil, J. M., & Turetsky, B. A. (1987). Is equal better? The relationship between marital equality and psychological symptomatology. In S. Oskamp (Ed.), *Family Processes and Problems: Social Psychological Aspects* (pp. 73–97). Newbury Park, CA: Sage.

Stein, C. H., Bush, E. G., Ross, R. R., & Ward, M. (1992). Mine, yours and ours: A configural analysis of the networks of married couples in relation to marital satisfaction and individual well-being. *Journal of Social and Personal Relationships, 9*, 365–383.

Steinberg, L. (1988). Reciprocal relation between parent–child distance and pubertal maturation. *Developmental Psychology, 24*, 122–128.

Steinberg, L., & Silverberg, S. B. (1986). The vicissitudes of autonomy in early adolescence. *Child Development, 57*, 841–851.

Stern, D. (1985). *The Interpersonal World of the Infant.* New York: Basic Books.

Sternberg, R. J. (1986). A triangular theory of love. *Psychological Review, 93*, 119–135.

Sternberg, R. J. (1988). Triangulating love. In R.J. Sternberg & M.L. Barnes (Eds.), *The Psychology of Love* (pp. 119–138). New Haven, CT: Yale University Press.

Sternberg, R. J., & Barnes, M. L. (Eds.). (1988). *The Psychology of Love.* New Haven, CT: Yale University Press.

Sternberg, R. J., & Grajek, S. (1984). The nature of love. *Journal of Personality and Social Psychology, 47*, 312–329.

Stiles, W. B., Shuster, P. L., & Harrigan, J. A. (1992). Disclosure and anxiety: A test of the fever model. *Journal of Personality and Social Psychology, 63*, 980–988.

Stinnett, N., & Sauer, K. (1977). Relationship characteristics of strong families. *Family Perspective, 11*, 3–11.

Stinson, L., & Ickes, W. (1992). Empathic accuracy in the interactions of male friends versus male strangers. *Journal of Personality and Social Psychology, 62*, 787–797.

Stokes, J., Childs, L., & Fuehrer, A. (1981). Gender and sex roles as predictors of self-disclosure. *Journal of Counseling Psychology, 28*, 510–514.

Stokes, J., Fuehrer, A., & Childs, L. (1980). Gender differences in self-disclosure to various target persons. *Journal of Counseling Psychology, 27*, 192–198.

Stoltz-Loike, M. (1992). *Dual-Career Couples: New Perspectives in Counseling.* Alexandria, VA: American Association for Counseling and Development.

Stover, L., Guerney, B., Ginsberg, B., & Schlein, S. (1977a). The Acceptance of Other Scale (AOS). In B. G. Guerney (Ed.), *Relationship Enhancement* (pp. 364–371). San Francisco: Jossey-Bass.

Stover, L., Guerney, B., Ginsberg, B., & Schlein, S. (1977b). The Self-Feeling Awareness Scale (SFAS). In B. G. Guerney (Ed.), *Relationship Enhancement* (pp. 371–377). San Francisco: Jossey-Bass.

Strassberg, D. S., & Anchor, K. (1975). Rating intimacy of self-disclosure. *Psychological Reports, 37*, 562.

Strayer, J., & Eisenberg, N. (1987). Empathy viewed in context. In N. Eisenberg & J. Strayer (Eds.), *Empathy and Its Development* (pp. 389–398). Cambridge, MA: Cambridge University Press.

Strayer, J., & Schroeder, M. (1989). Children's helping strategies: Influence of emotion, empathy, and age. In N. Eisenberg (Ed.), *Empathy and Related Emotional Responses* (pp. 85–105). San Francisco: Jossey-Bass.

Striegel-Moore, R. H., Silberstein, L. R., & Rodin, J. (1986). Toward an understanding of risk factors for bulimia. *American Psychologist, 41*, 246–263.

Stuart, R. B. (1980). *Helping Couples Change: A Social Learning Approach to Marital Therapy.* New York: Guilford Press.

Sullivan, H. S. (1953). *The Interpersonal Theory of Psychiatry.* New York: Norton.

Sunnafrank, M. (1988). Predicted outcome value in initial conversations. *Communication Research Reports, 5,* 169–172.

Suomi, S. J., & Harlow, H. F. (1978). Early experience and social development in rhesus monkeys. In M. Lamb (Ed.), *Social and Personality Development* (pp. 252–271). New York: Holt, Rinehart & Winston.

Suomi, S. J., & Harlow, H. F. (1972). Social rehabilitation of isolate-reared monkeys. *Developmental Psychology, 6,* 487–496.

Surra, C. A. (1985). Courtship types: Variations in interdependence between partners and social networks. *Journal of Personality and Social Psychology, 49,* 357–375.

Surra, C. A., & Bohman, T. (1991). The development of close relationships: A cognitive perspective. In G. J. O. Fletcher & F. D. Fincham (Eds.), *Cognition in Close Relationships* (pp. 281–306). Hillsdale, NJ: Erlbaum.

Surrey, J. L. (1991). The "self-in-relation": A theory of women's development. In J. V. Jordan, A. G. Kaplan, J. B. Miller, I. P. Stiver, & J. L. Surrey, *Women's Growth in Connection: Writings from the Stone Center* (pp. 51–66). New York: Guilford Press.

Swain, S. O. (1989). Covert intimacy: Closeness in men's friendships. In B. J. Risman & P. Schwartz (Eds.), *Gender in Intimate Relationships: A Microstructural Approach* (pp. 71–86). Belmont, CA: Wadsworth.

Swain, S. O. (1992). Men's friendships with women: Intimacy, sexual boundaries and the informant role. In P. M. Nardi (Ed.), *Men's Friendships* (pp. 153–171). Newbury Park, CA: Sage.

Swensen, C. H., Eskew, R. W., & Kohlhepp, K. A. (1981). Stage of family life cycle, ego development, and the marriage relationship. *Journal of Marriage and the Family, 43,* 841–853.

Szinovacz, M. (1989). Retirement, couples, and household work. In S. J. Bahr & E. T. Peterson (Eds.), *Aging and the Family* (pp. 33–58). Lexington, MA: Heath.

Tamir, L. M. (1982). *Men in their Forties: The Transition to Middle Age.* New York: Springer.

Tannen, D. (1990a). Gender differences in topical coherence: Creating involvement in best friends' talk. *Discourse Processes, 13,* 73–90.

Tannen, D. (1990b). *You Just Don't Understand: Women and Men in Conversation.* New York: Ballantine.

Taylor, D. A., & Altman, I. (1966). Intimacy-scaled stimuli for use in studies of interpersonal relations. *Psychological Reports, 19,* 729–730.

Tesch, S. A. (1984). Sex-role orientation and intimacy status in men and women. *Sex Roles, 11,* 451–465.

Tesch, S. A. (1985). The Psychosocial Intimacy Questionnaire: Validational studies and an investigation of sex roles. *Journal of Social and Personal Relationships, 2,* 471–488.

Tesch, S. A., & Martin, R. R. (1983). Friendship concepts of young adults in two age groups. *Journal of Psychology, 115,* 7–12.

Tesch, S. A., & Whitbourne, S. K. (1982). Intimacy and identity status in young adults. *Journal of Personality and Social Psychology, 43,* 1041–1051.

Tesser, A. (1980). Self-esteem maintenance in family dynamics. *Journal of Personality and Social Psychology, 39*, 77–91.

Thayer, S. (1986). Touch: Frontier of intimacy. *Journal of Nonverbal Behavior, 10*, 7–11.

Thayer, S. (1988). Close encounters. *Psychology Today, 22*, 31–36.

Thayer, S., & Schiff, W. (1975). Eye-contact, facial expression, and the experience of time. *Journal of Social Psychology, 95*, 117–124.

Thibaut, J. W., & Kelley, H. H. (1959). *The Social Psychology of Groups*. New York: Wiley.

Thiederman, S. (1991). *Bridging Cultural Barriers for Corporate Success*. New York: Lexington Books.

Thomas, A., & Chess, S. (1977). *Temperament and Development*. New York: Brunner/Mazel.

Thompson, S. K. (1975). Gender labels and early sex-role development. *Child Development, 46*, 339–347.

Thorbecke, W., & Grotevant, H. D. (1982). Gender differences in adolescent interpersonal identity formation. *Journal of Youth and Adolescence, 11*, 479–492.

Thorne, B., & Luria, Z. (1986). Sexuality and gender in children's daily worlds. *Social Problems, 33*, 176–190.

Tickle-Degnen, L., & Rosenthal, R. (1990). The nature of rapport and its nonverbal correlates. *Psychological Inquiry, 1*, 285–293.

Tobin-Richards, M. H., Boxer, A. M., & Petersen, A. C. (1983). The psychological significance of pubertal change. Sex differences in perceptions of self during early adolescence. In J. Brooks-Gunn & A. C. Petersen (Eds.), *Girls at Puberty* (pp. 127–154). New York: Plenum.

Todd, J. L., & Shapira, A. (1974). U.S. and British self-disclosure, anxiety, empathy and attitudes to psychotherapy. *Journal of Cross-Cultural Psychology, 5*, 364–369.

Tolstedt, B. E., & Stokes, J. P. (1983). Relation of verbal, affective, and physical intimacy to marital satisfaction. *Journal of Counseling Psychology, 30*, 573–580.

Tolstedt, B. E., & Stokes, J. P. (1984). Self-disclosure, intimacy and the depenetration process. *Journal of Personality and Social Psychology, 46*, 84–90.

Townsend, M. A. R., McCracken, H. F., & Wilton, K. M. (1981). Popularity and intimacy as determinants of psychological well-being in adolescent friendships. *Journal of Early Adolescence, 8*, 421–436.

Tracy, K. (1991). *Understanding Face-to-Face Interaction*. Hillsdale, NJ: Erlbaum.

Tschann, J. M. (1988). Self-disclosure in adult friendship: Gender and marital status differences. *Journal of Social and Personal Relationships, 5*, 65–81.

Unger, R. K. (1990). Imperfect reflections of reality: Psychology constructs gender. In R. T. Hare-Mustin & J. Marecek (Eds.), *Making a Difference: Psychology and the Construction of Gender* (pp. 102–149). New Haven, CT: Yale University Press.

Unger, R. K., & Crawford, M. (1992). *Women and Gender: A Feminist Psychology*. New York: McGraw-Hill.

U.S. Bureau of the Census (May 21, 1991). Monthly Vital Statistics Report. Washington, DC: U.S. Department of Commerce.

Vandell, D. L., Henderson, V. K., & Wilson, K. S. (1988). A longitudinal study of children with day-care experiences of varying quality. Child Development, 59, 1286–1292.

Vandell, D. L., Wilson, K. S., & Henderson, K. (1980). Peer interaction in the first year of life: An examination of its structure, content, and sensitivity to toys. Child Development, 51, 481–488.

Vangelisti, A. L. (1994). Family secrets: Forms, functions and correlates. Journal of Social and Personal Relationships, 11, 113–135.

Vanlear, C. A. (1987). The formation of social relationships. Human Communication Research, 13, 299–322.

Vernberg, E. M., Beery, S. H., Ewell, K. K., & Abwender, D. A. (1993). Parents' use of friendship facilitation strategies and the formation of friendships in early adolescence: A prospective study. Journal of Family Psychology, 7, 356–369.

Vinokur, A. D., & van Ryn, M. (1993). Social support and undermining in close relationships: Their independent effects on the mental health of unemployed persons. Journal of Personality and Social Psychology, 65, 350–359.

Vondra, J., & Belsky, J. (1993). Developmental origins of parenting: Personality and relationship factors. In T. Luster & L. Okagaki (Eds.), Parenting: An Ecological Perspective (pp. 1–33). Hillsdale, NJ: Erlbaum.

Vondracek, F. W. (1969). Behavioral measurement of self-disclosure. Psychological Reports, 25, 914.

Voydanoff, P. (1993). Work and family relationships. In T. Brubaker (Ed.), Family Relations: Challenges for the Future. Newbury Park, CA: Sage.

Wada, M. (1990). The effect of interpersonal distance change on nonverbal behaviors: Mediating effects of sex and intimacy levels in a dyad. Japanese Psychological Research, 32, 86–96.

Walker, A. J., & Thompson, L. (1983). Intimacy and intergenerational aid and contact among mothers and daughers. Journal of Marriage and the Family, 45, 841–849.

Walsh, V. L., Baucom, D. H., Tyler, S., & Sayers, S. L. (1993). Impact of message valence, focus, expressive style, and gender on communication patterns among maritally distressed couples. Journal of Family Psychology, 7, 163–175.

Waltz, M. (1986). Marital context and post-infarction quality of life: Is it social support or something more? Social Science Medicine, 22, 791–805.

Waltz, M., Badura, B., Pfaff, H., & Schott, T. (1988). Marriage and the psychological consequences of a heart attack: A longitudinal study of adaptation to chronic illness after 3 years. Social Science and Medicine, 27, 149–158.

Waring, E. M. (1981). Facilitating marital intimacy through self-disclosure. The American Journal of Family Therapy, 9, 33–42.

Waring, E. M., & Chelune, G. J. (1983). Marital intimacy and self-disclosure. Journal of Clinical Psychology, 39, 183–190.

Waring, E., McElrath, D., Lefcoe, D., & Weisz, G. (1981). Dimensions of intimacy in marriage. *Psychiatry, 44,* 169–175.

Waring, E. M., McElrath, D., Mitchell, P., & Derry, M. E. (1981). Intimacy and emotional illness in the general population. *Canadian Journal of Psychiatry, 26,* 167–172.

Waring, E. M., & Patton, D. (1984). Marital intimacy and depression. *British Journal of Psychiatry, 145,* 641–644.

Waring, E. M., & Reddon, J. R. (1983). The measurement of intimacy in marriage: The Waring Intimacy Questionnaire. *Journal of Clinical Psychology, 39,* 53–57.

Waring, E. M., & Russell, L. (1980). Family structure, marital adjustment, and intimacy in patients referred to a consultation–liaison service. *General Hospital Psychiatry, 3,* 198–203.

Waring, E. M., Tillman, M. P., Frelick, L., Russell, L., & Weisz, G. (1980). Concepts of intimacy in the general population. *Journal of Nervous and Mental Disease, 168,* 471–474.

Waterman, A. S., & Whitbourne, S. K. (1981). The Inventory of Psychosocial Development: A Review and Evaluation. *ISAS Catalog of Selected Documents in Psychology, 11,* 5.

Waters, E., Wippman, J., & Sroufe, L. A. (1979). Attachment, positive affect, and competence in the peer group: Two studies in construct validation. *Child Development, 50,* 821–829.

Weinberg, G. (1972). *Society and the Healthy Homosexual.* Boston: Alyson.

Weiner, M. F. (1980). Healthy and pathological love: Psychodynamic views. In K. S. Pope (Ed.), *On Love and Loving* (pp. 114–132). San Francisco: Jossey-Bass.

Weishaus, S., & Field, D. (1988). A half century of marriage: Continuity or change? *Journal of Marriage and the Family, 50,* 763–774.

Weiss, A. G. (1987). Privacy and intimacy: Apart and a part. *Journal of Humanistic Psychology, 27,* 118–125.

Weiss, L., & Lowenthal, M. F. (1973, August). Perceptions and complexities of friendship in four stages of the adult life cycle. Paper presented at the Annual Convention, American Psychological Association, Montreal, Canada.

Weiss, R. L., & Heyman, R. E. (1990). Observation of marital interaction. In F. D. Fincham & T. N. Bradbury (Eds.), *The Psychology of Marriage: Basic Issues and Applications* (pp. 87–117). New York: Guilford Press.

Weiss, R. S. (1973). *Loneliness: The Experience of Emotional and Social Isolation.* Cambridge, MA: MIT Press.

Weiss, R. S. (1986). Continuities and transformations in social relationships from childhood to adulthood. In W. W. Hartup & Z. Rubin (Eds.), *Relationships and Development* (pp. 95–110). Hillsdale, NJ: Erlbaum.

Wellman, B. (1992). Men in networks: Private communities, domestic friendships. In P. M. Nardi (Ed.), *Men's Friendships* (pp. 74–114). Newbury Park, CA: Sage.

West, C., & Zimmerman, D. (1991). Doing gender. In J. Lorder & S. A. Farrell

(Eds.), *The Social Construction of Gender* (pp. 13–37). Newbury Park, CA: Sage.

Wexler, D. A., & Rice, L. N. (Eds.). (1974). *Innovations in Client-Centered Therapy*. New York: Wiley.

Wheeler, L., & Nezlek, J. (1977). Sex differences in social participation. *Journal of Personality and Social Psychology, 35*, 742–754.

Wheeler, L., Reis, H. T., & Nezlek, J. (1983). Loneliness, social interaction, and sex roles. *Journal of Personality and Social Psychology, 45*, 943–953.

Whitbourne, S. K. (1986). *The Me I Know: A Study of Adult Identity*. New York: Springer-Verlag.

White, K. M., Speisman, J. C., & Costos, D. (1983). Young adults and their parents: Individuation to mutuality. In H. D. Grotevant & C. R. Cooper (Eds.), *Adolescent Development in the Family: New Directions for Child Development* (No. 22, pp. 61–76). San Francisco: Jossey-Bass.

White, K. M., Speisman, J. C., Jackson, D., Bartis, S., & Costos, D. (1986). Intimacy maturity and its correlates in young married couples. *Journal of Personality and Social Psychology, 50*, 152–162.

Wilkie, C. F., & Ames, E. W. (1986). The relationship of infant crying to parental stress in the transition to parenthood. *Journal of Marriage and the Family, 48*, 545–550.

Wilkie, J. R. (1988). Marriage, family life, and women's employment. In A. H. Stromberg & S. Harkness (Eds.), *Women Working: Theories and Facts in Perspective* (pp. 149–166). Mountain View, CA: Mayfield.

Wilks, J. (1986). The relative importance of parents and friends in adolescent decision-making. *Journal of Youth and Adolescence, 15*, 323–334.

Willer, D., & Anderson, B. (Eds.). (1981). *Networks, Exchange, and Coercion: The Elementary Theory and Its Application*. New York: Elsevier.

Williams, D. G. (1985). Gender, masculinity–femininity, and emotional intimacy in same-sex friendship. *Sex Roles, 12*, 587–600.

Williams, W. L. (1992). The relationship between male–male friendship and male–female marriage: American Indian and Asian comparisons. In P. M. Nardi (Ed.), *Men's Friendships* (pp. 186–200). Newbury Park, CA: Sage.

Williamson, D. S. (1991). *The Intimacy Paradox: Personal Authority in the Family System*. New York: Guilford Press.

Wilson, W. R. (1967). Correlates of avowed happiness. *Psychological Bulletin, 67*, 294–306.

Winnicott, D. W. (1953). Transitional objects and transitional phenomena: A study of the first not-me possession. *International Journal of Psycho-Analysis, 34*, 89–97. (Reprinted in Buckley, P. (Ed.). *Essential Papers on Object Relations* (pp. 254–271). New York: New York University Press.)

Winstead, B. A. (1986). Sex differences in same-sex friendships. In V. J. Derlega & B. Winstead (Eds.), *Friendship and Social Interaction* (pp. 81–99). New York: Springer-Verlag.

Winstead, B. A., Derlega, V. J., & Montgomery, M. J. (1995). The quality of friendships at work and job satisfaction. *Journal of Social and Personal Relationships, 12*, 199–215.

Winstead, B. A., Derlega, V. J., & Wong, P. T. P. (1984). Effects of sex-role orientation on behavioral self-disclosure. *Journal of Research in Personality, 18,* 541–553.

Wittgenstein, L. (1953). *Philosophical Investigations.* New York: Macmillan.

Wood, G. J., Barnes, S. M., & Waring, E. M. (1988). The criterion validity of the Waring Intimacy Questionnaire in a psychiatric inpatient sample. *Journal of Sex and Marital Therapy, 14,* 63–73.

Wood, J. T. (1993). Engendered relations: Interaction, caring, power, and responsibility in intimacy. In S. W. Duck (Ed.), *Social Context and Relationships* (pp. 26–54). Newbury Park, CA: Sage.

Wood, J. T. (1994). *Gendered Lives: Communication, Gender, and Culture.* Belmont, CA: Wadsworth.

Worthy, M., Gary, A. L., & Kahn, G. M. (1969). Self-disclosure as an exchange process. *Journal of Personality and Social Psychology, 13,* 59–63.

Wright, H., & Keple, W. (1981). Friends and parents of a sample of high school juniors: An explanatory study of relationship intensity and interpersonal rewards. *Journal of Marriage and the Family, 43,* 559–570.

Wright, P. H. (1982). Men's friendships, women's friendships, and the alleged inferiority of the latter. *Sex Roles, 8,* 1–20.

Wright, P. H. (1988). Interpreting research on gender differences in friendship: A case for moderation and a plea for caution. *Journal of Social and Personal Relationships, 5,* 367–373.

Wright, P. H. (1989). Gender differences in adults' same- and cross-gender friendships. In R. G. Adams & R. Blieszner (Eds.), *Older Adult Friendship: Structure and Process* (pp. 197–221). Newbury Park, CA: Sage.

Wright, P. H., & Scanlon, M. B. (1991). Gender role orientations and friendship: Some attenuation, but gender differences abound. *Sex Roles, 24,* 551–566.

Wynne, L. C., & Wynne, A. R. (1986). The quest for intimacy. *Journal of Marital and Family Therapy, 12,* 383–394.

Youniss, J. (1980). *Parents and Peers in Social Development: A Sullivan–Piaget Perspective.* Chicago: University of Chicago Press.

Youniss, J., & Ketterlinus, R. D. (1987). Communication and connectedness in mother– and father–adolescent relationships. *Journal of Youth and Adolescence, 3,* 265–280.

Youniss, J., & Smollar, J. (1985). *Adolescent Relations with Mothers, Fathers, and Friends.* Chicago: University of Chicago Press.

Zietlow, P. H., & Sillars, A. L. (1988). Life-stage differences in communication during marital conflicts. *Journal of Social and Personal Relationships, 5,* 223–245.

Index